ESSENTIAL PAPERS ON OBJECT LOSS

ESSENTIAL PAPERS IN PSYCHOANALYSIS

Essential Papers on Borderline Disorders
Edited by Michael D. Stone, M.D.

Essential Papers on Object Relations
Edited by Peter Buckley, M.D.

Essential Papers on Narcissism
Edited by Andrew P. Morrison, M.D.

Essential Papers on Depression
Edited by James C. Coyne

Essential Papers on Psychosis
Edited by Peter Buckley, M.D.

Essential Papers on Countertransference
Edited by Benjamin Wolstein

Essential Papers on Character Neurosis and Treatment
Edited by Ruth F. Lax

Essential Papers on the Psychology of Women
Edited by Claudia Zanardi

Essential Papers on Transference
Edited by Aaron H. Esman, M.D.

Essential Papers on Dreams
Edited by Melvin Lansky, M.D.

Essential Papers on Literature and Psychoanalysis
Edited by Emanuel Berman

Essential Papers on Object Loss
Edited by Rita V. Frankiel

ESSENTIAL PAPERS ON OBJECT LOSS

Edited by
Rita V. Frankiel

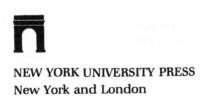

NEW YORK UNIVERSITY PRESS
New York and London

NEW YORK UNIVERSITY PRESS
New York and London

Library of Congress Cataloging-in-Publication Data
Essential papers on object loss / edited by Rita V. Frankiel
p. cm.—(Essential papers in psychoanalysis)
Includes bibliographical references and index.
ISBN 0-8147-2607-0 (cloth)—ISBN 0-8147-2621-6 (pbk.)
1. Object relations (Psychoanalysis)   2. Loss (Psychology)
3. Parents—Death.   4. Grief.   5. Bereavement.   I. Frankiel, Rita
V.   II. Series.
BF175.5.024E86   1994
155.9'37—dc20   93-37084
                        CIP

New York University Press books are printed on acid-free paper,
and their binding materials are chosen for strength and durability.

Manufactured in the United States of America

10   9   8   7   6   5   4   3   2

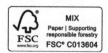

To Roy

Contents

Acknowledgments

A number of people have given me valuable assistance in assembling the material for this volume. I wish particularly to express my gratitude to David Tuckett, editor of the *International Journal of Psycho-Analysis*, for his helpfulness in facilitating the use of material from his journal. Special thanks go to the officers of the Melanie Klein Trust for their generosity in allowing Klein's paper "Mourning and Its Relation to Manic-Depressive States" to be reprinted here without the customary fees. Hanna Segal showed similar generosity in allowing her paper, "A Psychoanalytical Approach to Aesthetics," to be reprinted without fees.

Leo Goldberger, advisor to New York University Press, was intellectual "Dutch uncle" (actually, Danish-American uncle) to this project. Despina Papazoglou Gimbel, managing editor of New York University Press, has epitomized grace under pressure; her enthusiasm for this project and her professional skills added pleasure to my task and greatly facilitated its successful completion. Jason Renker, former editor of this series, and Katherine Gill, present editor, have done their best to speed it on its way. Lani Ting has been the organized, good-natured, intelligent gal Friday a writer hopes for.

My awareness of this vast literature began when I first became a teacher of psychoanalytic developmental theory in 1970, and was stimulated and encouraged by my mentor, the late David Schecter. The supervisees, students, and participants in the object loss study groups I have led over the past decade have made willing and open presentations of their clinical problems in treating those who have suffered early loss. They have helped me broaden my experience and deepen my understanding.

My husband, Roy Schafer, encouraged me to turn what was a passionate curiosity and involvement into a more permanent contribution to the psychoanalytic literature. His devotion to conceptual and clinical clarity have been a profound influence.

Introduction

Rita V. Frankiel

Anyone who has undertaken the treatment of an adult who suffered a major loss in childhood, or who has treated a child in the same situation, cannot escape awareness of the suffering and devastation such a loss can wreak on the inner world of the person. This devastation can disrupt future development as well as invade current reality. It is brought into the clinical situation in a variety of ways that can vastly complicate, if not derail, the therapist's attempt to initiate and develop a workable treatment.

Chances are good that the contemporary clinician undertaking the treatment of a patient—adult, adolescent, or child—who has suffered early object loss has not had any training specifically addressed to the technical difficulties that might be encountered in such a treatment or the difficulties of managing the intense countertransference feelings such patients can arouse in even the most seasoned clinician. The relative absence of special focus on this area in training programs is especially noteworthy since, on closer examination, many patients considered "hard to treat" are actually patients who have suffered early and often repeated object loss (Frankiel et al. 1989).

Furthermore, there is a substantial psychoanalytic literature in this area and also extensive epidemiological and medical studies that document the potentially dangerous health consequences of bereavement. This makes it all the more puzzling that the special problems in the effective treatment of those who have suffered early object loss and those adapting to object loss for the first time as adults have not yet received the attention they deserve in the curricula of most psychoanalytic training institutes and other programs offering training in psychoanalysis and psychotherapy.

In some situations, it is thought that the course or courses on depression typically offered will cover the essential issues of object loss. This notion is based, I think, on the assumption that once one has grasped the fundamental distinctions between mourning and depression carefully delineated by Freud

1

and Abraham, one is well on the road to understanding what needs to be understood about object loss. I do not question this assumption, with Freud and Abraham one *is* well underway, but the road has lengthened since its beginnings, and now includes many turnings, divergences, and detours. Technical issues that need to be considered and evaluated are not clearly in view until one takes a longer look. This collection has been assembled with the hope that recognizing the ubiquity of object loss trauma, as well as its nature, characteristics, and the specificity of obstacles to attachment that may ensure in its wake, will lead to more focused attention to this area in clinical work and teaching.

In recent years, there have been a number of edited books on the topic (Altschul 1988; J. and S. Bloom-Feshback et al., 1987; Dietrich and Shabad 1989). These are collections of papers that survey this extensive literature along a variety of lines, and from different theoretical points of view. They provide useful summaries of whole areas of the literature. Many of these summaries were prepared by recognized contributors to this area of interest. These books do not, however, provide the teacher and the student with primary sources, the original articles on which these later contributions are based. Searching discussion of clinical and theoretical matters can only benefit when the material studied also provides the student with a grounding in classical contributions. These contributions are the basis of our current understandings and misunderstandings of object loss and its consequences.

In this book, I have collected what I consider to be the most significant contributions to psychoanalytic and psychological understanding of the effect of object loss on adults and children. My choices are focused on those contributions most directly relevant to the clinical situation. Unfortunately, space limitations have required the omission of some equally important contributions. The contributions that I consider equally important but that could not be reprinted here are listed as highly recommended readings at the end of this collection of essays.

I have chosen *not* to add yet another review of the literature to the excellent reviews already available, since I feel it would not increase the clinical usefulness of this volume. Earlier reviews by Siggins (1966), Miller (1971), and E. Furman (1974, 233–96) are significant contributions and useful guides to the clinical implications of the literature on object loss as it has developed. I introduce my selections with discussions that outline their relevance to the practicing therapist; where it is pertinent to do so, I also summarize and comment on other contributions to the larger body of work in this area. Throughout, I approach these papers in the light of contemporary thought on the subject at hand. Although space does not permit exploration of all possible points of view, divergent viewpoints are not neglected.

This book shows that the consequences of object loss are determined by a combination of potentially devastating processes. These processes interact with individual differences in talent and endowment and with the presence or absence of suitable replacement objects and help at the time of the loss. This ensemble of factors can lead to potentially serious ego arrests and regressions. Also, either at the time of loss or later on, these victims may produce hysterical identifications with the sick and dying parent. Additionally, these losses can shape later object choice in adults.

No matter whether treatment is undertaken in childhood or adult life, the consequences of these losses are graphically displayed in, and profoundly influence, the unfolding of the clinical process. The unique individual story of each loss is reenacted in the clinical situation. These enactments may include utter conscious denial of death or complete unconscious denial covered by conscious acceptance, as well as accident proneness, disruptive anniversary reactions, compulsive wandering, and other indicators of unconscious preoccupations with traumatic absence and hoped-for reunion. Physical symptoms and illnesses provide yet another avenue for the expression of unacknowledged grief. This list is not exhaustive but does indicate the range of possible expressions in the treatment situation. Perhaps the most difficult to deal with is the tendency of these patients either to cling to the therapist without awareness of their separation anxiety or to deny attachment altogether.

We begin with two papers that describe and discuss adult responses to grief and the range of physiological and psychological consequences (Engel [1961], Lindemann [1944]). Both papers are considered classics in the field, providing thorough and careful clinical descriptions of the phenomena involved and their implications. Physiological responses to loss are by now well known. In children, asthma, sleep disturbances, and hyperactivity are often observed. We know that some bereaved spouses are vulnerable to alterations of their cardiovascular and/or immune systems and are more likely to experience a worsening of preexisting medical conditions. Some succumb to health-deteriorating dependencies—drugs, alcohol, food. In men, it is by now established that the first year of bereavement is associated with vastly increased death rates; in women, suicide rates increase in the second year after bereavement (Osterweis, Soloman, and Green 1984). The questions of how these phenomena are mediated and why some persons are more vulnerable than others are continuing areas of research. In adults, contemporary medical research work is attempting to track and specify immuno-suppressant activity set in train by loss (Stein, Miller, and Trestman 1991). Definitive results are not yet available.

The psychic effects and manifestations of object loss have intrigued psychoanalysts since the beginning of their literature. Freud's notice of and speculations about the meaning of patients' responses to loss dates from the earliest days of psychoanalysis (1887–1902, Draft G). The section below called "Theoretical Foundations" includes five of his discussions of the subject. Some of his papers are not reproduced in their entirety; only those aspects dealing with the sequelae and meaning of mourning are included here, whether that mourning follows a real loss in external reality or a loss in psychic reality, as in the changes necessitated around the dissolution of the Oedipus complex. Not all of Freud's writings that touch on mourning are included here. My effort has been to select the most meaningful materials for the practicing clinician today. Also included is an abridgment of Abraham's basic contribution to this area (1924). Originally a lengthy monograph dealing with a number of other topics, it has been edited to focus on those aspects that deal with object loss. The richness of Abraham's clinical observations and the fullness of his descriptions of clinical events are remarkable. He is a psychoanalytic writer of great clarity and accessibility. This contribution is essential to the clinician's understanding.

The other, to my mind, essential theoretical papers on object loss are those by Melanie Klein (1940), Loewald (1962), and Pollock (1961). In each instance the paper selected for this volume is preceded by an introduction indicating its importance and meaning in the unfolding of the literature.

The next section includes a series of papers describing aspects of pathological mourning and how it works. Included is Bowlby's seminal paper on similarities and differences between pathological mourning and what he considers to be mourning in childhood (1963). The section includes the often-cited paper by Helene Deutsch ("Absence of Grief" [1937]) along with similarly significant papers by Jacobson (1965) and Robert Tyson (1983).

Next come two papers dealing with technical issues in the treatment of pathological mourning. The classical and often-cited Fleming and Altschul paper of 1963 is followed by Volkan and Josephthal's (1980) description of re-grief therapy, a relatively recent therapeutic innovation with intriguing possibilities.

Any attempt to survey the literature on object loss must also explore an important area of controversy and disagreement: when does the capacity for mourning begin; is mourning possible before adolescence; if mourning is possible in childhood, what forms does it take? Several significant contributors to the literature on early object loss (J. Bowlby 1960, 1963, 1980; A. Freud 1960, 1973; E. Furman 1974, 1986; R. Furman 1964a, 1968, 1973) hold that whether or not the loss produces psychic devastation and consequent psychopathology may depend greatly on the conditions surrounding the loss and its aftermath such as the availability of sensitive supportive figures and replacement objects. Others (e.g., Nagera 1970; Wolfenstein 1966, 1969) insist that adolescence is the developmental line of demarcation for mourning. These writers claim that before adolescence there cannot be real decathexis of the lost object. The literature on this controversy will be summarized and discussed and a few papers that point to a position that seems promising for clinical understanding and prediction will be included along with Wolfenstein's very influential 1966 paper on the subject.

Three case reports are included in the next section. Each paper provides first-hand data on the vicissitudes of work with object loss patients. One patient is a young boy in treatment-via-the-parent (E. Furman 1981), one a preadolescent girl in a psychoanalytic treatment (McCann 1974). These two case reports originate in the work of the Cleveland Center for Research in Child Development, a group that has contributed substantially to our understanding of the effects of parent loss on children (E. Furman 1974, 1981, 1983, 1986; R. Furman 1964a, 1964b, 1968, 1973; Barnes 1964). Marie McCann's report (1974) of a creative and resourceful transference analysis of a deeply disturbed preadolescent girl who was in treatment until the age of eighteen records a remarkable accomplishment in a much less than optimal set of circumstances. Also included is a recent paper by Lerner (1990) that demonstrates adult patients' need to search for a representative of their lost object during treatment.

The often-mentioned correlation between early object loss and the creativity of writers, artists, and political leaders is the final aspect of the literature on object loss that is included here. This section begins with a seminal theoretical paper by Hanna Segal (1952) on the relation between processes of mourning in the inner world and acts of creation. The report of an intriguing research effort to establish whether or not the outstanding contributors to our civilization have suffered parent loss is included (Eisenstadt 1978). Unfortunately, space limitations preclude any sampling here of Pollock's significant work in this area.

I offer my selections and comments in the belief that they can be of value in the clinical practice of psychoanalysis and psychotherapy. I regret that I cannot include more of the vast and illuminating literature on this topic; the highly recommended readings listed at the end of the book are there for those whose interest is strongly aroused by the present collection.

PART I

GRIEF OBSERVED

Introductory Notes to Chapter 1

Rita V. Frankiel

This article is about grief and recovery from grief as causal entities in the etiology and course of disease and the maintenance of health, concepts that are hardly news to a contemporary professional. In the thirty years since this paper was published, there have been many efforts to specify the physiological components and sequelae of grief and the emotional reactions that have potential consequences for the development of disease (e.g., Hofer 1984; Osterweis, Soloman, and Green 1984; Stein, Miller and Trestman 1991). At the present time, the idea that loss *invariably* produces disruptive outcomes, physiological and/or psychological, has been challenged (e.g., E. Furman 1974, 1986; Wortman and Silver 1987). However, evidence accumulates that grief is implicated in vulnerability to a great range of diseases, and the morbidity statistics of the bereaved and recently widowed are by now well known (Osterweis, Solomon, and Green 1984; Parkes 1987).

Considering how entrenched by now—thirty years after Engel—are our ideas of what grief is *supposed* to be, it is relevant to quote him on our reluctance to change our views, since it may now be necessary to amend the socially and professionally accepted conviction that devastating disruption invariably follows object loss by including the view that takes individual differences more sharply into account:

The first response when confronted with news of a grievous loss is, "No, it can't be. I don't believe it; I won't believe it." I would call your attention to the fact that cherished ideas, even if false, are also psychic objects and as such are not easily given up. And only time and much work will establish whose cherished ideas are the false ones. (1961, 22).

1. Is Grief a Disease?

George L. Engel

This paper has perhaps more the qualities of a philosophic than a scientific discourse, but for this I offer no apology. I shall present no new data and shall speak of a quite familiar phenomenon, but I shall invite you to view it from a perspective perhaps somewhat different from that to which you are accustomed. In keeping with this philosophic approach I have written this in the form of a Socratic dialogue. I pose the question, "Is grief a disease?"

No doubt this seems a strange question, since grief has not usually been considered in such terms and, on first glance, there seems little reason to do so. Yet, a thoughtful consideration of the issues raised by such a question will, I believe, throw light on some deficiencies in currently held concepts of disease. And the concept of disease held by an investigator, whether or not consciously utilized, has an important influence on the choice of material and the design of clinical research.[1-3]

Grief is the characteristic response to the loss of a valued object, be it a loved person, a cherished possession, a job, status, home, country, an ideal, a part of the body, etc. *Uncomplicated* grief runs a consistent course, modified mainly by the abruptness of the loss, the nature of the preparation for the event, and the significance for the survivor of the lost object. Generally it includes an initial phase of shock and disbelief, in which the sufferer attempts to deny the loss and to insulate himself against the shock of the reality. This is followed by a stage of developing awareness of the loss, marked by the painful effects of sadness, guilt, shame, helplessness, or hopelessness; by crying; by a sense of loss and emptiness; by anorexia, sleep disturbance, sometimes somatic symptoms of pain or other discomfort, loss of interest in one's usual activities and associates, impairment of work performance, etc. Finally, there is a prolonged phase of restitution and recovery during which

Reprinted by permission of Williams and Wilkins from *Psychosomatic Medicine* 23 (1961): 18–22. © American Psychosomatic Society.

the work of mourning is carried on, the trauma of the loss is overcome, and a state of health and well-being re-established.[4-5]

In what respects does this correspond to other situations that we customarily regard as "disease"? Certainly it involves suffering and an impairment of the capacity to function, which may last for days, weeks, and even months. We can identify a consistent etiologic factor, namely, real, threatened, or even fantasied object loss. It fulfills all the criteria of a discrete syndrome, with relatively predictable symptomatology and course. The grieving person is often manifestly distressed and disabled to a degree quite evident to an observer.

The sceptic quickly raises some pointed questions: *Is not grief simply a natural reaction to a life experience? How can one put it into the same category as the pathological states we call disease?* To this we answer that it is "natural" or "normal" in the same sense that a wound or a burn is a natural or normal response to physical trauma. The designation "pathological" refers to the changed state and not to the fact of the response. That one responds to thermal radiation with a burn is natural or normal. The burn itself constitutes a pathological state and the concept is as appropriately applied to the state of grief as to a wound, burn, or infection.

Or it may be said: *Everyone experiences grief—it's part of life.* But that only emphasizes the ubiquity in life of the significant etiologic factor and the universal vulnerability of human beings to this particular stressful experience. The same may be said of many other disease states to which man is prone— measles, for example. Actually, the statement is not entirely correct. With a short life or under exceptionally favorable circumstances, one may escape both measles and grief.

Our sceptic resumes his argument: *Grief is a self-limited process, requiring no medical attention.* But so too are a great number of disease processes. Actually, many persons suffering primarily from grief do come to physicians but, because of cultural expectations and the role ascribed to or held by the physician, they do not complain to him of grief. Rather, they report some other, often somatic, symptom and the physician may not even learn of the grief. If he does, he may regard it either as not related to the complaint or not his concern. Besides, whether a condition requires medical attention is not relevant to the judgment as to whether it is to be regarded as a disease. The history of medicine provides innumerable examples of conditions that have come in time to be recognized as disease states but which had not been so regarded earlier. Epilepsy, alcoholism, and mental disease are examples.

We must not forget that in the prescientific era the roles of physician, magician, and priest were often embodied in the same person. It is the obligation of the physician of today to claim for scientific scrutiny all natural phenomena involving deviations in the individual's state of well-being, of which grief is one.

Grief is a purely subjective, psychological experience that does not involve any somatic changes. But, to my knowledge, no one has ever studied the bodily changes occurring during grief; hence, to begin with, there is no basis for such a statement. But even if it were true, one who holds such a view is, in essence, relegating to an extramedical and extrascientific status any kind of psychological or behavioral disturbance. As a matter of fact, many illnesses are largely subjective—at least, until we as observers discover the parameters and framework within which we can also make objective observations. Hyperparathyroidism, in many of its manifestations, was a purely subjective experience for many patients until we discovered what to look for and which instruments to use in the search. Again, the physician who is familiar with grief will recognize its occurrence through his systematic and ordered observations, even if the patient withholds or denies the necessary information.

No one ever dies of grief. Again, this is an irrelevant argument, even if true; but is it true? The newspapers repeatedly report persons collapsing and dying soon after learning of the death of a loved person. Have these cases been so carefully studied that we can say that the death represented pure coincidence, that the shock phase of the grief contributed in no way to this fatal outcome? I know of no such studies. Literature and folklore are replete with the notion that people fall ill and die "of grief." (I would prefer to say "during grief.") And few of the older physicians, from Hippocrates through the clinical giants of the late nineteenth century, failed to allude to grief as a factor in the causation of disease. While such views hardly constitute scientific evidence, the incidents are so common and the views so widely held that the cautious scientist will not be willing to say, without the benefit of scientific study, that it cannot be so. Actually, many recent investigations indicate that a wide variety of illnesses, including some that are fatal, may begin during a phase of grief. Schmale has recently surveyed a medical population and reviewed the modern as well as some of the older literature from this perspective.[6]

Perhaps one should speak of pathological grief and normal grief and restrict to the former the category of disease. This is a welcome concession, but it does not go far enough. At the outset I intentionally used the term "uncomplicated grief" rather than "normal grief." It is normal only in a statistical sense, meaning that it is the common, usual, and predictable response, as is an ecchymosis after a blow or measles after an infection with the measles virus. But it is not normal in the sense of total health. Predictable does not mean invariable and, in any situation, whether it be loss of an object or an exposure to physical trauma or a microorganism, we observe and define conditions under which the response may be different in degree or kind or where it may not occur at all. This is a widely accepted and familiar notion as applied to traditional disease states, but equally appropriate in respect to grief. We are familiar with such responses as the absence of grief, delayed grief, unresolved grief, depression, psychotic or neurotic reactions, pain or other conversion symptoms, and even organic disease occurring in the place of or in addition to the usual pattern of grief. As is true of the complications of a wound or an infection, we must also expect that other factors operate to account for these deviations from the usual course. Yet none of these considerations refutes the fact that the experience of uncomplicated grief also represents a manifest and gross departure from the dynamic state considered representative of health and well-being.

Is not grief really just a healthy, adaptive, and reparative process which corrects or overcomes a stress while the above-mentioned responses are the abnormal states that should be called diseases? The element of reparation is indeed to be found in grief, but so too is it found in every other disease; indeed, it always accounts for some of the symptoms and signs of a disease. If the adaptive or reparative processes involved in disease are successful, recovery occurs and the patient reachieves a state of health. If not, continued, progressive, or increased illness or death is the consequence.

Can it not be said that the person is really healthy and that he simply had the misfortune to suffer a loss and is now responding, naturally, with grief? This argument implies that all systems and levels of organization, actually and potentially, must be impaired by the stress before the condition can be considered disease. Actually, not only are health and disease relative concepts, but also at any time parts of the body and person may be more or less healthy, while other parts may be more or less impaired. Indeed, this is the usual situation. It is only in fatal disease, when the victim is near death, that we see total disorganization.

Perhaps by now the sceptic is ready to concede that grief can be considered a disease state. But what is gained by such a position? What are the implications for medical research and practice? They are, in my opinion, important and far reaching:

1. Grief, in all its forms and with all its ramifications, becomes a legitimate and proper subject for study by medical scientists. Research, utilizing the tools of the physical, biological, and behavioral sciences, must be directed to these sufferers no less than to those with other disorders. The occurrence of grief among animals is so well documented as to free the investigator from exclusive dependence on human subjects for such research.

2. The occurrence of grief, preceding or in the course of other illness, somatic and psychologic, as is so often reported by patients or their families, can no longer be passed off as irrelevant or coincidental until such data have been subjected to the same kind of rigorous and systematic exploration and examination that has been applied to other phenomena of disease. That grief in its various forms so often precedes the development of other disease states in itself constitutes no proof of a relationship. But the medical scientist is remiss if he does not subject all antecedent circumstances to examination as to whether they constitute contributing, necessary, or sufficient conditions for the development of a disease state. The obvious derangements in the functioning of the individual suffering from object loss and consequent grief make such inquiry all the more relevant. It is well to be reminded in this era of crash-program applied research that many fundamental discoveries elucidating the pathogenesis and mechanisms of disease states came about through the investigation of just such basic phenomena, often with grounds for anticipating a relationship far less than is the case with grief. One is reminded of the controversies concerning the role of miasmas in the pathogenesis of malaria. The investigation of the climatic and geographic conditions under which malaria occurred eventually provided the basis for elucidation of the disease even though the original theories concerning the miasmas were erroneous.

3. If the actual or threatened loss of an object so consistently disturbs the total adjustment of the organism, then we have identified an etiologic factor of such general importance as to put it in the same class as other major noxa, e.g., physical agents, microorganisms, etc. Until—and not until—much more is known about the biochemical, physiological, and psychological consequences of such losses, no one is justified in passing judgment as to how important this factor is in the genesis of the disease states that seem so often to follow close upon an episode of grief. To dismiss such inquiry as unnecessary or irrelevant at this stage of our knowledge is an expression of

prejudice (in its literal sense, a prejudgment, or forming a judgment without due knowledge or examination). Who now would be so rash as to dismiss the possibilities that biochemical or physiological processes occurring during the grief reaction may not constitute conditions conductive to other somatic changes of more serious consequence?

4. As a corollary of the above, we identify a ubiquitous *psychological stress,* meaning that the concept of objects and of object loss is only meaningful in terms of the existence and operation of the mental apparatus. This means that whatever the consequences of object loss and grief may be, whether manifest ultimately in biochemical, physiological, psychological, or social terms, they must first be initiated in the central nervous system. This imposes upon the medical scientist the necessity to pay more attention to the role of the central nervous system in the maintenance of the functional integrity of the organism as a whole as well as of its various parts. In spite of much lip service to the contrary, most physicians and clinical investigators think and work as if the central nervous system is the seat only of reflexes and of purely intellectual processes and really need not be considered when studying disease manifest elsewhere in the body. The reluctance and/or inability to consider psychological components of man and his illnesses actually has come to include the nervous system as well. But new knowledge of central integrating and regulating processes, as has been brought forth by recent work on the limbic and reticular activating systems, promises soon to dissipate this barrier.[7]

5. The concept of grief as a disease requires that we keep in view and in perspective aspects of the external environment other than what we have been accustomed to heretofore—namely, the environment made up of the significant psychic objects. This becomes one reason why the persons, job, home, goals, etc., in the life of our patients cannot be disregarded in our consideration of illness, at least not until it has been proven that the vicissitudes of object relations, including grief, the disorder consequent to object loss, plays no role in the pathogenesis of disease.

6. If object loss is a potential stress, then maintenance of objects or replacement of objects must be considered as important variables in sustaining health and adjustment. The physician, the hospital, the clinical investigator, indeed, even the experiment, may come to fulfill the requirements of a necessary and supporting psychic object for a patient. Everyone is aware of the therapeutic influence of the physician on the patient, but how many unwary clinical investigators have been observing physiologic or biochemical

changes in their experimental subjects, believing these to be the influence of some drug or other procedure when in fact these changes were secondary to the varying effects of the experimenter's unwitting role as a psychic object for the patient? For many varieties of clinical investigation it is necessary to regard the experimenter as part of the experiment.[8]

This does not exhaust the Pandora's box opened by such a perspective. Once opened, we cannot easily refute the real, yet unknown influences that must now come under our scrutiny. Yet the human mind, that wonderful instrument of discovery, has a disconcerting capacity to use denial, to turn away from that which is not easily comprehended or which has awesome implications, as I believe is true of this concept. The first response when confronted with news of a grievous loss is, "No, it can't be. I don't believe it; I won't believe it." I would call your attention to the fact that cherished ideas, even if false, are also psychic objects and as such are not easily given up. And only time and much work will establish whose cherished ideas are the false ones.

I close with a quotation ascribed to Albert Szent-Gyorgyi: "Research is to see what everybody else has seen and think what nobody else has thought." To this I would only add that Szent-Gyorgyi wisely refrained from claiming that this necessarily implied that the "new" thought is correct—at least, not until tested. And that is my challenge!

REFERENCES

1. Engel, G. L. "Homeostasis, Behavioral Adjustment and the Concept of Health and Disease." In Grinker, R. *Mid-Century Psychiatry,* Thomas, Springfield, Ill., 1953, pp. 33–59.
2. Engel, G. L. Selection of clinical material in psychosomatic medicine: The Need for a New physiology. *Psychosom. Med.* 16:368, 1954.
3. Engel, G. L. A unified concept of health and disease, *Perspectives in Biology and Medicine.* 3 No. 4, 1960.
4. Freud, S. "Mourning and Melancholia" (1917). Standard Edition, *Complete Works,* London, Vol. XIV, 237, 1957.
5. Lindemann, E. Symptomatology and management of acute grief. *Am. J. Psychiat.* 101:14, 1944.
6. Schmale, A. H. Relationship of separation and depression to disease. *Psychosom. Med.* 20:259, 1958.
7. Jasper, H. H., Ed. *Reticular Formation of the Brain,* Little, Boston, 1958.
8. Engel, G. L., Reichsman, F., and Segal, H. L. A study of an infant with a gastric fistula. I. Behavior and the rate of total HCl secretion, *Psychosom. Med.* 18:374, 1956.

Introductory Notes to Chapter 2

Rita V. Frankiel

This article, psychiatric—as distinct from psychoanalytic—in tone and outlook, was written during World War II. It presents a compassionate compendium of typical responses of adults to sudden, unexpected loss and is a significant contribution, even today, to our understanding of the nature of grief. It describes accurately and thoroughly the range of immediate responses in acute grief as observed in a sample of over one hundred cases. Excellent though it is in clinical description, the article shows its age in three respects. First, it is entirely centered on the psychiatrist as therapist for the bereaved. (Treatment by nonmedical practitioners—limited here to clergy and social workers—is seen as consisting exclusively in convincing the reluctant patient to continue in treatment with the psychiatrist. Psychologists and other caregivers are completely omitted. The field of clinical psychology only began in any serious or systematic way after the end of World War II, and so Lindeman's narrowness is understandable on historic grounds.) Second, a medication program is recommended for reducing emotional distress at bedtime; in the almost fifty years since this article was published, the range of medication available and sophistication about its use has made any universal prescription obsolete. Third, today we would not be surprised that in some families separation without death is traumatic and can produce symptoms in family members. Awareness and description of separation-individuation pathology has become one of our prominent clinical concerns.

2. Symptomatology and Management of Acute Grief

Erich Lindemann

INTRODUCTION

At first glance, acute grief would not seem to be a medical or psychiatric disorder in the strict sense of the word but rather a normal reaction to a distressing situation. However, the understanding of reactions to traumatic experiences, whether or not they represent clear-cut neuroses, has become of ever-increasing importance to the psychiatrist. Bereavement, or the sudden cessation of social interaction, seems to be of special interest because it is often cited among the alleged psychogenic factors in psychosomatic disorders. The enormous increase in grief reactions due to war casualties, furthermore, demands an evaluation of their probable effect on the mental and physical health of our population.

The points to be made in this paper are as follows:

1. Acute grief is a definite syndrome with psychological and somatic symptomatology.

2. This syndrome may appear immediately after a crisis; it may be delayed; it may be exaggerated or apparently absent.

3. In place of the typical syndrome there may appear distorted pictures, each of which represents one special aspect of the grief syndrome.

4. By appropriate techniques these distorted pictures can be successfully transformed into a normal grief reaction with resolution.

Our observations comprise 101 patients. Included are (1) psychoneurotic patients who lost a relative during the course of treatment, (2) relatives of patients who died in the hospital, (3) bereaved disaster victims (Cocoanut Grove Fire) and their close relatives, (4) relatives of members of the armed forces.

Reprinted by permission of the American Psychiatric Association from the *American Journal of Psychiatry* 101 (1944):141–48. Copyright 1944 American Psychiatric Association.

The investigation consisted of a series of psychiatric interviews. Both the timing and the content of the discussions were recorded. These records were subsequently analysed in terms of the symptoms reported and of the changes in mental status observed progressively through a series of interviews. The psychiatrist avoided all suggestions and interpretations until the picture of symptomatology and spontaneous reaction tendencies of the patients had become clear from the records. The somatic complaints offered important leads for objective study. Careful laboratory work on spirograms, g.-i. functions, and metabolic studies are in progress and will be reported separately. At present we wish to present only our psychological observations.

SYMPTOMATOLOGY OF NORMAL GRIEF

The picture shown by persons in acute grief is remarkably uniform. Common to all is the following syndrome: sensations of somatic distress occurring in waves lasting from twenty minutes to an hour at a time, a feeling of tightness in the throat, choking with shortness of breath, need for sighing, and an empty feeling in the abdomen, lack of muscular power, and an intense subjective distress described as tension or mental pain. The patient soon learns that these waves of discomfort can be precipitated by visits, by mentioning the deceased, and by receiving sympathy. There is a tendency to avoid the syndrome at any cost, to refuse visits lest they should precipitate the reaction, and to keep deliberately from thought all references to the deceased.

The striking features are (1) the marked tendency to sighing respiration; this respiratory disturbance was most conspicuous when the patient was made to discuss his grief. (2) The complaint about lack of strength and exhaustion is universal and is described as follows: "It is almost impossible to climb up a stairway." "Everything I lift seems so heavy." "The slightest effort makes me feel exhausted." "I can't walk to the corner without feeling exhausted." (3) Digestive symptoms are described as follows: "The food tastes like sand." "I have no appetite at all." "I stuff the food down because I have to eat." "My saliva won't flow." "My abdomen feels hollow." "Everything seems slowed up in my stomach."

The sensorium is generally somewhat altered. There is commonly a slight sense of unreality, a feeling of increased emotional distance from other people (sometimes they appear shadowy or small), and there is intense preoccupation with the image of the deceased. A patient who lost his daughter in the Cocoanut Grove disaster visualized his girl in the telephone booth calling for him and was much troubled by the loudness with which his name was called by her and was so vividly preoccupied with the scene that he became oblivious of his surroundings. A young navy pilot lost a close friend; he remained a vivid part of his imagery, not in terms of an imaginary companion. He ate with him and talked over problems with him, for instance, discussing with him his plan of joining the Air Corps. Up to the time of the study, six months later, he denied the fact that the boy was no longer with him. Some patients are much concerned about this aspect of their grief reaction because they feel it indicates approaching insanity.

Another strong preoccupation is with feelings of guilt. The bereaved searches the time before the death for evidence of failure to do right by the lost one. He accuses himself of negligence and exaggerates minor omissions. After the fire disaster the central topic of discussion for a young married woman was the fact that her husband died after he left her following a quarrel, and of a young man whose wife died that he fainted too soon to save her.

In addition, there is often disconcerting loss of warmth in relationship to other people, a tendency to respond with irritability and anger, a wish not to be bothered by others at a time when friends and relatives make a special effort to keep up friendly relationships.

These feelings of hostility, surprising and quite inexplicable to the patients, disturbed them and again were often taken as signs of approaching insanity. Great efforts are made to handle them, and the result is often a formalized, stiff manner of social interaction.

The activity throughout the day of the severely bereaved person shows remarkable changes. There is no retardation of action and speech; quite to the contrary, there is a push of speech, especially when talking about the deceased. There is restlessness, inability to sit still, moving about in an aimless fashion, continually searching for something to do. There is, however, at the same time, a painful lack of capacity to initiate and maintain organized patterns of activity. What is done is done with lack of zest, as though one were going through the motions. The bereaved clings to the daily routine of prescribed activities; but these activities do not proceed in the automatic, self-sustaining fashion which characterizes normal work but have to be carried on with effort, as though each fragment of the activity became a special task. The bereaved is surprised to find how large a part of his customary activity was done in some meaningful relationship to the deceased and has now lost its significance. Especially the habits of social interaction—

meeting friends, making conversation, sharing enterprises with others—
seem to have been lost. This loss leads to a strong dependency on anyone
who will stimulate the bereaved to activity and serve as the initiating agent.

These five points—(1) somatic distress, (2) preoccupation with the image
of the deceased, (3) guilt, (4) hostile reactions, and (5) loss of patterns of
conduct—seem to be pathognomonic for grief. There may be added a sixth
characteristic, shown by patients who border on pathological reactions,
which is not so conspicuous as the others but nevertheless often striking
enough to color the whole picture. This is the appearance of traits of the
deceased in the behavior of the bereaved, especially symptoms shown during
the last illness, or behavior which may have been shown at the time of the
tragedy. A bereaved person is observed or finds himself walking in the
manner of his deceased father. He looks in the mirror and believes that his
face appears just like that of the deceased. He may show a change of
interests in the direction of the former activities of the deceased and may start
enterprises entirely different from his former pursuits. A wife who lost
her husband, an insurance agent, found herself writing to many insurance
companies offering her services with somewhat exaggerated schemes. It
seemed a regular observation in these patients that the painful preoccupation
with the image of the deceased described above was transformed into preoccupation with symptoms or personality traits of the lost person, but now
displaced to their own bodies and activities by identification.

COURSE OF NORMAL GRIEF REACTIONS

The duration of a grief reaction seems to depend upon the success with which
a person does the *grief work*, namely emancipation from the bondage to the
deceased, readjustment to the environment in which the deceased is missing,
and the formation of new relationships. One of the big obstacles to this work
seems to be the fact that many patients try to avoid the intense distress
connected with the grief experience and to avoid the expression of emotion
necessary for it. The men victims after the Cocoanut Grove fire appeared in
the early psychiatric interviews to be in a state of tension with tightened
facial musculature, unable to relax for fear they might "break down." It
required considerable persuasion to yield to the grief process before they
were willing to accept the discomfort of bereavement. One assumed a hostile
attitude toward the psychiatrist, refusing to allow any references to the
deceased and rather rudely asking him to leave. This attitude remained

throughout his stay on the ward, and the prognosis for his condition is not good in the light of other observations. Hostility of this sort was encountered on only occasional visits with the other patients. They became willing to accept the grief process and to embark on a program of dealing in memory with the deceased person. As soon as this became possible there seemed to be a rapid relief of tension and the subsequent interviews were rather animated conversations in which the deceased was idealized and in which misgivings about the future adjustment were worked through.

Examples of the psychiatrist's rôle in assisting patients in their readjustment after bereavement are contained in the following case histories. The first shows a very successful readjustment.

A woman, aged forty, lost her husband in the fire. She had a history of good adjustment previously. One child, ten years old. When she heard about her husband's death she was extremely depressed, cried bitterly, did not want to live, and for three days showed a state of utter dejection.

When seen by the psychiatrist, she was glad to have assistance and described her painful preoccupation with memories of her husband and her fear that she might lose her mind. She had a vivid visual image of his presence, picturing him as going to work in the morning and herself as wondering whether he would return in the evening, whether she could stand his not returning, then, describing to herself how he does return, plays with the dog, receives his child, and gradually tried to accept the fact that he is not there any more. It was only after ten days that she succeeded in accepting his loss and then only after having described in detail the remarkable qualities of her husband, the tragedy of his having to stop his activities at the pinnacle of his success, and his deep devotion to her.

In the subsequent interviews she explained with some distress that she had become very much attached to the examiner and that she waited for the hour of his coming. This reaction she considered disloyal to her husband but at the same time she could accept the fact that it was a hopeful sign of her ability to fill the gap he had left in her life. She then showed a marked drive for activity, making plans for supporting herself and her little girl, mapping out the preliminary steps for resuming her old profession as secretary, and making efforts to secure help from the occupational therapy department in reviewing her knowledge of French.

Her convalescence, both emotional and somatic, progressed smoothly, and she made a good adjustment immediately on her return home.

A man of fifty-two, successful in business, lost his wife, with whom he had lived in happy marriage. The information given him about his wife's death confirmed his suspicions of several days. He responded with a severe grief reaction, with which he was unable to cope. He did not want to see visitors, was ashamed of breaking down, and asked to be permitted to stay in the hospital on the psychiatric service, when his physical condition would have permitted his discharge, because he wanted further assistance. Any mention of his wife produced a severe wave of depressive reaction, but with psychiatric assistance he gradually became willing to go through this painful process, and after three days on the psychiatric service he seemed well enough to go home.

He showed a high rate of verbal activity, was restless, needed to be occupied continually, and felt that the experience had whipped him into a state of restless overactivity.

As soon as he returned home he took an active part in his business, assuming a post in which he had a great many telephone calls. He also took over the rôle of amateur psychiatrist to another bereaved person, spending time with him and comforting him for his loss. In his eagerness to start anew, he developed a plan to sell all his former holdings, including his house, his furniture, and giving away anything which could remind him of his wife. Only after considerable discussion was he able to see that this would mean avoiding immediate grief at the price of an act of poor judgment. Again he had to be encouraged to deal with his grief reactions in a more direct manner. He has made good adjustment.

With eight to ten interviews in which the psychiatrist shares the grief work, and with a period of from four to six weeks, it was ordinarily possible to settle an uncomplicated and undistorted grief reaction. This was the case in all but one of the thirteen Cocoanut Grove fire victims.

MORBID GRIEF REACTIONS

Morbid grief reactions represent distortions of normal grief. The conditions mentioned here were transformed into "normal reactions" and then found their resolution.

a. *Delay of Reaction.* The most striking and most frequent reaction of this sort is *delay* and *postponement*. If the bereavement occurs at a time when the patient is confronted with important tasks and when there is necessity for maintaining the morale of others, he may show little or no reaction for weeks or even much longer. A brief delay is described in the following example.

A girl of seventeen lost both parents and her boy friend in the fire and was herself burned severely, with marked involvement of the lungs. Throughout her stay in the hospital her attitude was that of cheerful acceptance without any sign of adequate distress. When she was discharged at the end of three weeks she appeared cheerful, talked rapidly, with a considerable flow of ideas, seemed eager to return home and to assume the rôle of parent for her two younger siblings. Except for slight feelings of "lonesomeness" she complained of no distress.

This period of griefless acceptance continued for the next two months, even when the household was dispersed and her younger siblings were placed in other homes. Not until the end of the tenth week did she begin to show a true state of grief with marked feelings of depression, intestinal emptiness, tightness in her throat, frequent crying, and vivid preoccupation with her deceased parents.

That this delay may involve years became obvious first by the fact that patients in acute bereavement about a recent death may soon upon exploration be found preoccupied with grief about a person who died many years ago. In this manner a woman of thirty-eight, whose mother had died recently and who had responded to the mother's death with a surprisingly severe reaction, was found to be but mildly concerned with her mother's death but deeply engrossed with unhappy and perplexing fantasies concerning the death of her brother, who died twenty years ago under dramatic circumstances from metastasizing carcinoma after amputation of his arm had been postponed too long. The discovery that a former unresolved grief reaction may be precipitated in the course of the discussion of another recent event was soon demonstrated in psychiatric interviews by patients who showed all the traits of a true grief reaction when the topic of a former loss arose.

The precipitating factor for the delayed reaction may be a deliberate recall of circumstances surrounding the death or may be a spontaneous occurrence in the patient's life. A peculiar form of this is the circumstance that a patient develops the grief reaction at the time when he himself is as old as the person who died. For instance, a railroad worker, aged forty-two appeared in the psychiatric clinic with a picture which was undoubtedly a grief reaction for which he had no explanation. It turned out that when he was twenty-two his mother, then forty-two, had committed suicide.

b. *Distorted Reactions.* The delayed reactions may occur after an interval which was not marked by any abnormal behavior or distress, but in which there developed an *alteration* in the patient's *conduct* perhaps not conspicuous or serious enough to lead him to a psychiatrist. These alterations may be considered as the surface manifestations of an unresolved grief reaction, which may respond to fairly simple and quick psychiatric management if recognized. They may be classified as follows: (1) *overactivity without a sense of loss,* rather with a sense of well-being and zest, the activities being of an expansive and adventurous nature and bearing semblance to the activities formerly carried out by the deceased, as described above: (2) *the acquisition of symptoms belonging to the last illness of the deceased.* This type of patient appears in medical clinics and is often labelled hypochondriasis or hysteria. To what extent actual alterations of physiological functions occur under these circumstances will have to be a field of further careful inquiry. I owe to Dr. Chester Jones a report about a patient whose electrocardiogram showed a definite change during a period of three weeks, which started two weeks after the time her father died of heart disease.

While this sort of symptom formation "by identification" may still be considered as conversion symptoms such as we know from hysteria, there is another type of disorder doubtlessly presenting (3) a recognized *medical disease,* namely, a group of psychosomatic conditions, predominantly ulcerative colitis, rheumatoid arthritis, and asthma. Extensive studies in ulcerative colitis have produced evidence that thirty-three out of forty-one patients with ulcerative colitis developed their disease in close time relationship to the loss of an important person. Indeed, it was this observation which first gave the impetus for the present detailed study of grief. Two of the patients developed bloody diarrhea at funerals. In the others it developed within a few weeks after the loss. The course of the ulcerative colitis was strikingly benefited when this grief reaction was resolved by psychiatric technique.

At the level of social adjustment there often occurs a conspicuous (4) *alteration in relationship to friends and relatives.* The patient feels irritable, does not want to be bothered, avoids former social activities, and is afraid he might antagonize his friends by his lack of interest and his critical attitudes. Progressive social isolation follows, and the patient needs considerable encouragement in re-establishing his social relationship.

While overflowing hostility appears to be spread out over all relationships it may also occur as (5) *furious hostility against specific persons;* the docto: or the surgeon are accused bitterly for neglect of duty and the patient may assume that foul play has led to the death. It is characteristic that while patients talk a good deal about their suspicions and their bitter feelings, they are not likely to take any action against the accused, as a truly paranoic person might do.

(6) Many bereaved persons struggled with much effort against these feel ings of hostility, which to them seem absurd, representing a vicious change in their characters and to be hidden as much as possible. Some patient: succeed in hiding their hostility but become wooden and formal, with affec tivity and conduct *resembling schizophrenic pictures.* A typical report is this "I go through all the motions of living. I look after my children. I do my errands. I go to social functions, but it is like being in a play; it doesn't really concern me. I can't have any warm feelings. If I were to have any feelings a all I would be angry with everybody." This patient's reaction to therapy was characterized by growing hostility against the therapist, and it require considerable skill to make her continue interviews in spite of the discon certing hostility which she had been fighting so much. The absence o emotional display in this patient's face and actions was quite striking. He face had a mask-like appearance, her movements were formal, stilted, robot like, without the fine play of emotional expression.

(7) Closely related to this picture is a *lasting loss of patterns of socia interaction.* The patient cannot initiate any activity, is full of eagerness to b active—restless, can't sleep—but throughout the day he will not start an: activity unless "primed" by somebody else. He will be grateful at sharin: activities with others but will not be able to make up his mind to do anythin alone. The picture is one of lack of decision and initiative. Organize activities along social lines occur only if a friend takes the patient along an shares the activity with him. Nothing seems to promise reward; only th ordinary activities of the day are carried on, and these in a routine manner falling apart into small steps, each of which has to be carried out with muc effort and without zest.

(8) There is, in addition, a picture in which a patient is active but i which most of his activities attain a coloring which is *detrimental to his ow social and economic existence.* Such patients, with uncalled for generosity give away their belongings, are easily lured into foolish economic dealings lose their friends and professional standing by a series of "stupid acts," an

find themselves finally without family, friends, social status or money. This protracted self-punitive behavior seems to take place without any awareness of excessive feelings of guilt. It is a particularly distressing grief picture because it is likely to hurt other members of the family and drag down friends and business associates.

(9) This leads finally to the picture in which the grief reaction takes the form of a straight *agitated depression* with tension, agitation, insomnia, feelings of worthlessness, bitter self-accusation, and obvious need for punishment. Such patients may be dangerously suicidal.

A young man aged thirty-two had received only minor burns and left the hospital apparently well on the road to recovery just before the psychiatric survey of the disaster victims took place. On the fifth day he had learned that his wife had died. He seemed somewhat relieved of his worry about her fate; impressed the surgeon as being unusually well-controlled during the following short period of his stay in the hospital.

On January 1st he was returned to the hospital by his family. Shortly after his return home he had become restless, did not want to stay at home, had taken a trip to relatives trying to find rest, had not succeeded, and had returned home in a state of marked agitation, appearing preoccupied, frightened, and unable to concentrate on any organized activity. The mental status presented a somewhat unusual picture. He was restless, could not sit still or participate in any activity on the ward. He would try to read, drop it after a few minutes, or try to play pingpong, give it up after a short time. He would try to start conversations, break them off abruptly, and then fall into repeated murmured utterances: "Nobody can help me. When is it going to happen? I am doomed, am I not?" With great effort it was possible to establish enough rapport to carry on interviews. He complained about his feeling of extreme tension, inability to breathe, generalized weakness and exhaustion, and his frantic fear that something terrible was going to happen. "I'm destined to live in insanity or I must die. I know that it is God's will. I have this awful feeling of guilt." With intense morbid guilt feelings, he reviewed incessantly the events of the fire. His wife had stayed behind. When he tried to pull her out, he had fainted and was shoved out by the crowd. She was burned while he was saved. "I should have saved her or I should have died too." He complained about being filled with an incredible violence and did not know what to do about it. The rapport established with him lasted for only brief periods of time. He then would fall back into his state of intense agitation and muttering. He slept poorly even with large sedation. In the course of four days he became somewhat more composed, had longer periods of contact with the psychiatrist, and seemed to feel that he was being understood and might be able to cope with his morbid feelings of guilt and violent impulses. On the sixth day of his hospital stay, however, after skillfully distracting the attention of his special nurse, he jumped through a closed window to a violent death.

If the patient is not conspicuously suicidal, it may nevertheless be true that he has a strong desire for painful experiences, and such patients are likely to desire shock treatment of some sort, which they picture as a cruel experience, such as electrocution might be.

A twenty-eight-year-old woman whose twenty-months-old son was accidentally smothered developed a state of severe agitated depression with self-accusation, inability to enjoy anything, hopelessness about the future, overflow of hostility against the husband and his parents, also with excessive hostility against the psychiatrist. She insisted upon electric-shock treatment and was finally referred to another physician who treated her. She responded to the shock treatments very well and felt relieved of her sense of guilt.

It is remarkable that agitated depressions of this sort represent only a small fraction of the pictures of grief in our series.

PROGNOSTIC EVALUATION

Our observations indicate that to a certain extent the type and severity of the grief reaction can be predicted. Patients with obsessive personality make-up and with a history of former depressions are likely to develop an agitated depression. Severe reactions seem to occur in mothers who have lost young children. The intensity of interaction with the deceased before his death seems to be significant. It is important to realize that such interaction does not have to be of the affectionate type; on the contrary, the death of a person who invited much hostility, especially hostility which could not well be expressed because of his status and claim to loyalty, may be followed by a severe grief reaction in which hostile impulses are the most conspicuous feature. Not infrequently the person who passed away represented a key person in a social system, his death being followed by disintegration of this social system and by a profound alteration of the living and social conditions for the bereaved. In such cases readjustment presents a severe task quite apart from the reaction to the loss incurred. All these factors seem to be more important than a tendency to react with neurotic symptoms in previous life. In this way the most conspicuous forms of morbid identification were found in persons who had no former history of a tendency to psychoneurotic reactions.

MANAGEMENT

Proper psychiatric management of grief reactions may prevent prolonged and serious alterations in the patient's social adjustment, as well as potential medical disease. The essential task facing the psychiatrist is that of sharing the patient's grief work, namely, his efforts at extricating himself from the bondage to the deceased and at finding new patterns of rewarding interaction. It is of the greatest importance to notice that not only over-reaction but under-reaction of the bereaved must be given attention, because delayed responses may occur at unpredictable moments and the dangerous distortions of the grief reaction, not conspicuous at first, be quite destructive later, and these may be prevented.

Religious agencies have led in dealing with the bereaved. They have provided comfort by giving the backing of dogma to the patient's wish for continued interaction with the deceased, have developed rituals which maintain the patient's interaction with others, and have counteracted the morbid guilt feelings of the patient by Divine Grace and by promising an opportunity for "making up" to the deceased at the time of a later reunion. While these measures have helped countless mourners, comfort alone does not provide adequate assistance in the patient's grief work. He has to accept the pain of the bereavement. He has to review his relationship with the deceased, and has to become acquainted with the alterations in his own modes of emotional reaction. His fear of insanity, his fear of accepting the surprising changes in his feelings, especially the overflow of hostility, have to be worked through. He will have to express his sorrow and sense of loss. He will have to find an acceptable formulation of his future relationship to the deceased. He will have to verbalize his feelings of guilt, and he will have to find persons around him whom he can use as "primers" for the acquisition of new patterns of conduct. All this can be done in eight to ten interviews.

Special techniques are needed if hostility is the most marked feature of the grief reaction. The hostility may be directed against the psychiatrist, and the patient will have such guilt over his hostility that he will avoid further interviews. The help of a social workers or a minister, or if these are not available, a member of the family, to urge the patient to continue coming to see the psychiatrist may be indispensable. If the tension and the depressive features are too great, a combination of benzedrine sulphate, 5–10 mgm. b.i.d., and sodium amytal, 3 gr. before retiring, may be useful in first reducing emotional distress to a tolerable degree. Severe agitated depressive reactions may defy all efforts to psychotherapy and may respond well to shock treatment.

Since it is obvious that not all bereaved persons, especially those suffering because of war casualties, can have the benefit of expert psychiatric help, much of this knowledge will have to be passed on to auxiliary workers. Social workers and ministers will have to be on the look-out for the more ominous pictures, referring these to the psychiatrist while assisting the more normal reactions themselves.

ANTICIPATORY GRIEF REACTIONS

While our studies were at first limited to reactions to actual death, it must be understood that grief reactions are just one form of separation reactions. Separation by death is characterized by its irreversibility and finality. Separation may, of course, occur for other reasons. We were at first surprised to find genuine grief reactions in patients who had not experienced a bereavement but who had experienced separation, for instance with the departure of a member of the family into the armed forces. Separation in this case is not due to death but is under the threat of death. A common picture hitherto not appreciated is a syndrome which we have designated *anticipatory grief*. The patient is so concerned with her adjustment after the potential death of father or son that she goes through all the phases of grief—depression, heightened preoccupation with the departed, a review of all the forms of death which might befall him, and anticipation of the modes of readjustment which might be necessitated by it. While this reaction may well form a safeguard against the impact of a sudden death notice, it can turn out to be of a disadvantage at the occasion of reunion. Several instances of this sort came to our attention when a soldier just returned from the battlefront complained that his wife did not love him anymore and demanded immediate divorce. In such situations apparently the grief work had been done so effectively that the patient has emancipated herself and the readjustment must now be directed towards new interaction. It is important to know this because many family disasters of this sort may be avoided through prophylactic measures.

BIBLIOGRAPHY

Many of the observations are, of course, not entirely new. Delayed reactions were described by Helene Deutsch (1). Shock treatment in agitated depressions due to bereavement has recently been advocated by Myerson (2). Morbid identification has been stressed at many points in the psychoanalytic literature and recently by H. A. Murray (3). The relation of mourning and depressive psychoses has been discussed by Freud (4), Melanie Klein (5), and Abraham (6). Bereavement reactions in war time were discussed by Wilson (7). The reactions after the Cocoanut Grove fire were described in some detail in a chapter of the monograph on this civilian disaster (8). The effect of wartime separations was reported by Rosenbaum (9). The incidence of grief reactions among the psychogenic factors in the asthma and rheumatoid arthritis has been mentioned by Cobb, *et al.* (10, 11).

1. Deutsch, Helene. Absence of grief. Psychoanalyt. Quart., 6:12, 1937.
2. Myerson, Abraham. The use of shock therapy in prolonged grief reactions. New England J. Med., 230:9, Mar. 2, 1944.
3. Murray, H. A. Visual manifestations of personality. Jr. Abn. & Social Psychol., 32:161–184, 1937.
4. Freud, Sigmund. Mourning and melancholia. Collected Papers IV, 288–317; 152–170.
5. Klein, Melanie. Mourning and its relation to manic-depressive states. Internat. J. Psychoan., 21:125–153, 1940.
6. Abraham, K. Notes on the psycho-analytical investigation and treatment of the libido, viewed in the light of mental disorder. Selected Papers.
7. Wilson, A. T. M. Reactive emotional disorders. Practitioner, 146:254–258.
8. Cobb, S., and Lindemann, E. Neuropsychiatric observations after the Cocoanut Grove fire. Ann. Surg., June 1943.
9. Rosenbaum, Milton. Emotional aspects of wartime separations. Family, 24:337–341, 1944.
10. Cobb, S., Bauer, W., and Whitney. I. Environmental factors in rheumatoid arthritis. J. A. M. A., 113:668–670, 1939.
11. McDermott, N., and Cobb, S. Psychogenic factors in asthma. Psychosom. Med. 1:204–341. 1939.

PART II

THEORETICAL FOUNDATIONS

Introductory Notes to Chapters 3, 4, 5, and 6

Rita V. Frankiel

In psychoanalysis, all roads begin with Freud. In the study of object loss, "Mourning and Melancholia" (1917) is usually taken to be the beginning of the road, although Abraham had already published a major paper in this area several years before Freud (Abraham 1911). It is, however, Freud's publication that is the one best known to all who work in this area, and it is the one we all begin with. In this paper, Freud describes mourning in adults, contrasts it with depressive states, and explicates the relation between the two conditions. He begins to develop his ideas about the difference between normal mourning and its pathological counterpart. He formulates the idea that pathological mourning is founded on profound unconscious ambivalence toward the lost object. In the process, he adds to his developing body of thought about the relation between identification and object loss. Freud makes an explicit connection between narcissism, narcissistic object choice, and the tendency to experience repeated depressive states and unresolvable—that is, pathological—mourning.

The concept of mourning has played a significant part in the development of psychoanalysis. Starting from his earliest clinical contributions, Freud described patients in acute and chronic states of mourning, but his thoughts on the subject were not made explicit until the publication of "Mourning and Melancholia." For example, of the five treatments reported in detail in Freud's first purely clinical treatise, "Studies on Hysteria" (Breuer and Freud 1893–95), three patients fell ill subsequent to the death of someone close to them: the father in two instances, the husband in the third. In the fourth case, the symptoms followed on the patient discovering that her hopes for winning her employer's love were unrealistic: also a loss, though of quite another kind. Only one of the cases does not involve symptoms originating in some form of mourning. At that time in the development of psychoanalysis, Freud was immersed in understanding hysteria and symptom formation; consequently, although grief reactions are described, their relation to the causation of the disturbances under study (through identification with and ambivalence toward the lost object), are not discussed in those terms. In fact, in "Mourning and Melancholia," Freud begins an examination of the whole question of identification, seeing it as a "preliminary stage of object-choice . . . the first way in which the ego picks out an object" (249–50). In depression, the object-choice is replaced by an identification, and the person abuses his or her object by abusing himself or herself.

In his treatment of the Rat Man, Freud makes a clear distinction between pathological and normal mourning. The Rat Man's obsessional symptoms worsened significantly after the death of his father. In the initial phase of the treatment, Freud told him that although normally one to two years would suffice for the work of grieving to be completed, in the Rat Man's case, since the mourning had taken a pathological course, it could last indefinitely (1909, 186).

With the formulation of the structural theory in "The Ego and the Id" (1923), Freud was in a position to describe further how the lost object is represented in the development and ongoing life of the ego. In the passage from that work included here, Freud argues that object loss and identification in mourning are paralleled by identifications leading to the formation of the super-ego and the ego ideal. Now fully recognizing the part that object loss or shifts in relation to objects play in all development, he shows that in the dissolution of the Oedipus complex, relations with the feared, loved, and hated objects are forever continued in the form of personal similarities based on identification and aversive inhibitions that carry forward the real and imagined prohibitions imposed by the object in the past. Recognition of these processes is essential in understanding the lifelong deviations of personality and character that are set in train by losses either before identification is developmentally possible or at a time when satisfactory replacement objects are not available.

In "Inhibitions, Symptoms, and Anxiety" (1926), Freud picks up the question, pondered but unanswered in "Mourning and Melancholia": "Why is mourning so painful?" He formulates an answer in terms of psychic energy: "Mourning is entrusted with the task of carrying out this retreat from the object in all those situations in which it was the recipient of a high degree of cathexis. That this separation should be painful fits in with what we have just said, in view of the high and unsatisfiable cathexis of longing which is concentrated on the object by the bereaved person during the reproduction of the situations in which he must undo the ties that bind him to it" (172). The papers by Klein and Segal later in this volume present a different way of accounting for the pain of mourning. Their formulations rest on the notion that the loss of a loved figure in external reality has a profound effect on the sense of well-being because the loss puts the internal object world into disarray. The pain of mourning is related to the collapse and rebuilding of the inner world and the restoration of the internal good object, which is the source of optimism and good feeling about self and the world.

In "Fetishism" (1927), Freud describes the splitting of the ego in relation to the unacceptable perception that women have no penis. Freud mentions but does not here focus on an analogous psychic operation: two of his patients had disavowed the death of a beloved father (one at the age two, the other at age ten) in such a way that while in one aspect of their mental life they did not recognize the father's death, in other aspects they fully affirmed it (156). These patients were not psychotic. In general, they could and did affirm reality, but in some aspect of their inner lives and behavior, they acted as if the dead father was still a living force.

The splitting of the ego implied in these cases held Freud's interest to the point where he was working on them at the end of his life. His last, unfinished, posthumously published paper is "The Splitting of the Ego in the Process of Defense" (1938b). The interpretation of splitting was also clearly stated in another of his last works, "An Outline of Psycho-Analysis" (1938a). In that work he reiterated that splitting of the ego is by no means restricted to fetishism; he saw it as expressing the need to fend off distressing demands from the external world. The denial of these demands is effected through a disavowal of perceptions originating in reality. Freud calls these disavowals, "half measures, incomplete attempts at detachment from reality. The disavowal is always supplemented by an acknowledgment; two contrary and independent attitudes always arise and result in the situation of there being a splitting of the ego . . . the issue depends on which of the two can seize hold of the greater intensity" ("Outline," 204). In these works, we have the fundamental descriptions of the conscious avowal and unconscious disavowal of the death of a loved one that is the source of so much of the psychopathology developed by the bereaved—no matter whether their bereavement happens early in life or late.

3. Mourning and Melancholia

Sigmund Freud

Dreams having served us as the prototype in normal life of narcissistic mental disorders, we will now try to throw some light on the nature of melancholia by comparing it with the normal affect of mourning.[1] This time, however, we must begin by making an admission, as a warning against any over-estimation of the value of our conclusions. Melancholia, whose definition fluctuates even in descriptive psychiatry, takes on various clinical forms the grouping together of which into a single unity does not seem to be established with certainty; and some of these forms suggest somatic rather than psy-chogenic affections. Our material, apart from such impressions as are open to every observer, is limited to a small number of cases whose psychogenic nature was indisputable. We shall, therefore, from the outset drop all claim to general validity for our conclusions, and we shall console ourselves by reflecting that, with the means of investigation at our disposal to-day, we could hardly discover anything that was not typical, if not a whole class of disorders, at least of a small group of them.

The correlation of melancholia and mourning seems justified by the general picture of the two conditions.[2] Moreover, the exciting causes due to environmental influences are, so far as we can discern them at all, the same for both conditions. Mourning is regularly the reaction to the loss of a loved person, or to the loss of some abstraction which has taken the place of one, such as one's country, liberty, an ideal, and so on. In some people the same influences produce melancholia instead of mourning and we consequently suspect them of a pathological disposition. It is also well worth notice that, although mourning involves grave departures from the normal attitude to life, it never occurs to us to regard it as a pathological condition and to refer it to medical treatment. We rely on its being overcome after a certain lapse of time, and we look upon any interference with it as useless or even harmful.

The distinguishing mental features of melancholia are a profoundly painful dejection, cessation of interest in the outside world, loss of the capacity to love, inhibition of all activity, and a lowering of the self-regarding feelings to a degree that finds utterance in self-reproaches and self-revilings, and culminates in a delusional expectation of punishment. This picture becomes a little more intelligible when we consider that, with one exception, the same traits are met with in mourning. The disturbance of self-regard is absent in mourning; but otherwise the features are the same. Profound mourning, the reaction to the loss of someone who is loved, contains the same painful frame of mind, the same loss of interest in the outside world—in so far as it does not recall him—the same loss of capacity to adopt any new object of love (which would mean replacing him) and the same turning away from any activity that is not connected with thoughts of him. It is easy to see that this inhibition and circumscription of the ego is the expression of an exclusive devotion to mourning which leaves nothing over for other purposes or other interests. It is really only because we know so well how to explain it that this attitude does not seem to us pathological.

We should regard it as an appropriate comparison, too, to call the mood of mourning a "painful" one. We shall probably see the justification for this when we are in a position to give a characterization of the economics of pain.

In what, now, does the work which mourning performs consist? I do not think there is anything far-fetched in presenting it in the following way. Reality-testing has shown that the loved object no longer exists, and it proceeds to demand that all libido shall be withdrawn from its attachments to that object. This demand arouses understandable opposition—it is a matter of general observation that people never willingly abandon a libidinal position, not even, indeed, when a substitute is already beckoning to them. This opposition can be so intense that a turning away from reality takes place and a clinging to the object through the medium of a hallucinatory wishful psychosis. Normally, respect for reality gains the day. Nevertheless its orders cannot be obeyed at once. They are carried out bit by bit, at great expense of time and cathectic energy, and in the meantime the existence of the lost object is psychically prolonged. Each single one of the memories and expectations in which libido is bound to the object is brought up and hyper-cathected, and detachment of the libido is accomplished in respect of it. Why this compromise by which the command of reality is carried out piecemeal should be so extraordinarily painful is not at all easy to explain in terms of economics. It is remarkable that this painful unpleasure is taken as a matter of course by us. The fact is, however, that when the work of mourning is completed the ego becomes free and uninhibited again.

Let us now apply to melancholia what we have learnt about mourning. In one set of cases it is evident that melancholia too may be the reaction to the loss of a loved object. Where the exciting causes are different one can recognize that there is a loss of a more ideal kind. The object has not perhaps actually died, but has been lost as an object of love (e.g. in the case of a betrothed girl who has been jilted). In yet other cases one feels justified in maintaining the belief that a loss of this kind has occurred, but one cannot see clearly what it is that has been lost, and it is all the more reasonable to suppose that the patient cannot consciously perceive what he has lost either. This, indeed, might be so even if the patient is aware of the loss which has given rise to his melancholia, but only in the sense that he knows *whom* he has lost but not *what* he has lost in him. This would suggest that melancholia is in some way related to an object-loss which is withdrawn from consciousness, in contradistinction to mourning, in which there is nothing about the loss that is unconscious.

In mourning we found that the inhibition and loss of interest are fully accounted for by the work of mourning in which the ego is absorbed. In melancholia, the unknown loss will result in a similar internal work and will therefore be responsible for the melancholic inhibition. The difference is that the inhibition of the melancholic seems puzzling to us because we cannot see what it is that is absorbing him so entirely. The melancholic displays something else besides which is lacking in mourning—an extraordinary diminution in his self-regard, an impoverishment of his ego on a grand scale. In mourning it is the world which has become poor and empty; in melancholia it is the ego itself. The patient represents his ego to us as worthless, incapable of any achievement and morally despicable; he reproaches himself, vilifies himself and expects to be cast out and punished. He abases himself before everyone and commiserates with his own relatives for being connected with anyone so unworthy. He is not of the opinion that a change has taken place in him, but extends his self-criticism back over the past; he declares that he was never any better. This picture of a delusion of (mainly moral) inferiority is completed by sleeplessness and refusal to take nourishment, and—what is psychologically very remarkable—by an overcoming of the instinct which compels every living thing to cling to life.

It would be equally fruitless from a scientific and a therapeutic point of view to contradict a patient who brings these accusations against his ego. He must surely be right in some way and be describing something that is as it seems to him to be. Indeed, we must at once confirm some of his statements without reservation. He really is as lacking in interest and as incapable of love and achievement as he says. But that, as we know, is secondary; it is the effect of the internal work which is consuming his ego—work which is unknown to us but which is comparable to the work of mourning. He also seems to us justified in certain other self-accusations; it is merely that he has a keener eye for the truth than other people who are not melancholic. When in his heightened self-criticism he describes himself as petty, egoistic, dishonest, lacking in independence, one whose sole aim has been to hide the weakness of his own nature, it may be, so far as we know, that he has come pretty near to understanding himself; we only wonder why a man has to be ill before he can be accessible to a truth of this kind. For there can be no doubt that if anyone holds and expresses to others an opinion of himself such as this (an opinion which Hamlet held both of himself and of everyone else),[3] he is ill, whether he is speaking the truth or whether he is being more or less unfair to himself. Nor is it difficult to see that there is no correspondence, so far as we can judge, between the degree of self-abasement and its real justification. A good, capable, conscientious woman will speak no better of herself after she develops melancholia than one who is in fact worthless; indeed, the former is perhaps more likely to fall ill of the disease than the latter, of whom we too should have nothing good to say. Finally, it must strike us that after all the melancholic does not behave in quite the same way as a person who is crushed by remorse and self-reproach in a normal fashion. Feelings of shame in front of other people, which would more than anything characterize this latter condition, are lacking in the melancholic, or at least they are not prominent in him. One might emphasize the presence in him of an almost opposite trait of insistent communicativeness which finds satisfaction in self-exposure.

The essential thing, therefore, is not whether the melancholic's distressing self-denigration is correct, in the sense that his self-criticism agrees with the opinion of other people. The point must rather be that he is giving a correct description of his psychological situation. He has lost his self-respect and he must have good reason for this. It is true that we are then faced with a contradiction that presents a problem which is hard to solve. The analogy with mourning led us to conclude that he had suffered a loss in regard to an object; what he tells us points to a loss in regard to his ego.

Before going into this contradiction, let us dwell for a moment on the view which the melancholic's disorder affords of the constitution of the human ego. We see how in him one part of the ego sets itself over against the other, judges it critically, and, as it were, takes it as its object. Our suspicion that the critical agency which is here split off from the ego might also show its independence in other circumstances will be confirmed by every further observation. We shall really find grounds for distinguishing this agency from the rest of the ego. What we are here becoming acquainted with is the agency commonly called ''conscience''; we shall count it, along with the censorship of consciousness and reality-testing, among the major institutions of the ego, and we shall come upon evidence to show that it can become diseased on its own account. In the clinical picture of melancholia, dissatisfaction with the ego on moral grounds is the most outstanding feature. The patient's self-evaluation concerns itself much less frequently with bodily infirmity, ugliness or weakness, or with social inferiority; of this category, it is only his fears and asseverations of becoming poor that occupy a prominent position.

There is one observation, not at all difficult to make, which leads to the explanation of the contradiction mentioned above. If one listens patiently to a melancholic's many and various self-accusations, one cannot in the end avoid the impression that often the most violent of them are hardly at all applicable to the patient himself, but that with insignificant modifications they do fit someone else, someone whom the patient loves or has loved or should love. Every time one examines the facts this conjecture is confirmed. So we find the key to the clinical picture: we perceive that the self-reproaches are reproaches against a loved object which have been shifted away from it on to the patient's own ego.

The woman who loudly pities her husband for being tied to such an incapable wife as herself is really accusing her *husband* of being incapable, in whatever sense she may mean this. There is no need to be greatly surprised that a few genuine self-reproaches are scattered among those that have been transposed back. These are allowed to obtrude themselves, since they help to mask the others and make recognition of the true state of affairs impossible. Moreover, they derive from the *pros* and *cons* of the conflict of love that has led to the loss of love. The behaviour of the patients, too, now becomes much more intelligible. Their complaints are really "plaints" in the old sense of the word. They are not ashamed and do not hide themselves, since everything derogatory that they say about themselves is at bottom said about someone else. Moreover, they are far from evincing towards those around them the attitude of humility and submissiveness that would alone befit such worthless people. On the contrary, they make the greatest nuisance of themselves, and always seem as though they felt slighted and had been treated with great injustice. All this is possible only because the reactions expressed in their behaviour still proceed from a mental constellation of revolt, which has then, by a certain process, passed over into the crushed state of melancholia.

There is no difficulty in reconstructing this process. An object-choice, an attachment of the libido to a particular person, had at one time existed; then, owing to a real slight or disappointment coming from this loved person, the object-relationship was shattered. The result was not the normal one of a withdrawal of the libido from this object and a displacement of it on to a new one, but something different, for whose coming-about various conditions seem to be necessary. The object-cathexis proved to have little power of resistance and was brought to an end. But the free libido was not displaced on to another object; it was withdrawn into the ego. There, however, it was not employed in any unspecified way, but served to establish an *identification* of the ego with the abandoned object. Thus the shadow of the object fell upon the ego, and the latter could henceforth be judged by a special agency, as though it were an object, the forsaken object. In this way an object-loss was transformed into an ego-loss and the conflict between the ego and the loved person into a cleavage between the critical activity of the ego and the ego as altered by identification.

One or two things may be directly inferred with regard to the preconditions and effects of a process such as this. On the one hand, a strong fixation to the loved object must have been present; on the other hand, in contradiction to this, the object-cathexis must have had little power of resistance. As Otto Rank has aptly remarked, this contradiction seems to imply that the object-choice has been effected on a narcissistic basis, so that the object-cathexis, when obstacles come in its way, can regress to narcissism. The narcissistic identification with the object then becomes a substitute for the erotic cathexis, the result of which is that in spite of the conflict with the loved person the love-relation need not be given up. This substitution of identification for object-love is an important mechanism in the narcissistic affections; Karl Landauer (1914) has lately been able to point to it in the process of recovery in a case of schizophrenia. It represents, of course, a *regression* from one type of object-choice to original narcissism. We have elsewhere shown that identification is a preliminary stage of object-choice, that it is the first way—and one that is expressed in an ambivalent fashion— in which the ego picks out an object. The ego wants to incorporate this object into itself, and, in accordance with the oral or cannibalistic phase of libidinal development in which it is, it wants to do so by devouring it. Abraham is undoubtedly right in attributing to this connection the refusal of nourishment met with in severe forms of melancholia.

The conclusion which our theory would require—namely, that the disposition to fall ill of melancholia (or some part of that disposition) lies in the predominance of the narcissistic type of object-choice—has unfortunately not yet been confirmed by observation. In the opening remarks of this paper, I admitted that the empirical material upon which this study is founded is insufficient for our needs. If we could assume an agreement between the results of observation and what we have inferred, we should not hesitate to include this regression from object-cathexis to the still narcissistic oral phase of the libido in our characterization of melancholia. Identifications with the object are by no means rare in the transference neuroses either; indeed, they are a well-known mechanism of symptom-formation, especially in hysteria. The difference, however, between narcissistic and hysterical identification may be seen in this: that, whereas in the former the object-cathexis is abandoned, in the latter it persists and manifests its influence, though this is usually confined to certain isolated actions and innervations. In any case, in the transference neuroses, too, identification is the expression of there being something in common, which may signify love. Narcissistic identification is the older of the two and it paves the way to an understanding of hysterical identification, which has been less thoroughly studied.

Melancholia, therefore, borrows some of its features from mourning, and the others from the process of regression from narcissistic object-choice to narcissism. It is on the one hand, like mourning, a reaction to the real loss of a loved object; but over and above this, it is marked by a determinant which is absent in normal mourning or which, if it is present, transforms the latter into pathological mourning. The loss of a love-object is an excellent opportunity for the ambivalence in love-relationships to make itself effective and come into the open. Where there is a disposition to obsessional neurosis the conflict due to ambivalence gives a pathological cast to mourning and forces it to express itself in the form of self-reproaches to the effect that the mourner himself is to blame for the loss of the loved object, i.e. that he has willed it. These obsessional states of depression following upon the death of a loved person show us what the conflict due to ambivalence can achieve by itself when there is no regressive drawing-in of libido as well. In melancholia, the occasions which give rise to the illness extend for the most part beyond the clear case of a loss by death, and include all those situations of being slighted, neglected or disappointed, which can import opposed feelings of love and hate into the relationship or reinforce an already existing ambivalence. This conflict due to ambivalence, which sometimes arises more from real experiences, sometimes more from constitutional factors, must not be overlooked among the preconditions of melancholia. If the love for the object—a love which cannot be given up though the object itself is given up—takes refuge in narcissistic identification, then the hate comes into operation on this substitutive object, abusing it, debasing it, making it suffer and deriving sadistic satisfaction from its suffering. The self-tormenting melancholia, which is without doubt enjoyable, signifies, just like the corresponding phenomenon in obsessional neurosis, a satisfaction of trends of sadism and hate[4] which relate to an object, and which have been turned around upon the subject's own self in the ways we have been discussing. In both disorders the patients usually still succeed, by the circuitous path of self-punishment, in taking revenge on the original object and in tormenting their loved one through their illness, having resorted to it in order to avoid the need to express their hostility to him openly. After all, the person who has occasioned the patient's emotional disorder, and on whom his illness is centred, is usually to be found in his immediate environment. The melancholic's erotic cathexis in regard to his object has thus undergone a double vicissitude: part of it has regressed to identification, but the other part, under the influence of the conflict due to ambivalence, has been carried back to the stage of sadism which is nearer to that conflict.

It is this sadism alone that solves the riddle of the tendency to suicide which makes melancholia so interesting—and so dangerous. So immense is the ego's self-love, which we have come to recognize as the primal state from which instinctual life proceeds, and so vast is the amount of narcissistic libido which we see liberated in the fear that emerges at a threat to life, that we cannot conceive how that ego can consent to its own destruction. We have long known, it is true, that no neurotic harbours thoughts of suicide which he has not turned back upon himself from murderous impulses against others, but we have never been able to explain what interplay of forces can carry such a purpose through to execution. The analysis of melancholia now shows that the ego can kill itself only if, owing to the return of the object-cathexis, it can treat itself as an object—if it is able to direct against itself the hostility which relates to an object and which represents the ego's original reaction to objects in the external world.[5] Thus in regression from narcissistic object-choice the object has, it is true, been got rid of, but it has nevertheless proved more powerful than the ego itself. In the two opposed situations of being most intensely in love and of suicide the ego is overwhelmed by the object, though in totally different ways.

As regards one particular striking feature of melancholia that we have mentioned, the prominence of the fear of becoming poor, it seems plausible to suppose that it is derived from anal erotism which has been torn out of its context and altered in a regressive sense.

Melancholia confronts us with yet other problems, the answer to which in part eludes us. The fact that it passes off after a certain time has elapsed without leaving traces of any gross changes is a feature it shares with mourning. We found by way of explanation that in mourning time is needed for the command of reality-testing to be carried out in detail, and that when this work has been accomplished the ego will have succeeded in freeing its libido from the lost object. We may imagine that the ego is occupied with analogous work during the course of a melancholia; in neither case have we any insight into the economics of the course of events. The sleeplessness in melancholia testifies to the rigidity of the condition, the impossibility of effecting the general drawing-in of cathexes necessary for sleep. The complex of melancholia behaves like an open wound, drawing to itself cathectic energies—which in the transference neuroses we have called "anticathexes"—from all directions, and emptying the ego until it is totally impoverished. It can easily prove resistant to the ego's wish to sleep.

What is probably a somatic factor, and one which cannot be explained psychogenically, makes itself visible in the regular amelioration in the condition that takes place towards evening. These considerations bring up the question whether a loss in the ego irrespectively of the object—a purely narcissistic blow to the ego—may not suffice to produce the picture of melancholia and whether an impoverishment of ego-libido directly due to toxins may not be able to produce certain forms of the disease.

The most remarkable characteristic of melancholia, and the one in most need of explanation, is its tendency to change round into mania—a state which is the opposite of it in its symptoms. As we know, this does not happen to every melancholia. Some cases run their course in periodic relapses, during the intervals between which signs of mania may be entirely absent or only very slight. Others show the regular alternation of melancholic and manic phases which has led to the hypothesis of a circular insanity. One would be tempted to regard these cases as non-psychogenic, if it were not for the fact that the psycho-analytic method has succeeded in arriving at a solution and effecting a therapeutic improvement in several cases precisely of this kind. It is not merely permissible, therefore, but incumbent upon us to extend an analytic explanation of melancholia to mania as well.

I cannot promise that this attempt will prove entirely satisfactory. It hardly carries us much beyond the possibility of taking one's initial bearings. We have two things to go upon: the first is psycho-analytic impression, and the second what we may perhaps call a matter of general economic experience. The impression which several psycho-analytic investigators have already put into words is that the content of mania is no different from that of melancholia, that both disorders are wrestling with the same "complex," but that probably in melancholia the ego has succumbed to the complex whereas in mania it has mastered it or pushed it aside. Our second pointer is afforded by the observation that all states such as joy, exultation or triumph, which give us the normal model for mania, depend on the same economic conditions. What has happened here is that, as a result of some influence, a large expenditure of physical energy, long maintained or habitually occurring, has at last become unnecessary, so that it is available for numerous applications and possibilities of discharge—when, for instance, some poor wretch, by winning a large sum of money, is suddenly relieved from chronic worry about his daily bread, or when a long and arduous struggle is finally crowned with success, or when a man finds himself in a position to throw off at a single blow some oppressive compulsion, some false position which he has long had to keep up, and so on. All such situations are characterized by high spirits, by the signs of discharge of joyful emotion and by increased readiness for all kinds of action—in just the same way as in mania, and in complete contrast to the depression and inhibition of melancholia. We may venture to assert that mania is nothing other than a triumph of this sort, only that here again what the ego has surmounted and what it is triumphing over remain hidden from it. Alcoholic intoxication, which belongs to the same class of states, may (in so far as it is an elated one) be explained in the same way; here there is probably a suspension, produced by toxins, of expenditures of energy in repression. The popular view likes to assume that a person in a manic state of this kind finds such delight in movement and action because he is so "cheerful." This false connection must of course be put right. The fact is that the economic condition in the subject's mind referred to above has been fulfilled, and this is the reason why he is in such high spirits on the one hand and so uninhibited in action on the other.

If we put these two indications together, what we find is this. In mania, the ego must have got over the loss of the object (or its mourning over the loss, or perhaps the object itself), and thereupon the whole quota of anticathexis which the painful suffering of melancholia had drawn to itself from the ego and "bound" will have become available. Moreover, the manic subject plainly demonstrates his liberation from the object which was the cause of his suffering, by seeking like a ravenously hungry man for new object-cathexes.

This explanation certainly sounds plausible, but in the first place it is too indefinite, and, secondly, it gives rise to more new problems and doubts than we can answer. We will not evade a discussion of them, even though we cannot expect it to lead us to a clear understanding.

In the first place, normal mourning, too, overcomes the loss of the object, and it, too, while it lasts, absorbs all the energies of the ego. Why, then, after it has run its course, is there no hint in its case of the economic condition for a phrase of triumph? I find it impossible to answer this objection straight away. It also draws our attention to the fact that we do not even know the economic means by which mourning carries out its task. Possibly, however, a conjecture will help us here. Each single one of the memories and situations of expectancy which demonstrate the libido's attachment to the lost object is met by the verdict of reality that the object no longer exists; and the ego, confronted as it were with the question whether it shall share this fate, is persuaded by the sum of the narcissistic satisfactions it derives from being alive to sever its attachment to the object that has been abolished. We may perhaps suppose that this work of severance is so slow and gradual that by the time it has been finished the expenditure of energy nesessary for it is also dissipated.[6]

It is tempting to go on from this conjecture about the work of mourning and try to give an account of the work of melancholia. Here we are met at the outset by an uncertainty. So far we have hardly considered melancholia from the topographical point of view, nor asked ourselves in and between what psychical systems the work of melancholia goes on. What part of the mental processes of the disease still takes place in connection with the unconscious object-cathexes that have been given up, and what part in connection with their substitute, by identification, in the ego?

The quick and easy answer is that "the unconscious (thing-) presentation [7] of the object has been abandoned by the libido." In reality, however, this presentation is made up of innumerable single impressions (or unconscious traces of them), and this withdrawal of libido is not a process that can be accomplished in a moment, but must certainly, as in mourning, be one in which progress is long-drawn-out and gradual. Whether it begins simultaneously at several points or follows some sort of fixed sequence is not easy to decide; in analyses it often becomes evident that first one and then another memory is activated, and that the laments which always sound the same and are wearisome in their monotony nevertheless take their rise each time in some different unconscious source. If the object does not possess this great significance for the ego—a significance reinforced by a thousand links— then, too, its loss will not be of a kind to cause either mourning or melancholia. This characteristic of detaching the libido bit by bit is therefore to be ascribed alike to mourning and to melancholia; it is probably supported by the same economic situation and serves the same purposes in both.

As we have seen, however, melancholia contains something more than normal mourning. In melancholia the relation to the object is no simple one; it is complicated by the conflict due to ambivalence. The ambivalence is either constitutional, i.e. is an element of every love-relation formed by this particular ego, or else it proceeds precisely from those experiences that involved the threat of losing the object. For this reason the exciting causes of melancholia have a much wider range than those of mourning, which is for the most part occasioned only by a real loss of the object, by its death. In melancholia, accordingly, countless separate struggles are carried on over the object, in which hate and love contend with each other; the one seeks to detach the libido from the object, the other to maintain this position of the libido against the assault. The location of these separate struggles cannot be assigned to any system but the *Ucs.*, the region of the memory-traces of *things* (as contrasted with *word*-cathexes). In mourning, too, the efforts to detach the libido are made in this same system; but in it nothing hinders these processes from proceeding along the normal path through the *Pcs.* to consciousness. This path is blocked for the work of melancholia, owing perhaps to a number of causes or a combination of them. Constitutional ambivalence belongs by its nature to the repressed; traumatic experiences in connection with the object may have activated other repressed material. Thus everything to do with these struggles due to ambivalence remains withdrawn from consciousness, until the outcome characteristic of melancholia has set in. This, as we know, consists in the threatened libidinal cathexis at length abandoning the object, only, however, to draw back to the place in the ego from which it had proceeded. So by taking flight into the ego love escapes extinction. After this regression of the libido the process can become conscious, and it is represented to consciousness as a conflict between one part of the ego and critical agency.

What consciousness is aware of in the work of melancholia is thus not the essential part of it, nor is it even the part which we may credit with an influence in bringing the ailment to an end. We see that the ego debases itself and rages against itself, and we understand as little as the patient what this can lead to and how it can change. We can more readily attribute such a function to the *unconscious* part of the work, because it is not difficult to perceive an essential analogy between the work of melancholia and of mourning. Just as mourning impels the ego to give up the object by declaring the object to be dead and offering the ego the inducement of continuing to live, so does each single struggle of ambivalence loosen the fixation of the libido to the object by disparaging it, denigrating it and even as it were killing it. It is possible for the process in the *Ucs,* to come to an end, either after the fury has spent itself or after the object has been abandoned as valueless. We cannot tell which of these two possibilities is the regular or more usual one in bringing melancholia to an end, nor what influence this termination has on the future course of the case. The ego may enjoy in this the satisfaction of knowing itself as the better of the two, as superior to the object.

Even if we accept this view of the work of melancholia, it still does not supply an explanation of the one point on which we were seeking light. It was our expectation that the economic condition for the emergence of mania after the melancholia has run its course is to be found in the ambivalence which dominates the latter affection; and in this we found support from analogies in various other fields. But there is one fact before which that expectation must bow. Of the three preconditions of melancholia—loss of the object, ambivalence, and regression of libido into the ego—the first two are also found in the obsessional self-reproaches arising after a death has occurred. In those cases it is unquestionably the ambivalence which is the motive force of the conflict, and observation shows that after the conflict has come to an end there is nothing left over in the nature of the triumph of a manic state of mind. We are thus led to the third factor as the only one responsible for the result. The accumulation of cathexis which is at first bound and then, after the work of melancholia is finished, becomes free and makes mania possible must be linked with regression of the libido to narcissism. The conflict within the ego, which melancholia substitutes for the struggle over the object, must act like a painful wound which calls for an extraordinarily high anticathexis.—But here once again, it will be well to call a halt and to postpone any further explanation of mania until we have gained some insight into the economic nature, first, of physical pain, and then of the mental pain which is analogous to it. As we already know, the interdependence of the complicated problems of the mind forces us to break off every enquiry before it is completed—till the outcome of some other enquiry can come to its assistance.[8]

NOTES

1. The German *"Trauer,"* like the English "mourning," can mean both the affect of grief and its outward manifestation. Throughout the present paper, the word has been rendered "mourning."
2. Abraham (1912), to whom we owe the most important of the few analytic studies on this subject, also took this comparison as his starting point.
3. "Use every man after his desert, and who shall scape whipping?" (Act II, Scene 2).
4. For the distinction between the two, see my paper on "Instincts and their Vicissitudes."
5. Cf. "Instincts and their Vicissitudes."
6. The economic standpoint has hitherto received little attention in psycho-analytic writings. I would mention as an exception a paper by Victor Tausk (1913) on motives for repression devalued by recompenses.
7. [*"Dingvorstellung."*]
8. [*Footnote added* 1925:] Cf. a continuation of this discussion of mania in *Group Psychology and the Analysis of the Ego* (1921).

4. The Ego and the Id: Part III (Abridged): The Ego and the Super-Ego (Ego Ideal)

Sigmund Freud

. . . We succeeded in explaining the painful disorder of melancholia by supposing that [in those suffering from it] an object which was lost has been set up again inside the ego—that is, that an object-cathexis has been replaced by an identification.[1] At that time, however, we did not appreciate the full significance of this process and did not know how common and how typical it is. Since then we have come to understand that this kind of substitution has a great share in determining the form taken by the ego and that it makes an essential contribution towards building up what is called its "character." . . .

At the very beginning, in the individual's primitive oral phase, object-cathexis and identification are no doubt indistinguishable from each other. We can only suppose that later on object-cathexes proceed from the id, which feels erotic trends as needs. The ego, which to begin with is still feeble, becomes aware of the object-cathexes, and either acquiesces in them or tries to fend them off by the process of repression.

When it happens that a person has to give up a sexual object, there quite often ensues an alteration of his ego which can only be described as a setting up of the object inside the ego, as it occurs in melancholia; the exact nature of this substitution is as yet unknown to us. It may be that by this introjection, which is a kind of regression to the mechanism of the oral phase, the

Reprinted from *The Ego and The Id Part III: The Ego and The Super-Ego (Ego Ideal)* by Sigmund Freud, translated by Joan Riviere, revised and edited by James Strachey by permission of W. W. Norton & Company, Inc., copyright © 1960 by James Strachey (Copyright renewed 1988 by Alix Strachey), and by permission of Sigmund Freud Copyrights, The Institute of Psycho-Analysis and The Hogarth Press to quote from *The Standard Edition of Complete Psychological Works of Sigmund Freud,* translated and edited by James Strachey, 1957, vol. 19: (1923) 28–39. The above selection is an abridgment required by the publisher.

ego makes it easier for the object to be given up or renders that process possible. It may be that this identification is the sole condition under which the id can give up its objects. At any rate the process, especially in the early phases of development, is a very frequent one, and it makes it possible to suppose that the character of the ego is a precipitate of abandoned object-cathexes and that it contains the history of those object-choices. . . .

Whatever the character's later capacity for resisting the influences of abandoned object-cathexes may turn out to be, the effects of the first identifications made in earliest childhood will be general and lasting. This leads us back to the origin of the ego ideal; for behind it there lies hidden an individual's first and most important identification, his identification with the father in his own personal prehistory.[2] This is apparently not in the first instance the consequence or outcome of an object-cathexis; it is a direct and immediate identification and takes place earlier than any object-cathexis. But the object-choices belonging to the first sexual period and relating to the father and mother seem normally to find their outcome in an identification of this kind, and would thus reinforce the primary one.

The whole subject, however, is so complicated that it will be necessary to go into it in greater detail. The intricacy of the problem is due to two factors: the triangular character of the Oedipus situation and the constitutional bisexuality of each individual.

In its simplified form the case of a male child may be described as follows. At a very early age the little boy develops an object-cathexis for his mother, which originally related to the mother's breast and is the prototype of an object-choice on the anaclitic model; the boy deals with his father by identifying himself with him. For a time these two relationships proceed side by side, until the boy's sexual wishes in regard to his mother become more intense and his father is perceived as an obstacle to them; from this the Oedipus complex originates. His identification with his father then takes on a hostile colouring and changes into a wish to get rid of his father in order to take his place with his mother. Henceforward his relation to his father is ambivalent; it seems as if the ambivalence inherent in the identification from the beginning had become manifest. An ambivalent attitude to his father and an object-relation of a solely affectionate kind to his mother make up the content of the simple positive Oedipus complex in a boy.

Along with the demolition of the Oedipus complex, the boy's object-cathexis of his mother must be given up. Its place may be filled by one of two things: either an identification with his mother or an intensification of his identification with his father. We are accustomed to regard the latter outcome as the more normal; it permits the affectionate relation to the mother to be in a measure retained. In this way the dissolution of the Oedipus complex would consolidate the masculinity in a boy's character. In a precisely analogous way,[3] the outcome of the Oedipus attitude in a little girl may be an intensification of her identification with her mother (or the setting up of such an identification for the first time)—a result which will fix the child's feminine character.

These identifications are not what we should have expected since they do not introduce the abandoned object into the ego; but this alternative outcome may also occur, and is easier to observe in girls than in boys. Analysis very often shows that a little girl, after she has had to relinquish her father as a love-object, will bring her masculinity into prominence and identify herself with her father (that is, with the object which has been lost), instead of with her mother. This will clearly depend on whether the masculinity in her disposition—whatever that may consist in—is strong enough.

It would appear, therefore, that in both sexes the relative strength of the masculine and feminine sexual dispositions is what determines whether the outcome of the Oedipus situation shall be an identification with the father or with the mother. This is one of the ways in which bisexuality takes a hand in the subsequent vicissitudes of the Oedipus complex. The other way is even more important. For one gets an impression that the simple Oedipus complex is by no means its commonest form, but rather represents a simplification or schematization which, to be sure, is often enough justified for practical purposes. Closer study usually discloses the more complete Oedipus complex, which is twofold, positive and negative, and is due to the bisexuality originally present in children: that is to say, a boy has not merely an ambivalent attitude towards his father and an affectionate object-choice towards his mother, but at the same time he also behaves like a girl and displays an affectionate feminine attitude to his father and a corresponding jealousy and hostility towards his mother. It is this complicating element introduced by bisexuality that makes it so difficult to obtain a clear view of the facts in connection with the earliest object-choices and identifications, and still more difficult to describe them intelligibly. It may even be that the ambivalence displayed in the relations to the parents should be attributed entirely to bisexuality and that it is not, as I have represented above, developed out of identification in consequence of rivalry.

In my opinion it is advisable in general, and quite especially where neurotics are concerned, to assume the existence of the complete Oedipus complex. Analytic experience then shows that in a number of cases one or the other constituent disappears, except for barely distinguishable traces; so that the result is a series with the normal positive Oedipus complex at one end and the inverted negative one at the other, while its intermediate members exhibit the complete form with one or other of its two components preponderating. At the dissolution of the Oedipus complex the four trends of which it consists will group themselves in such a way as to produce a father-identification and a mother-identification. The father-identification will preserve the object-relation to the mother which belonged to the positive complex and will at the same time replace the object-relation to the father which belonged to the inverted complex: and the same will be true, *mutatis mutandis,* of the mother-identification. The relative intensity of the two identifications in any individual will reflect the preponderance in him of one or other of the two sexual dispositions.

The broad general outcome of the sexual phase dominated by the Oedipus complex may, therefore, be taken to be the forming of a precipitate in the ego, consisting of these two identifications in some way united with each other. This modification of the ego retains its special position; it confronts the other contents of the ego as an ego ideal or super-ego.

The super-ego is, however, not simply a residue of the earliest object-choices of the id; it also represents an energetic reaction-formation against those choices. Its relation to the ego is not exhausted by the precept: "You *ought to be* like this (like your father)." It also comprises the prohibition: "You *may not be* like this (like your father)—that is, you may not do all that he does; some things are his prerogative." This double aspect of the ego ideal derives from the fact that the ego ideal had the task of repressing the Oedipus complex; indeed, it is to that revolutionary event that it owes its existence. Clearly the repression of the Oedipus complex was no easy task. The child's parents, and especially his father, were perceived as the obstacle to a realization of his Oedipus wishes; so his infantile ego fortified itself for the carrying out of the repression by erecting this same obstacle within itself. It borrowed strength to do this, so to speak, from the father, and this loan was an extraordinarily momentous act. The super-ego retains the character of the father, while the more powerful the Oedipus complex was and the more rapidly it succumbed to repression (under the influence of authority, religious teaching, schooling and reading), the stricter will be the domination of the super-ego over the ego later on—in the form of conscience or perhaps of an unconscious sense of guilt. . . .

If we consider once more the origin of the super-ego as we have described it, we shall recognize that it is the outcome of two highly important factors, one of a biological and the other of a historical nature: namely, the lengthy duration in man of his childhood helplessness and dependence, and the fact of his Oedipus complex, the repression of which we have shown to be connected with the interruption of libidinal development by the latency period and so with the diphasic onset of man's sexual life. . . .

Psycho-analysis has been reproached time after time with ignoring the higher, moral, supra-personal side of human nature. The reproach is doubly unjust, both historically and methodologically. For, in the first place, we have from the very beginning attributed the function of instigating repression to the moral and aesthetic trends in the ego, and secondly, there has been a general refusal to recognize that psycho-analytic research could not, like a philosophical system, produce a complete and ready-made theoretical structure, but had to find its way step by step along the path towards understanding the intricacies of the mind by making an analytic dissection of both normal and abnormal phenomena. So long as we had to concern ourselves with the study of what is repressed in mental life, there was no need for us to share in any agitated apprehensions as to the whereabouts of the higher side of man. But now that we have embarked upon the analysis of the ego we can give an answer to all those whose moral sense has been shocked and who have complained that there must surely be a higher nature in man: "Very true," we can say, "and here we have that higher nature, in this ego ideal or super-ego, the representative of our relation to our parents. When we were little children we knew these higher natures, we admired them and feared them; and later we took them into ourselves."

The ego ideal is therefore the heir of the Oedipus complex, and thus it is also the expression of the most powerful impulses and most important libidinal vicissitudes of the id. By setting up this ego ideal, the ego has mastered the Oedipus complex and at the same time placed itself in subjection to the id. Whereas the ego is essentially the representative of the external world, of reality, the super-ego stands in contrast to it as the representative of the internal world, of the id. Conflicts between the ego and the ideal will, as we are now prepared to find, ultimately reflect the contrast between what is real and what is psychical, between the external world and the internal world.

Through the forming of the ideal, what biology and the vicissitudes of the human species have created in the id and left behind in it is taken over by the ego and re-experienced in relation to itself as an individual. Owing to the way in which the ego ideal is formed, it has the most abundant links with the phylogenetic acquisition of each individual—his archaic heritage. What has belonged to the lowest part of the mental life of each of us is changed, through the formation of the ideal, into what is highest in the human mind by our scale of values. It would be vain, however, to attempt to localize the ego ideal, even in the sense in which we have localized the ego, or to work it into any of the analogies with the help of which we have tried to picture the relation between the ego and the id.

It is easy to show that the ego ideal answers to everything that is expected of the higher nature of man. As a substitute for a longing for the father, it contains the germ from which all religions have evolved. The self-judgement which declares that the ego falls short of its ideal produces the religious sense of humility to which the believer appeals in his longing. As a child grows up, the role of father is carried on by teachers and others in authority; their injunctions and prohibitions remain powerful in the ego ideal and continue, in the form of conscience, to exercise the moral censorship. The tension between the demands of conscience and the actual performances of the ego is experienced as a sense of guilt. Social feelings rest on identifications with other people, on the basis of having the same ego ideal.

Religion, morality, and a social sense—the chief elements in the higher side of man[4]—were originally one and the same thing. According to the hypothesis which I put forward in *Totem and Taboo* they were acquired phylogenetically out of the father-complex: religion and moral restraint through the process of mastering the Oedipus complex itself, and social feeling through the necessity for overcoming the rivalry that then remained between the members of the younger generation. The male sex seems to have taken the lead in all these moral acquisitions; and they seem to have then been transmitted to women by cross-inheritance. Even to-day the social feelings arise in the individual as a superstructure built upon impulses of jealous rivalry against his brothers and sisters. Since the hostility cannot be satisfied, an identification with the former rival develops. The study of mild cases of homosexuality confirms the suspicion that in this instance, too, the identification is a substitute for an affectionate object-choice which has taken the place of the aggressive, hostile attitude. . . .

The way in which the super-ego came into being explains how it is that the early conflicts of the ego with the object-cathexes of the id can be continued in conflicts with their heir, the super-ego. If the ego has not succeeded in properly mastering the Oedipus complex, the energic cathexis of the latter, springing from the id, will come into operation once more in the reaction-formation of the ego ideal. The abundant communication between the ideal and these *Ucs.* instinctual impulses solves the puzzle of how it is that the ideal itself can to a great extent remain unconscious and inaccessible to the ego. The struggle which once raged in the deepest strata of the mind, and was not brought to an end by rapid sublimation and identification, is now continued in a higher region. . . .

NOTES

1. "Mourning and Melancholia" (1917).
2. Perhaps it would be safer to say "with the parents"; for before a child has arrived at definite knowledge of the difference between the sexes, the lack of a penis, it does not distinguish in value between its father and its mother. I recently came across the instance of a young married woman whose story showed that, after noticing the lack of a penis in herself, she had supposed it to be absent not in all women, but only in those whom she regarded as inferior, and had still supposed that her mother possessed one. . . . In order to simplify my presentation I shall discuss only identification with the father.
3. The idea that the outcome of the Oedipus complex was 'precisely analogous' in girls and boys was abandoned by Freud not long after this. . . .
4. I am at the moment putting science and art on one side.

5. Inhibitions, Symptoms, and Anxiety: Addendum C: Anxiety, Pain, and Mourning

Sigmund Freud

So little is known about the psychology of emotional processes that the tentative remarks I am about to make on the subject may claim a very lenient judgement. The problem before us arises out of the conclusion we have reached that anxiety comes to be a reaction to the danger of a loss of an object. Now we already know one reaction to the loss of an object, and that is mourning. The question therefore is, when does that loss lead to anxiety and when to mourning? In discussing the subject of mourning on a previous occasion I found that there was one feature about it which remained quite unexplained. This was its peculiar painfulness.[1] And yet it seems self-evident that separation from an object should be painful. Thus the problem becomes more complicated: when does separation from an object produce anxiety, when does it produce mourning and when does it produce, it may be, only pain?

Let me say at once that there is no prospect in sight of answering these questions. We must content ourselves with drawing certain distinctions and adumbrating certain possibilities.

Our starting-point will again be the one situation which we believe we understand—the situation of the infant when it is presented with a stranger instead of its mother. It will exhibit the anxiety which we have attributed to the danger of loss of object. But its anxiety is undoubtedly more complicated than this and merits a more thorough discussion. That it does have anxiety there can be no doubt; but the expression of its face and its reaction of crying indicate that it is feeling pain as well. Certain things seem to be joined

Reprinted by permission of Sigmund Freud Copyrights, The Institute of Psycho-Analysis and The Hogarth Press from *The Standard Edition of Complete Psychological Works of Sigmund Freud,* translated and edited by James Strachey, 1959, vol. 20: (1926) 169–72.

together in it which will later on be separated out. It cannot as yet distinguish between temporary absence and permanent loss. As soon as it loses sight of its mother it behaves as if it were never going to see her again; and repeated consoling experiences to the contrary are necessary before it learns that her disappearance is usually followed by her re-appearance. Its mother encourages this piece of knowledge which is so vital to it by playing the familiar game of hiding her face from it with her hands and then, to its joy, uncovering it again. In these circumstances it can, as it were, feel longing unaccompanied by despair.

In consequence of the infant's misunderstanding of the facts, the situation of missing its mother is not a danger-situation but a traumatic one. Or, to put it more correctly, it is a traumatic situation if the infant happens at the time to be feeling a need which its mother should be the one to satisfy. It turns into a danger-situation if this need is not present at the moment. Thus, the first determinant of anxiety, which the ego itself introduces, is loss of perception of the object (which is equated with loss of the object itself). There is as yet no question of loss of love. Later on, experience teaches the child that the object can be present but angry with it; and then loss of love from the object becomes a new and much more enduring danger and determinant of anxiety.

The traumatic situation of missing the mother differs in one important respect from the traumatic situation of birth. At birth no object existed and so no object could be missed. Anxiety was the only reaction that occurred. Since then repeated situations of satisfaction have created an object out of the mother; and this object, whenever the infant feels a need, receives an intense cathexis which might be described as a "longing" one. It is to this new aspect of things that the reaction of pain is referable. Pain is thus the actual reaction to loss of object, while anxiety is the reaction to the danger which that loss entails and, by a further displacement, a reaction to the danger of the loss of object itself.

We know very little about pain either. The only fact we are certain of is that pain occurs in the first instance and as a regular thing whenever a stimulus which impinges on the periphery breaks through the devices of the protective shield against stimuli and proceeds to act like a continuous instinctual stimulus, against which muscular action, which is as a rule effective because it withdraws the place that is being stimulated from the stimulus, is powerless. If the pain proceeds not from a part of the skin but from an internal organ, the situation is still the same. All that has happened is that a portion of the inner periphery has taken the place of the outer periphery. The child obviously has occasion to undergo experiences of pain of this sort, which are independent of its experiences of need. This determinant of the generating of pain seems, however, to have very little similarity with the loss of an object. And besides, the element which is essential to pain, peripheral stimulation, is entirely absent in the child's situation of longing. Yet it cannot be for nothing that the common usage of speech should have created the notion of internal, mental pain and have treated the feeling of loss of object as equivalent to physical pain.

When there is physical pain, a high degree of what may be termed narcissistic cathexis of the painful place occurs. This cathexis continues to increase and tends, as it were, to empty the ego. It is well known that when internal organs are giving us pain we receive spatial and other presentations of parts of the body which are ordinarily not represented at all in conscious ideation. Again, the remarkable fact that, when there is a physical diversion brought about by some other interest, even the most intense physical pains fail to arise (I must not say "remain unconscious" in this case) can be accounted for by there being a concentration of cathexis on the physical representative of the part of the body which is giving pain. I think it is here that we shall find the point of analogy which has made it possible to carry sensations of pain over to the mental sphere. For the intense cathexis of longing which is concentrated on the missed or lost object (a cathexis which steadily mounts up because it cannot be appeased) creates the same economic conditions as are created by the cathexis of pain which is concentrated on the injured part of the body. Thus the fact of the peripheral causation of physical pain can be left out of account. The transition from physical pain to mental pain corresponds to a change from narcissistic cathexis to object-cathexis. An object-presentation which is highly cathected by instinctual need plays the same role as a part of the body which is cathected by an increase of stimulus. The continuous nature of the cathectic process and the impossibility of inhibiting it produce the same state of mental helplessness. If the feeling of unpleasure which then arises has the specific character of pain (a character which cannot be more exactly described) instead of manifesting itself in the reactive form of anxiety, we may plausibly attribute this to a factor which we have not sufficiently made use of in our explanations—the high level of cathexis and "binding" that prevails while these processes which lead to a feeling of unpleasure take place.

We know of yet another emotional reaction to the loss of an object, and that is mourning. But we have no longer any difficulty in accounting for it. Mourning occurs under the influence of reality-testing; for the latter function demands categorically from the bereaved person that he should separate himself from the object, since it no longer exists. Mourning is entrusted with the task of carrying out this retreat from the object in all those situations in which it was the recipient of a high degree of cathexis. That this separation should be painful fits in with what we have just said, in view of the high and unsatisfiable cathexis of longing which is concentrated on the object by the bereaved person during the reproduction of the situations in which he must undo the ties that bind him to it.

NOTES

1. "Mourning and Melancholia" (1917).

6. Fetishism

Sigmund Freud

In the last few years I have had an opportunity of studying analytically a number of men whose object-choice was dominated by a fetish. There is no need to expect that these people came to analysis on account of their fetish. For though no doubt a fetish is recognized by its adherents as an abnormality, it is seldom felt by them as the symptom of an ailment accompanied by suffering. Usually they are quite satisfied with it, or even praise the way in which it eases their erotic life. As a rule, therefore, the fetish made its appearance in analysis as a subsidiary finding.

For obvious reasons the details of these cases must be withheld from publication; I cannot, therefore, show in what way accidental circumstances have contributed to the choice of a fetish. The most extraordinary case seemed to me to be one in which a young man had exalted a certain sort of "shine on the nose" into a fetishistic precondition. The surprising explanation of this was that the patient had been brought up in an English nursery but had later come to Germany, where he forgot his mother-tongue almost completely. The fetish, which originated from his earliest childhood, had to be understood in English, not German. The "shine on the nose" [in German *"Glanz auf der Nase"*]—was in reality a *"glance* at the nose." The nose was thus the fetish, which, incidentally, he endowed at will with the luminous shine which was not perceptible to others.

In every instance, the meaning and the purpose of the fetish turned out, in analysis, to be the same. It revealed itself so naturally and seemed to me so compelling that I am prepared to expect the same solution in all cases of fetishism. When now I announce that the fetish is a substitute for the penis, I shall certain create disappointment; so I hasten to add that it is not a substitute

Reprinted by permission of Sigmund Freud Copyrights, The Institute of Psycho-Analysis and the Hogarth Press for permission to quote from *The Standard Edition of the Complete Psychological Works of Sigmund Freud,* translated and edited by James Strachey, 1961, vol. 21: (1921) 149–57.

for any chance penis, but for a particular and quite special penis that had been extremely important in early childhood but had later been lost. That is to say, it should normally have been given up, but the fetish is precisely designed to preserve it from extinction. To put it more plainly: the fetish is a substitute for the woman's (the mother's) penis that the little boy once believed in and—for reasons familiar to us—does not want to give up.[1]

What happened, therefore, was that the boy refused to take cognizance of the fact of his having perceived that a woman does not posses a penis. No, that could not be true: for if a woman had been castrated, then his own possession of a penis was in danger; and against that there rose in rebellion the portion of his narcissism which Nature has, as a precaution, attached to that particular organ. In later life a grown man may perhaps experience a similar panic when the cry goes up that Throne and Altar are in danger, and similar illogical consequences will ensure. If I am not mistaken, Laforgue would say in this case that the boy "scotomizes" his perception of the woman's lack of a penis.[2] A new technical term is justified when it describes a new fact or emphasizes it. This is not so here. The oldest word in our psycho-analytic terminology, "repression," already relates to this pathological process. If we wanted to differentiate more sharply between the vicissitude of the *idea* as distinct from that of the *affect,* and reserve the word *"Verdrängung"* ["repression"] for the affect, then the correct German word for the vicissitude of the idea would be *"Verleugnung"* ["disavowal"]. "Scotomization" seems to me particularly unsuitable, for it suggests that the perception is entirely wiped out, so that the result is the same as when a visual impression falls on the blind spot in the retina. In the situation we are considering, on the contrary, we see that the perception has persisted, and that a very energetic action has been undertaken to maintain the disavowal. It is not true that, after the child has made his observation of the woman, he has preserved unaltered his belief that women have a phallus. He has retained that belief, but he has also given it up. In the conflict between the weight of the unwelcome perception and the force of his counter-wish, a compromise has been reached, as is only possible under the dominance of the unconscious laws of thought—the primary processes. Yes, in his mind the woman *has* got a penis, in spite of everything; but this penis is no longer the same as it was before. Something else has taken its place, has been appointed its substitute, as it were, and now inherits the interest which was formerly directed to its predecessor. But this interest suffers an extraordinary increase as well, because the horror of castration has set up a memorial to itself in the creation of this substitute. Furthermore, an aversion, which is never absent in any fetishist, to the real female genitals remains a *stigma indelebile* of the repression that has taken place. We can now see what the fetish achieves and what it is that maintains it. It remains a token of triumph over the threat of castration and a protection against it. It also saves the fetishist from becoming a homosexual, by endowing women with the characteristic which makes them tolerable as sexual objects. In later life, the fetishist feels that he enjoys yet another advantage from his substitute for a genital. The meaning of the fetish is not known to other people, so the fetish is not withheld from him: it is easily accessible and he can readily obtain the sexual satisfaction attached to it. What other men have to woo and make exertions for can be had by the fetishist with no trouble at all.

Probably no male human being is spared the fright of castration at the sight of a female genital. Why some people become homosexual as a consequence of that impression, while others fend it off by creating a fetish, and the great majority surmount it, we are frankly not able to explain. It is possible that, among all the factors at work, we do not yet know those which are decisive for the rare pathological results. We must be content if we can explain what has happened, and may for the present leave on one side the task of explaining why something has *not* happened.

One would expect that the organs or objects chosen as substitutes for the absent female phallus would be such as appear as symbols of the penis in other connections as well. This may happen often enough, but is certainly not a deciding factor. It seems rather that when the fetish is instituted some process occurs which reminds one of the stopping of memory in traumatic amnesia. As in this latter case, the subject's interest comes to a halt half-way, as it were; it is as though the last impression before the uncanny and traumatic one is retained as a fetish. Thus the foot or shoe owes its preference as a fetish—or a part of it—to the circumstance that the inquisitive boy peered at the woman's genitals from below from her legs up; fur and velvet—as has long been suspected—are a fixation of the sight of the pubic hair, which should have been followed by the longed-for sight of the female member; pieces of underclothing, which are so often chosen as a fetish, crystallize the moment of undressing, the last moment in which the woman could still be regarded as phallic. But I do not maintain that it is invariably possible to discover with certainty how the fetish was determined.

An investigation of fetishism is strongly recommended to anyone who still doubts the existence of the castration complex or who can still believe that fright at the sight of the female genital has some other ground—for instance, that it is derived from a supposed recollection of the trauma of birth.

For me, the explanation of fetishism had another point of theoretical interest as well. Recently, along quite speculative lines, I arrived at the proposition that the essential difference between neurosis and psychosis was that in the former the ego, in the service of reality, suppresses a piece of the id, whereas in a psychosis it lets itself be induced by the id to detach itself from a piece of reality. I returned to this theme once again later on.[3] But soon after this I had reason to regret that I had ventured so far. In the analysis of two young men I learned that each—one when he was two years old and the other when he was ten—had failed to take cognizance of the death of his beloved father—had "scotomized" it—and yet neither of them had developed a psychosis. Thus a piece of reality which was undoubtedly important had been disavowed by the ego, just as the unwelcome fact of women's castration is disavowed in fetishists. I also began to suspect that similar occurrences in childhood are by no means rare, and I believed that I had been guilty of an error in my characterization of neurosis and psychosis. It is true that there was one way out of the difficulty. My formula needed only to hold good where there was a higher degree of differentiation in the psychical apparatus; things might be permissible to a child which would entail severe injury to an adult.

But further research led to another solution of the contradiction. It turned out that the two young men had no more "scotomized" their father's death than a fetishist does the castration of women. I was only one current in their mental life that had not recognized their father's death; there was another current which took full account of that fact. The attitude which fitted in with the wish and the attitude which fitted in with reality existed side by side. In one of my two cases this split had formed the basis of a moderately severe obsessional neurosis. The patient oscillated in every situation in life between two assumptions: the one, that his father was still alive and was hindering his activities; the other, opposite one, that he was entitled to regard himself as his father's successor. I may thus keep to the expectation that in a psychosis the one current—that which fitted in with reality—would have in fact been absent.

Returning to my description of fetishism, I may say that there are many and weighty additional proofs of the divided attitude of fetishists to the question of the castration of women. In very subtle instances both the disavowal and the affirmation of the castration have found their way into the construction of the fetish itself. This was so in the case of a man whose fetish was an athletic support-belt which could also be worn as bathing drawers. This piece of clothing covered up the genitals entirely and concealed the distinction between them. Analysis showed that it signified that women were castrated and that they were not castrated; and it also allowed of the hypothesis that men were castrated, for all these possibilities could equally well be concealed under the belt—the earliest rudiment of which in his childhood had been the fig-leaf on a statue. A fetish of this sort, doubly derived from contrary ideas, is of course especially durable. In other instances the divided attitude shows itself in what the fetishist does with his fetish, whether in reality or in his imagination. To point out that he reveres his fetish is not the whole story; in many cases he treats it in a way which is obviously equivalent to a representation of castration. This happens particularly if he has developed a strong identification with his father and plays the part of the latter; for it is to him that as a child he ascribed the woman's castration. Affection and hostility in the treatment of the fetish—which run parallel with the disavowal and the acknowledgment of castration—are mixed in unequal proportions in different cases, so that the one or the other is more clearly recognizable. We seem here to approach an understanding, even if a distant one, of the behavior of the *"coupeur de nattes."* [4] In him the need to carry out the castration which he disavows has come to the front. His action contains in itself the two mutually incompatible assertions: "the woman has still got a penis" and "my father has castrated the woman." Another variant, which is also a parallel to fetishism in social psychology, might be seen in the Chinese custom of mutilating the female foot and then revering it like a fetish after it has been mutilated. It seems as though the Chinese male wants to thank the woman for having submitted to being castrated.

In conclusion we may say that the normal prototype of fetishes is a man's penis, just as the normal prototype of inferior organs is a woman's real small penis, the clitoris.

NOTES

1. This interpretation was made as early as 1910, in my study on Leonardo da Vinci, without any reasons being given for it.
2. I correct myself, however, by adding that I have the best reasons for supposing that Laforgue would not say anything of the sort. It is clear from his own remarks that "scotomization" is a term which derives from descriptions of dementia praecox, which does not arise from a

carrying-over of psycho-analytic concepts to the psychoses and which has no application to developmental processes or to the formation of neuroses. In his exposition in the text of his paper, the author has been at pains to make this incompatibility clear.

3. "Neurosis and Psychosis" (1924) and "The Loss of Reality in Neurosis and Psychosis" (1924).

4. [A pervert who enjoys cutting off the hair of females.]

Introductory Notes to Chapter 7

Rita V. Frankiel

This tender letter to Ludwig Binswanger was written after Freud learned that Binswanger had suffered the death of a son for the second time in his life;[1] this time it was the son to whom he was most attached. In the letter, Freud emerges as a deeply caring friend, meanwhile adding significantly to our understanding of mourning. First, he offers support by mentioning his admiration for Binswanger's courage (in coping with a malignant tumor eleven or twelve years before), his own infirmity, and his ongoing thoughts of his own dead daughter (Sophie Halberstadt), and then he presents his understanding of the fact that, following certain losses, there is no way to completely replace a lost love, even when the work of mourning has been done. When you compare the last paragraph of this letter to the message of "Mourning and Melancholia," you must amend Freud's notion that, after a finite period of time, mourning is over and one goes on to new attachments. All losses are not the same; all replacements are not equal. One can go on, but there is no way to replace the uniqueness of the one who is gone and the special quality and meaning of the attachment. Years later, reflecting on Freud's letter, Binswanger remarked, and we join him: "The concluding passage of the above letter, when compared with Freud's discussion in his 'Mourning and Melancholia,' suffices by itself to show how far Freud the man surpasses Freud the scientist in largeness and depth of humanity" (Binswanger 1957).

I include Freud's letter in this collection of essential papers in order to bring these humane thoughts into interaction with Freud's scientific contributions so that we may be better prepared to modify where necessary our understanding of completed and healthy mourning. That I am not alone in this point of view will be evident by reference to E. Furman 1974, Bowlby 1980, Parkes and Weiss 1983, and Wortman and Silver, 1987, among others.

NOTES

1. Biographical data from Gay (1988, 422–23) and L. Binswanger (1957).

7. Letter to Ludwig Binswanger

Sigmund Freud

Vienna IX, Berggasse 19
April 11, 1929

Dear Dr. Binswanger

I don't know whether it was in 1912 or 1913 that I paid you a visit and was so impressed by your courage that it has gained for you ever since a high place in my estimation. The intervening years, as you know, have made a rather frail old man of me. I can no longer travel to shake your hand.

April 12, 1939

My daughter who died would have been thirty-six years old today.

Yesterday I nearly committed a serious blunder. I began reading your letter, deciphered some isolated friendly words which I would have been sorry to miss, but I was unable to fit them into a sentence, and the further I got the more enigmatic your handwriting became. I considered returning the letter to you with a jocular expression of my indignation and the suggestion that you send it back to me rewritten. Then my sister-in-law offered her assistance and gave me the deeply moving news contained in the latter part of the letter, whereupon I understood why you had not dictated it into the machine.

Although we know that after such a loss the acute state of mourning will subside, we also know we shall remain inconsolable and will never find a substitute. No matter what may fill the gap, even if it be filled completely, it nevertheless remains something else. And actually this is how it should be. It is the only way of perpetuating that love which we do not want to relinquish.

Please give my warm regards to your wife.

In old friendship
Your old
Freud

Reprinted by permission of Chatto & Windus and Basic Books, a division of Harper Collins Publishers, Inc., from *The Letters of Sigmund Freud,* selected and edited by Ernst L. Freud, translated and edited by Tania and James Stern. Copyright © 1960 by Sigmund Freud Copyrights, London.

Introductory Notes to Chapter 8

Rita V. Frankiel

Abraham enriched Freud's formulation of the stages of the libido by elaborating and explicating the complexity of the libidinal stages. It was his special contribution that he described the characteristic mode of relating to the object characteristic of each libidinal stage. In essence, he took a theory focused on cathexis and libidinal investment and showed that embedded in it were processes dictating how connections to and interactions with objects will be elaborated.

In the paper condensed and reprinted here he amplifies Freud's observations stated in "Mourning and Melancholia" by demonstrating that (1) ambivalence is not restricted to cases of pathological mourning and is not completely absent in normal mourning; and (2) introjection of the lost person is not restricted to the mourning of the melancholic (those with severe depression) but can be found at times in the mourning of normal persons as well. The paper is rich in clinical examples that demonstrate the vicissitudes of normal and pathological object relations and reactions to object loss.

Of Abraham's several contributions touching on this subject (1911, 1916, 1924), we only have room for one, and this one—which ranges over many topics—has been abridged to focus entirely on object loss and mourning. The reader is urged to consult the original text for more far-reaching discussions of the role of introjection in depression, the psychogenesis of depression and mania, and the growth of object love.

8. A Short Study of the Development of the Libido, Viewed in the Light of Mental Disorders (Abridged)

Karl Abraham

. . . Freud's paper, "Mourning and Melancholia," confirmed my view[1] that melancholia stood in the same relation to normal mourning for a loss as did morbid anxiety to ordinary fear. And we may now regard as definitely established the psychological affinity between melancholia and obsessional neuroses. Furthermore, these two illnesses show similarities in regard to the process of the disengagement of the libido from the external world. . . .

Freud had been led by the analysis of obsessional neuroses to postulate a pre-genital phase in the development of the libido which he called the sadistic-anal phase. A little later[2] he gave a detailed description of a still earlier phase, the oral or cannibalistic one. Basing my views on a large and varied collection of empiric material I was able[3] to show that certain psychoneuroses contain clear traces of that earliest phase in the organization of the libido; and I ventured the suggestion that what we saw in melancholia was the result of a regression of the patient's libido to that same primitive oral level. . . .

At about the same time Freud approached the problem of melancholia from another angle, and he made the first real step towards the discovery of the mechanism of that illness. He showed that the patient, after having lost his love-object, regains it once more by a process of introjection (so that, for instance, the self-reproaches of a melancholiac are really directed towards his lost object).

Subsequent experience has confirmed in my mind the importance of both processes—the regression of the libido to the oral stage and the mechanism

Reprinted by permission of Basic Books, a division of Harper Collins Publishers Inc., and Chatto & Windus from *Selected Papers of Karl Abraham*, translated by Douglas Bryan and Alix Strachey. Copyright © 1960 by Basic Books, Inc.

of introjection. And more than that, it has shown that there is an intimate connection between the two. . . . As I hope to be able to make quite clear, the introjection of the love-object is an incorporation of it, in keeping with the regression of the libido to the cannibalistic level. . . .

I. MELANCHOLIA AND OBSESSIONAL NEUROSIS: TWO STAGES OF THE SADISTIC-ANAL PHASE OF THE LIBIDO

. . . As early as 1911, . . . I pointed out that obsessional symptoms were very frequently present in cases of melancholia and that obsessional neurotics were subject to states of depression. I went on to say that in both kinds of illness a high degree of ambivalence was found in the patient's instinctual life; and that this was most clearly seen in the want of adjustment between his emotions of love and of hate, and between his homosexual and heterosexual tendencies. . . .

From the point of view of the clinical observer manic-depressive states run an intermittent course, whereas obsessional states are on the whole chronic in character. . . . Careful observation spread over a long period of time shows us that here, as in so many other cases, the one condition shades off into the other, whereas at first we only saw an absolute cleavage between the two. . . . In their "free interval" patients suffering from circular insanity exhibit the same characteristics as psycho-analysis has made us acquainted with in the obsessional neuroses—the same peculiarities in regard to cleanliness and order; the same tendency to take up an obstinate and defiant attitude alternating with exaggerated docility and an excess of "goodness"; the same abnormalities of behaviour in relation to money and possessions. These character-traits furnish important evidence that these two pathological conditions have a close psychological relationship with one and the same pregenital phase of the libido. If we assume the existence of such an extensive agreement in the characterological constitution of persons who incline to melancholia and of those who incline to an obsessional neurosis, it is quite incomprehensible to us why an illness which takes its inception from the same character-formation should be now of the one type, now of the other. It is true that we have come to the conclusion that in melancholia the patient gives up his psycho-sexual relations to his object, whereas the obsessional neurotic does in the end manage to escape that fate. But we are then faced with the problem why the object-relation is so much more labile in the one class of patients than in the other. . . .

In spite of their common relation to the anal-sadistic organization of the libido, melancholia and obsessional neuroses exhibit certain fundamental differences not only in respect of the phase to which the libido regresses at the onset of the illness, but also in respect of the attitude of the individual to his object, since the melancholiac gives it up, while the obsessional patient retains it. If, therefore, it appears that such widely divergent pathological processes can take their inception from the sadistic-anal stage, it follows that *this stage contains heterogeneous elements which we have not been able to separate out hitherto*. . . .

Up till now we have been acquainted with three stages in the development of the libido, in each of which we were able to observe that one particular erotogenic zone was of preponderant importance. These erotogenic zones are, in order of time, the oral, the anal, and the genital. We found that the libidinal excitations belonging to anal erotism had close and manifold connections in that stage with sadistic impulses. . . . We have learnt from the psycho-analysis of neurotic patients that excretory processes are employed for sadistic purposes, and have found this fact confirmed by observation of the psychology of children. We have also seen that a single character-trait—defiance, for instance—proceeds from sadistic as well as from anal sources. But these observations and others like them have not enabled us to understand the reason of that combination of sadistic and anal activities.

We can get a step nearer to the solution of the problem if we take into consideration another piece of well-ascertained psycho-analytic knowledge. . . . This is, that a complete capacity for love is only achieved when the libido has reached its genital stage. Thus we have on the one hand anal erotic processes combined with sadistic behaviour, in especial with unkind and hostile emotions which are destructive to their object; and on the other, a genital erotism combined with tendencies which are friendly to their object.

But this comparison only serves, as I have said, to bring us a step nearer to our problem, which remains unanswered so long as we do not know why, at a certain level of development, the sadistic impulses exhibit a special affinity precisely for anal erotism and not, for instance, for oral or genital erotism. Here again the empirical data of psycho-analysis may be of use to us. For they show us

1. That anal erotism contains two opposite pleasurable tendencies.
2. That similarly two opposite tendencies exist in the field of sadistic impulses.

The evacuation of the bowels calls forth a pleasurable excitation of the anal zone. To this primitive form of pleasurable experience there is presently added another, based on a reverse process—the retention of the faeces.

Psycho-analytic experience has shown beyond a doubt that in the middle stage of his libidinal development the individual regards the person who is the object of his desire as something over which he exercises ownership, and that he consequently treats that person in the same way as he does his earliest piece of private property, *i.e.* the contents of his body, his faeces. Whereas on the genital level "love" means the transference of his positive feeling on to the object and involves a psycho-sexual adaptation to that object, on the level below it means that he treats his object as though it belonged to him. And since the ambivalence of feelings still exists in full force on this inferior level, he expresses his positive attitude towards his object in the form of retaining his property, and his negative attitude in the form of *rejecting* it. Thus when the obsessional neurotic is threatened with the loss of his object, and when the melancholiac actually does lose his, it signifies to the unconscious mind of each an expulsion of that object in the sense of a physical expulsion of faeces. . . .

Many neurotic persons react in an anal way to every loss, whether it is the death of a person or the loss of a material object. They will react with constipation or diarrhoea according as the loss is viewed by their unconscious mind—whose attitude, in agreement with the ambivalence of their emotional life, is itself naturally a variable one. Their unconscious denies or affirms the loss by means of the "organ-speech" with which we are familiar. News of the death of a near relative will often set up in a person a violent pressure in his bowels as if the whole of his intestines were being expelled, or as if something was being torn away inside him and was going to come out through his anus. Without forgetting that a reaction like this is over-determined, I should like in this place to single out this one cause with which we are concerned. We must regard the reaction as an archaic form of mourning which has been conserved in the unconscious; and we can set it side by side with a primitive ritual, described by Róheim,[4] in which the relatives of the deceased man defaecate on his new-made grave. . . .

As an illustration I should like to relate the following curious ceremonial performed by a neurotic woman. . . . This woman, who presented anal character-traits of an extreme kind, was as a rule unable to throw away disused objects. Nevertheless she felt impelled from time to time to get rid of one or other of them. And so she had invented a way of cheating herself, as it were. She used to go out into the wood close by, and before she left the house she would take the object that was to be thrown away—an old garment, for instance—and tuck a corner of it under her petticoat strings behind. Then she would "lose" the thing on her walk in the wood. She would come home by another way so as not to come across it again. Thus in order to be able to give up the possession of an object she had to let it drop from the back of her body.

Moreover, nothing is so eloquent in confirmation of our view as the utterances of children. A small Hungarian boy, whose family lived in Buda-Pesth, once threatened his nurse with these words: "If you make me angry I'll ka-ka you across to Ofen" (a district on the other side of the Danube). According to the child's view the way to get rid of a person one no longer liked was by means of defaecation. . . .

The removal or loss of an object can be regarded by the unconscious either as a sadistic process of destruction or as an anal one of expulsion. . . .

Certain forms of speech show how closely are united in the unconscious mind anal and sadistic tendencies to abolish an object. The most widely different languages tend to express only by indirect allusion or metaphor behaviour which is based on sadistic impulses. But those metaphors are derived from activities which psycho-analytic experience has taught us to trace back to anal erotic and coprophilic instincts. A good example of this is to be found in the military reports and despatches which appeared on both sides during the late war. In them places were *"gesäubert"* ("cleaned") of the enemy, trenches were *"aufgeräumt"* ("cleared out"); in the French accounts the word used was *"nettoyer"* ("to clean"), and in the English, "cleaning up" or "mopping up" was the expression.

The analysis of neurotic patients has taught us that the second, *conserving* set of tendencies that spring from anal and sadistic sources—tendencies to retain and to control the object—combine in many ways and reinforce one another. And in the same way there is a close alliance between the *destructive* tendencies coming from those two sources—tendencies to expel and to destroy the object. The way in which these latter tendencies co-operate will become especially clear in the psychology of states of melancholia. And we shall enter into this point in greater detail later on.

What I should like to do in this place is to discuss briefly the convergent action of anal and sadistic instincts in the obsessional character. We have hitherto accounted for the excessive love of cleanliness shown by such characters as being a reaction formation against coprophilic tendencies, and for their marked love of order as a repressed or sublimated anal erotic instinct. This view, though correct and supported by a great mass of empirical data, is in some ways one-sided. It does not take sufficiently into consideration the over-determination of psychological phenomena.

For we are able to detect in our patients' compulsive love of order and cleanliness the co-operation of sublimated *sadistic* instincts as well. . . . Compulsive orderliness is at the same time an expression of the patient's desire for domination. He exerts power over things. He forces them into a rigid and pedantic system. And it not seldom happens that he makes people themselves enter into a system of this kind. We have only to think of the compulsion for cleaning everything from which some housewives suffer. They very often behave in such a way that nothing and no one is left in peace. They turn the whole house upside down and compel other persons to submit to their pathological impulses. In extreme cases of an obsessional character, as it is met with in housewife's neurosis and in neurotic exaggerations of the bureaucratic mind, this craving for domination becomes quite unmistakable. Or again, we need only think of the sadistic elements that go to make up the well-known anal character-trait of obstinacy to realize how anal and sadistic instinctual forces act together. . . .

As soon as something special occurs to threaten the "loss" of their object in the sense already used, both classes of neurotics react with great violence. The patient summons up the whole energy of his positive libidinal fixations to combat the danger that the current of feeling hostile to his object will grow too strong. If the conserving tendencies—those of retaining and controlling his object—are the more powerful, this conflict around the love-object will call forth phenomena of psychological compulsion. But if the opposing sadistic-anal tendencies are victorious—those which aim at destroying and expelling the object—then the patient will fall into a state of melancholic depression. . . .

Psycho-analytic experience and the direct observation of children have established the fact that that set of instincts which aims at the destruction and expulsion of the object is ontogenetically the elder of the two. In the normal development of his psycho-sexual life the individual ends by being capable of loving his object. . . .

Psycho-analytic experience has already obliged us to assert the existence of a pre-genital, anal-sadistic stage of libidinal development; and we now find ourselves led to assume that that stage includes two different levels within itself. On the later level the conserving tendencies of retaining and controlling the object predominate, whereas on the earlier level those hostile to their object—those of destroying and losing it—come to the fore. The obsessional neurotic regresses to the later of these two levels, and so he is able to maintain contact with his object. . . .

This differentiation of the anal-sadistic stage into a primitive and a later phase seems to be of radical importance. For at the dividing line between those two phases there takes place a decisive change in the attitude of the individual to the external world. Indeed, we may say that this dividing line is where "object-love" in the narrower sense begins, for it is at this point that the tendency to preserve the object begins to predominate. . . .

II. OBJECT-LOSS AND INTROJECTION IN NORMAL MOURNING AND IN ABNORMAL STATES OF MIND

Having taken as the starting-point of our investigations the "free interval" in periodical depressive and manic states, we may now proceed to inquire into the event which ushers in the actual melancholic illness—that event which Freud has called the "loss of object"—and into the process, so closely allied to it, of the introjection of the lost love-object. . . .

Dr. Elekes of Klausenburg has recently communicated to me the following peculiarly instructive case from his psychiatric practice in an asylum. A female patient was brought to the asylum on account of a melancholic depression. She repeatedly accused herself of being a thief. In reality she had never stolen anything. But her father, with whom she lived, and to whom she clung with all an unmarried daughter's love, had been arrested a short while before for a theft. This event, which not only removed her father from her in the literal meaning of the word but also called forth a profound psychological reaction in the sense of estranging her from him, was the beginning of her attack of melancholia. The loss of the loved person was immediately succeeded by an act of introjection; and now it was the patient herself who had committed the theft. This instance once more bears out

Freud's view that the self-reproaches of melancholia are in reality reproaches directed against the loved person.

It is easy enough to see in certain cases that object-loss and introjection have taken place. But we must remember that our knowledge of these facts is purely superficial, for we can give no explanation of them whatever. It is only by means of a regular psycho-analysis that we are able to perceive that there is a relationship between object-loss and tendencies, based on the earlier phase of the anal-sadistic stage, to lose and destroy things; and that the process of introjection has the character of a physical incorporation by way of the mouth. Furthermore, a superficial view of this sort misses the whole of the ambivalence conflict that is inherent in melancholia. The material which I shall bring forward in these pages will, I hope, help to some extent to fill in this gap in our knowledge. I should like to point out at once, however, that our knowledge of what takes place in normal mourning is equally superficial; for psycho-analysis has thrown no light on that mental state in healthy people and in cases of transference-neurosis. True, Freud has made the very significant observation that the serious conflict of ambivalent feelings from which the melancholiac suffers is absent in the normal person. But how exactly the process of mourning is effected in the normal mind we do not at present know. . . . I have had a case of this sort which has at last enabled me to gain some knowledge of this till now obscure subject, and which shows that in the normal process of mourning, too, the person reacts to a real object-loss by effecting a temporary introjection of the loved person. The case was as follows:

The wife of one of my analyzands became became very seriously ill while he was still under treatment. She was expecting her first child. At last it became necessary to put an end to her pregnancy by a Caesarian section. My analyzand was hurriedly called to her bedside and arrived after the operation had been performed. But neither his wife nor the prematurely born child could be saved. After some time the husband came back to me and continued his treatment. His analysis, and in especial a dream he had shortly after its resumption, made it quite evident that he had reacted to his painful loss with an act of introjection of an oral-cannibalistic character.

One of the most striking mental phenomena exhibited by him at this time was a dislike of eating, which lasted for weeks. This feature was in marked contrast to his usual habits, and was reminiscent of the refusal to take nourishment met with in melancholiacs. One day his disinclination for food disappeared, and he ate a good meal in the evening. That night he had a dream in which he was present at the *post-mortem* on his late wife. The dream was divided into two contrasting scenes. In the one, the separate parts of the body grew together again, the dead woman began to show signs of life, and he embraced her with feelings of the liveliest joy. In the other scene the dissecting-room altered its appearance, and the dreamer was reminded of slaughtered animals in a butcher's shop.

The scene of the dissection, twice presented in the dream, was associated with his wife's operation *(sectio Caesaris)*. In the one part it turned into the re-animation of the dead body; in the other it was connected with cannibalistic ideas. The dreamer's association to the dream in analysis brought out the remarkable fact that the sight of the dissected body reminded him of his meal of the evening before, and especially of a meat dish he had eaten.

We see here, therefore, that a single event has had two different sequels in the dream, set side by side with one another, as is so often the case when a parallel has to be expressed. Consuming the flesh of the dead wife is made equivalent to restoring her to life. Now Freud has shown that by introjecting the lost object the melancholiac does indeed recall it to life: he sets it up in his ego. In the present case the widowed man had abandoned himself to his grief for a certain period of time as though there were no possible escape from it. His disinclination for food was in part a playing with his own death; it seemed to imply that now that the object of his love was dead life had no more attraction for him. He then began to work off the traumatic effect of his loss by means of an unconscious process of introjection of the loved object. While this was going on he was once more able to take nourishment, and at the same time his dream announced the fact that the work of mourning had succeeded. The process of mourning thus brings with it the consolation: "My loved object is not gone, for now I carry it within myself and can never lose it."

This psychological process is, we see, identical with what occurs in melancholia. I shall try to make it clear later on that melancholia is an archaic form of mourning. But the instance given above leads us to the conclusion that the work of mourning in the healthy individual also assumes an archaic form in the lower strata of his mind.

At the time of writing I find that the fact that introjection takes place in normal mourning has already come near discovery from another quarter. Groddeck[5] cites the case of a patient whose hair went grey at the time of his father's death, and he attributes it to an unconscious tendency on the part of the patient to become like his father, and thus as it were to absorb him in himself and to take his place with his mother.

And here I find myself obliged to contribute an experience out of my own life. When Freud published his "Mourning and Melancholia," so often quoted in these pages, I noticed that I felt a quite unaccustomed difficulty in following his train of thought. I was aware of an inclination to reject the idea of an introjection of the loved object. I combated this feeling in myself, thinking that the fact that the genius of Freud had made a discovery in a field of interest so much my own had called forth in me an affective "no." It was not till later that I realized that this obvious motive was only of secondary importance compared with another. The facts were these:

Towards the end of the previous year my father had died. During the period of mourning which I went through certain things occurred which I was not at the time able to recognize as the consequence of a process of introjection. The most striking event was that my hair rapidly turned very grey and then went black again in a few months' time. At the time I attributed this to the emotional crisis I had been through. But I am now obliged to accept Groddeck's view, quoted above, concerning the deeper connection between my hair turning grey and my state of mourning. For I had seen my father for the last time a few months before his death, when I was home from the war on a short leave. I had found him very much aged and not at all strong, and I had especially noticed that his hair and his beard were almost white and were longer than usual on account of his having been confined to his bed. My recollection of my last visit to him was closely associated with this impression. Certain other features in the situation, which I am unfortunately unable to describe here, lead me to attribute my temporary symptom of turning grey to a process of introjection. It thus appears that my principal motive in being averse to Freud's theory of the pathological process of melancholia at first was my own tendency to employ the same mechanism during mourning.

Nevertheless, although introjection occurs in mourning in the healthy person and in the neurotic no less than in the melancholiac, we must not overlook the important differences between the process in the one and in the other. In the normal person it is set in motion by real loss (death); and its main purpose is to preserve the person's relations to the dead object, or—what comes to the same thing—to compensate for his loss. Furthermore, his conscious knowledge of his loss will never leave the normal person, as it does the melancholiac. The process of introjection in the melancholiac, moreover, is based on a radical disturbance of his libidinal relations to his object. It rests on a severe conflict of ambivalent feelings, from which he can only escape by turning against himself the hostility he originally felt towards his object.

Recent observations, those of Freud in the first instance, have shown that introjection is a far commoner psychological process than has hitherto been supposed. I should like to refer in particular to a remark of Freud's[6] concerning the psycho-analysis of homosexuality.

He expresses the view (though he does not support it with any clinical material) that we should be able to trace certain cases of homosexuality to the fact that the subject has introjected the parent of the opposite sex. Thus a young man will feel an inclination towards male persons because he has assimilated his mother by means of a psychological process of incorporation and consequently reacts to male objects in the way that she would do. Up till now we have been chiefly acquainted with another aetiology of homosexuality. The analysis of such cases has shown that as a rule the person has had a disappointment in his love for his mother and has left her and gone over to his father, towards whom he henceforward adopts the attitude usually taken by the daughter, identifying himself like her with his mother. A short time ago I had a case in which I was able to establish the presence of both these possible lines of mental development. The patient had a bisexual libidinal attitude, but was in a homosexual phase at the time he came to me for analysis. Twice before—once in early childhood and once during puberty—he had passed through a homosexual phase. It was only the second of these that set in with what must be described as a complete process of introjection. On that occasion the patient's ego was really submerged by the introjected object. I shall give a short abstract of his analysis, for it seems to me that the material is not only important for an understanding of the process of introjection, but also throws light on certain phenomena of mania and melancholia.

The patient was the younger of two children and had been a spoilt child in every sense of the word in his infancy. His mother had continued to suckle him well on into his second year, and even in his third year she still occasionally gave way to his desire, vehemently urged, to be fed at the breast. She did not wean him till he was three years old. At the same time as he was being weaned—a process which was achieved with great difficulty—a succession of events took place which robbed the spoilt child all at once of the paradise he had lived in. Up till then he had been the darling of his parents, of his sister, who was three years his senior, and of his nurse. Then his sister died. His mother withdrew into an abnormally severe and long period of mourning and thus became still more estranged from him than the weaning had already made her. The nurse left them. His parents could not bear to go on living in the same house, where they were constantly being reminded of their dead child, and they moved into an hotel and then into a new house. This series of events deprived the patient of all the things he had hitherto enjoyed in the way of maternal solicitude. First his mother had withdrawn the breast from him. Then she had shut herself off from him psychologically in mourning for her other child. His elder sister and his nurse were gone. Finally the house, that important symbol of the mother, was given up. It is not surprising that the small boy should have turned towards his father for love at this point. Besides this, he fixed his inclinations on a friendly neighbour, a woman who lived near their new house, and he made a great show of his preference for her over his mother. The splitting up of his libido—one part going to his father, the other to a woman who was a mother-surrogate—had already become evident. In the years following this period he became attached by a strong erotic interest to boys older than himself who resembled his father in their physical characteristics.

In his later childhood, as his father began to give way to drink more and more, the boy withdrew his libido from him and once more directed it towards his mother. He maintained this position for several years. Then his father died, and he lived alone with his mother, to whom he was devoted. But after a short period of widowhood she married again and went travelling with her husband for quite a long time. In doing this she had once more repulsed her son's love. And at the same time the boy's feelings of hatred were aroused against his step-father.

A new wave of homosexual feeling came over the half-grown boy. But this time he was attracted by a different type of young man, one which closely resembled that of his mother in certain physical qualities. The kind of youth he had loved on the first occasion, and the kind he loved now, exactly represented the contrast between his father and his mother in respect of their determining physical characteristics. It must be mentioned that the patient was himself entirely of his mother's type. His attitude towards this second type of young man for whom he now had a preference was, in his own words, tender, loving, and full of solicitude, like a mother.

Several years later the patient's mother died. He was with her during her last illness and she died in his arms. The very great effect which this experience had on him was caused by the fact that in a deeper stratum of his mind it represented the complete reversal of that unforgotten situation in which he, as an infant, had lain at his mother's breast and in her arms.

No sooner was his mother dead than he hurried back to the neighbouring town where he lived. His state of feeling, however, was by no means that of a sorrowing son; he felt, on the contrary, elated and blissful. He described to me how he was filled with the feeling that now he carried his mother safely in himself, his own for ever. The only thing that caused him uneasiness was the thought of her burial. It was as if he was disturbed by the knowledge that her body was still visible and lying in the house she had died in. It was not till the funeral was over that he could give himself up to the feeling that he possessed his mother for evermore.

If it were possible for me to publish more details from the analysis of this patient, I could make this process of incorporating the mother still more evident. But enough has been said to make its occurrence quite clear.

In this instance the process of introjecting the loved object began when the patient lost his mother through her second marriage. He was unable to move his libido away on to his father, as he had done in his fourth year; and his step-father was not qualified to attach his libido to himself. The last object of his infantile love that was left—his mother—was also the first. He strove against this heaviest loss that could befall him by employing the mechanism of introjection.

It is astonishing to find this process of introjection should have resulted in such a feeling of happiness, in direct contradiction to its effect on the melancholiac upon whose mind it weighs so heavily. But our surprise is lessened when we recollect Freud's explanation of the mechanism of melancholia. We have only to reverse his statement that "the shadow of the lost love-object falls upon the ego" and say that in this case it was not the shadow but the bright radiance of his loved mother which was shed upon her son. In the normal person, too, feelings of affection easily oust the hostile ones in regard to an object he has (in reality) lost. But it is otherwise in the case of the melancholiac. For here we find so strong a conflict based on libidinal ambivalence that every feeling of love is at once threatened by its opposite emotion. A "frustration," a disappointment from the side of the loved object, may at any time let loose a mighty wave of hatred which will sweep away his all too weakly-rooted feelings of love. Such a removal of the positive libidinal cathexes will have a most profound effect: it will lead to the giving up of the object. In the above-cited case, which was not one of melancholia, however, the loss *in reality* of the object was the primary event, and the alteration in the libido only a necessary consequence of it.

III. THE PROCESS OF INTROJECTION IN
MELANCHOLIA: TWO STAGES OF THE ORAL PHASE
OF THE LIBIDO

The following particularly instructive example may serve as a starting-point for further inquiry into the process of introjection.

The patient in question had already had several typical attacks of melancholia when he first came to me, and I began his analysis just as he was recovering from an attack of this kind. It had been a severe one, and had set in under rather curious circumstances. The patient had been fond of a young girl for some time back and had become engaged to her. Certain events, which I will not go into here, had caused his inclinations to give place to a violent resistance. It had ended in his turning away completely from his love-object—whose identification with his mother became quite evident in his analysis—and succumbing to a depressive condition accompanied by marked delusions. During his convalescence a *rapprochement* took place between him and his fiancée, who had remained constant to him in spite of his having left her. But after some time he had a brief relapse, the onset and termination of which I was able to observe in detail in his analysis.

His resistance to his fiancée re-appeared quite clearly during his relapse, and one of the forms it took was the following transitory symptom: During the time when his state of depression was worse than usual, he had a compulsion to contract his *sphincter ani*. This symptom proved to be over-determined. What is of most interest here is its significance as a convulsive holding fast to the contents of the bowels. As we know, such a retention symbolizes possession, and is its prototype in the unconscious. Thus the patient's transitory symptom stood for a retention, in the physical sense, of the object which he was once more in danger of losing. It had another determinant which I shall briefly notice. This was his passive homosexual attitude towards his father. Whenever he turned away from his mother or from a mother-substitute he was in danger of adopting this attitude; and his symptom was a defence not only against an object-loss but against a move towards homosexuality.

We have followed Freud in assuming that after he has lost his object the melancholiac attempts some kind of restitution of it. In paranoia this restitution is achieved by the specific mechanism of projection. In melancholia the mechanism of introjection is adopted, and the results are different. In the case of my patient the transitory symptom mentioned above, which was formed at the beginning of a brief remission of his illness, was not the end of the matter. A few days later he told me, once more of his own accord, that he had a fresh symptom which had, as it were, stepped into the shoes of the first one. As he was walking along the street he had had a compulsive phantasy of eating the excrements that were lying about. This phantasy turned out to be the expression of a desire to take back into his body the love-object which he had expelled from it in the form of excrement. We have here, therefore, a literal confirmation of our theory that the unconscious regards the loss of an object as an anal process, and its introjection as an oral one.

The tendency to coprophagia seems to me to contain a symbolism which is typical for melancholia. My own observations on a number of cases have always shown that the patient makes his love-object the target of certain impulses which correspond to the lower level of his anal-sadistic libidinal development. These are the impulses of expelling (in an anal sense) and of destroying (murdering). The product of such a murder—the dead body— becomes identified with the product of expulsion—with excrement. We can now understand that the patient's desire to eat excrement is a cannibalistic impulse to devour the love-object which he has killed. In one of my patients the idea of eating excrement was connected with the idea of being punished for a great sin. Psychologically speaking, he was right. For it was in this way that he had to make up for a certain crime whose identity with the deed of Oedipus we shall presently learn to understand.[7] I should like in this place to mention Róheim's interesting remarks[8] on the subject of necrophagia. What he has said makes it very probable that in their archaic form mourning rites consisted in the eating of the dead person.

The example given above is unusual in the easy and simple way in which it discloses the meaning of melancholic symptoms as an expulsion and a re-incorporation of the love-object. To show to what a degree these impulses can be rendered unrecognizable, I will give a second instance, taken from the psycho-analysis of another patient.

This patient told me one day that he had noticed a curious tendency that he had during his states of depression. At the beginning of those states he used to go about with his head lowered, so that his eyes were fixed on the ground rather than on the people about him. He would then begin to look with compulsive interest to see whether any mother-of-pearl buttons were lying in the street. If he found one he would pick it up and put it in his pocket. He rationalized this habit by saying that at the beginning of his depression he had such a feeling of inferiority that he had to feel glad if he even so much as found a button in the street; for he did not know whether he would ever again be capable of earning enough money to buy the least thing for himself. In the wretched condition he was in, he said, even those objects which other people left about must have a considerable value for him.

This explanation was contradicted by the fact that he passed by other objects, especially buttons made of other material, with a certain feeling of contempt. His free associations gradually led us to the deeper motives of his strange inclination. They showed that he connected the mother-of-pearl of which the buttons were made with the idea of brightness and cleanness, and then of special worth. We had thus arrived at his repressed coprophilic interests. I may remind my readers of Ferenczi's excellent paper on this subject.[9] In it he shows how the child first takes pleasure in substance that is soft and yielding, then in hard and granular material, and finally in small, solid objects with a clean and shining surface. In the unconscious these objects all remain equivalent to excrement.

The mother-of-pearl buttons stood, then, for excrement. Having to pick them up from the road reminds us of the obsessional impulse in the case described before, in which there was a direct compulsion to pick up excrement from the street and eat it. A further point of similarity between the two may be noted, namely, that people lose buttons off clothes just as they let faeces drop.[10] In both instances, therefore, the action is concerned with taking up and keeping a lost object.

In one of his next analytic hours the patient resumed his theme and said that what he had told me was not the only strange impulse he had had in his states of depression. During his first attack of this kind he had gone to Professor Y's nursing home at X. One day two relatives of his had come to take him out for a walk. They had shown him the public gardens and buildings and other things, but he had been utterly uninterested in them. But on his way back he had stopped in front of a shop-window in which he saw some pieces of Johannis bread.[11] He felt a strong desire to buy some of it, and had done so.

The patient at once had an association to this story, which was as follows: In the little town in which he lived as a child there was a small shop opposite his house. The shop was owned by a widow, whose son was a playmate of his. He recollected that this woman used to give him Johannis bread. At that time he had already had the fateful experience which was the origin of his later illness—a profound disappointment in his love-relations from the side of his mother. In his childhood memories this woman across the road was set up as a model and contrasted with his "wicked" mother. His automatic impulse to buy Johannis bread in a shop and to eat it had as its immediate significance his desire for maternal love and care. That he should have selected precisely Johannis bread as a symbol for this was because its long shape and brown colour reminded him of faeces. Thus we once more meet with the impulse to eat excrement as an expression of the desire for a lost love-object.

The patient had another association that went back to his childhood days. A road was being constructed in his native town and the workmen had dug up some shells. One side of them was covered with earth and looked dirty, but the other side glistened like mother-of-pearl. Here again the patient's associations took him back to his native place, which he undoubtedly identified with his mother. These shells were the precursors of the mother-of-pearl buttons about which he had his obsession. The idea of mother-of-pearl shells, moreover, proved in analysis to be a means of representing his ambivalent attitude towards his mother. The world "mother-of-pearl" expressed his high esteem for his mother as a "pearl." But the smooth, shining surface was deceptive—the other side was not so beautiful. In likening this other side, which was covered with dirt (excrement), to his "wicked" mother, from whom he had had to withdraw his libido, he was abusing her and holding her up to scorn.[12]

The instances given above may suffice for the present. They help us to understand psycho-analytically the course run by melancholia in its two phases—the loss and the re-incorporation of the love-object. Each of these phases, however, calls for further examination.

We have already said that the tendency to give up the love-object has its source in the fixation of the libido on the earlier phase of the anal-sadistic level. But if we find that the melancholiac is inclined to give up that position in favour of a yet more primitive one, namely, the oral level, then we must suppose that there are also certain fixation points in his libidinal development which date back to the time when his instinctual life was still mainly centred in the oral zone. And psycho-analytic observations bear out this supposition fully. A few examples may serve as an illustration.

In dealing with the melancholic cases I have repeatedly come across strong perverse cravings which consisted in using the mouth in place of the genitals. The patients satisfied these cravings in part by practising *cunnilinctus*. But they chiefly used to indulge in very vivid phantasies based on cannibalistic impulses. They used to phantasy about biting into every possible part of the body of their love-object—breast, penis, arm, buttocks, and so on. In their free associations they would very frequently have the idea of devouring the loved person or of biting pieces off his body; or they would occupy themselves with necrophagic images. They sometimes produced these various phantasies in an uninhibited and infantile way, sometimes concealed them behind feelings of disgust and terror. They also often exhibited a violent resistance against using their teeth. One of them used to speak of "chewing laziness" as one of the phenomena of his melancholic depression. . . .

In their pathological symptoms, their phantasies and their dreams, melancholic patients supply us with a great number and variety of oral-sadistic tendencies both conscious and repressed. These tendencies are one of the main sources of the mental suffering of depressive patients, especially in the case where they are turned against the subject's ego in the shape of a tendency to self-punishment. It is to be noticed that this situation is in contrast to some neurotic conditions of mind in which particular symptoms can be seen to be substitutive forms of gratification of the oral zone. . . . And there are besides certain perversions in which oral erotism provides a considerable amount of pleasure. Even taking into account the masochistic pleasure-value of its symptoms, we must nevertheless lay stress upon the fact that melancholia brings with it a very high degree of displeasure compared to other mental illnesses. If we observe attentively the depressive patient's chain of associations we shall discover that the excessive amount of displeasure he feels is allied to that stage of libidinal development to which he has regressed after he has lost his object. For we shall notice that he has a peculiar longing to use his mouth in a manner quite at variance with the biting and eating phantasies mentioned above. I will give you an instance.

At a time when he was recovering from his depression a patient told me about his day-dreams. In these he was at times impelled to imagine that he had a female body. He would employ all sorts of devices to create in himself the illusion that he had a woman's breasts, and would take special pleasure in the phantasy that he was suckling an infant. Although he played the part of the mother in this phantasy, he would sometimes exchange his rôle for that of the child at her breast. His fixation on the mother's breast found expression in two ways—in a great number of symptoms connected with the oral zone, and in a very marked desire to lean his head against something soft like a woman's breast. Thus, for instance, he used to behave in a very curious way with the cushion on the sofa during analysis. Instead of leaving it where it was and laying his head on it, he used to take it up and put it over his face. His associations showed that the cushion represented the breast being brought close to his head from above. The scene with the cushion repeated a pleasurable situation in his infancy. He had, moreover, seen his younger brother in this position later on and had connected feelings of intense jealousy with that spectacle.

Another melancholic patient I had said that during his deepest fits of depression he had the feeling that a woman might free him from his suffering if she expended on him a special maternal love and solicitude. The same type of conative idea was present here. I have repeatedly been able to analyse the meaning of an idea like this, and I can remember a case in point which I described in an earlier paper. A young man suffering from depression— though not a melancholic one—used to feel himself almost miraculously soothed by drinking a glass of milk which his mother handed to him. The milk gave him a sensation of something warm, soft, and sweet, and reminded him of something he had known long ago. In this instance the patient's longing for the breast was unmistakable.

All my psycho-analytic observations up till now lead me to the conclusion that the melancholiac is trying to escape from his oral-sadistic impulses. Beneath these impulses, whose manifestations colour the clinical picture, there lurks the desire for a pleasurable, sucking activity.

We are thus obliged to assume that there is a differentiation within the oral phase of the libido, just as there is within the anal-sadistic phase. On the primary level of that phase the libido of the infant is attached to the act of sucking. This act is one of incorporation, but one which does not put an end to the existence of the object. The child is not yet able to distinguish between its own self and the external object. Ego and object are concepts which are incompatible with that level of development. There is as yet no differentiation made between the sucking child and the suckling breast. Moreover, the child has as yet neither feelings of hatred nor of love. Its mental state is consequently free from all manifestations of ambivalence in this stage.

The secondary level of this phase differs from the first in that the child exchanges its sucking activity for a biting one. . . . What we call the sadistic impulses spring from a number of different sources, among which we may mention in especial the excremental ones. We must also bear in mind the close association of sadism with the muscular system. But there is no doubt that in small children far and away the most powerful muscles of the body are the jaw muscles. And, besides, the teeth are the only organs they possess that are sufficiently hard to be able to injure objects around them.

In the biting stage of the oral phase the individual incorporates the object in himself and in so doing destroys it. One has only to look at children to see how intense the impulse to bite is—an impulse in which the eating instinct and the libido still co-operate. This is the stage in which cannibalistic impulses predominate. As soon as the child is attracted by an object, it is liable, indeed bound, to attempt its destruction. It is in this stage that the ambivalent attitude of the ego to its object begins to grow up. We may say, therefore, that in the child's libidinal development the second stage of the oral-sadistic phase marks the beginning of its ambivalence conflict; whereas the first (sucking) stage should still be regarded as pre-ambivalent.

The libidinal level, therefore, to which the melancholiac regresses after the loss of his object contains in itself a conflict of ambivalent feelings in its most primitive and therefore most unmodified form. On that level the individual threatens to destroy his libidinal object by devouring it. It is only gradually that the ambivalence conflict assumes a milder aspect and that the libido consequently adopts a less violent attitude towards its object. Nevertheless this ambivalent attitude remains inherent in the tendencies of the libido during the subsequent phases of its development. We have already discussed its importance in the anal-sadistic phase. But even in the structure of neuroses based on the genital phase we meet this ambivalence everywhere in the patient's emotional life. It is only the normal person—the person who is relatively far removed from the infantile forms of sexuality—who is in the main without ambivalence. His libido has, as it were, reached a post-ambivalent stage and has thus achieved a full capacity for adapting itself to the external world.

It now becomes evident that we ought also to distinguish two stages within the genital phase of the libido, just as we did within its two pre-genital phases. And this leads us to a result which seems to coincide perfectly with Freud's recently published view[13] that there exists an early stage of the genital phase—what he calls a "phallic" stage. Thus it would seem that the libido passes through six stages of development in all. But I should like to state explicitly that I do not consider the above classification either as final or exhaustive. It only presents a general picture of the continuous evolution of the libido in so far as our present-day psycho-analytic knowledge has been able to throw light on that slow and laborious process. Nevertheless in my opinion the transition from the earlier stage to the later one within each of the three main developmental phases of the libido is by no means a process of minor importance. We have long since become acquainted with the significance that the change from one preponderating erotogenic zone to another has for the normal psychosexual development of the individual and for the formation of his character. We now see that within each of those three main periods a process takes place which is of great importance for the gradual attainment by the individual of complete object-love. Within the first—the oral—period, the child exchanges its pre-ambivalent libidinal attitude, which is free from conflict, for one which is ambivalent and preponderantly hostile towards its object. Within the second—the anal-sadistic—period, the transition from the earlier to the later stage means that the individual has begun to spare his object from destruction. Finally, within the third—the genital—period, he overcomes his ambivalent attitude and his libido attains to its full capacity both from a sexual and a social point of view.

The above account does not by any means cover the whole of the changes that take place in the relations between the individual and the external world. Those changes will have to form the subject of a thorough investigation in a later part of my study. . . .

NOTES

1. Abraham, K. (1911). Notes on the psycho-analytical investigation and treatment of Manic-Depressive insanity and allied conditions. In K. Abraham, *Selected Papers on Psycho-Analysis*. London: Hogarth, 1942. 137–56.
2. In the third edition of his *Drei Abhandlungen zur Sexualtheorie*.
3. Abraham, K. (1916). The first pregenital stage of the libido. *Op. cit.* 248–79.
4. "Nach dem Tode des Urvaters" (1923).
5. In his *Buch vom Es* (1923), p. 24.
6. Cf. his *Group Psychology*, p. 66.
7. Dr. J. Hárnik has pointed out that in Egypt a prayer is often put on gravestones in which the dead man asks that he may be spared the punishment of having to eat excrement. Cf. Erman, *Religion der Ägypter*.
8. Communicated to the Psycho-Analytical Congress in 1922.
9. "On the Ontogenesis of an Interest in Money" (1914).
10. Regarding this assimilation of ideas, cf. the case described in Section I of this chapter.
11. [A fancy bread.—*Trans.*]
12. Before leaving this subject I should like to add that the shell is a universal female symbol.
    We learn from Róheim that in many places shells are employed as money. This use of

them is once more connected with them as a symbol of the female genitals. It is worth noting that they are never used in this way in the place in which they are found. Only shells coming from a distance can be used as money. This fact seems to be the expression of a widely extended fear of incest, and parallel to the law of exogamy. A woman belonging to the same tribe or a shell found on the shore nearby both represent the forbidden genitals of the mother.

Moreover, shells are also likened to excrement, since they are cast up by the sea as are sea-amber and other substances. (These notes are taken in part from a discussion that took place at a meeting of the Berlin Psycho-Analytical Society.)

13. "The Infantile Genital Organization of the Libido" (1923).

Introductory Notes to Chapter 9

Rita V. Frankiel

In this paper, which is one of a group of papers central to the development and exposition of Melanie Klein's theory of psychic life, she develops and supports the idea that the extreme painfulness of mourning in adults has its basis in the fact that the loss of a loved object in adult life reactivates in the mourner the extremely painful affects and fantasies characteristic of the "depressive position" of early life. The resolution of the depressive position is the essential prerequisite for the development of the capacity to grieve; with this resolution comes the creation and maintenance of what Freudians call "post-ambivalent" relationship.

Klein posits that the loss of the *external* good object through death brings with it the profound unconscious fear that the *internal* good object is gone as well. The reason why the loss is so painful is that the person often feels total despair and helplessness—the object is gone, guilt and persecutory anxiety may prevail, and the person feels powerless to restore or recreate the loved one's image and is unable to pine after him or her. Reinstating the sense of once again possessing the internal good object despite the loss of the external object is the outcome of a process of mourning carried to a healthy resolution.

Pathological mourning involves processes of reparation of fantasied damage to the object that have destructive consequences; manic and omnipotent reparation are examples of pathological need to repair the damaged object. The intense feeling of having triumphed over the dead one by surviving, if more than a transitory phase, is, on Klein's view, symptomatic of a mourning process gone astray. Here she differs from Freud, who sees triumph as a common constituent of the end phase of mourning. Klein's theory here offers what seems a cogent approach to the problem that continued to preoccupy Freud: why is mourning so painful and why does it take so long?

9. Mourning and Its Relation to Manic-Depressive States

Melanie Klein

An essential part of the work of mourning is, as Freud points out in "Mourning and Melancholia," the testing of reality. He says that "in grief this period of time is necessary for detailed carrying out of the behest imposed by the testing of reality, and . . . by accomplishing this labour the ego succeeds in freeing its libido from the lost object." [1] And again: "Each single one of the memories and hopes which bound the libido to the object is brought up and hyper-cathected, and the detachment of the libido from it accomplished. Why this process of carrying out the behest of reality bit by bit, which is in the nature of a compromise, should be so extraordinarily painful is not at all easy to explain in terms of mental economics. It is worth noting that this pain seems natural to us." [2] And, in another passage: "We do not even know by what economic measures the work of mourning is carried through; possibly, however, a conjecture may help us here. Reality passes its verdict—that the object no longer exists—upon each single one of the memories and hopes through which the libido was attached to the lost object, and the ego, confronted as it were with the decision whether it will share this fate, is persuaded by the sum of its narcissistic satisfactions in being alive to sever its attachment to the non-existent object. We may imagine that, because of the slowness and the gradual way in which this severance is achieved, the expenditure of energy necessary for it becomes somehow dissipated by the time the task is carried through." [3]

In my view there is a close connection between the testing of reality in normal mourning and early processes of the mind. My contention is that the child goes through states of mind comparable to the mourning of the adult,

Reprinted by permission of *The International Journal of Psycho-Analysis* 21 (1940):125–53. Permission granted by the Melanie Klein Trust. Copyright© The Institute of Psycho-Analysis and The Melanie Klein Trust 1975.

or rather, that this early mourning is revived whenever grief is experienced in later life. The most important of the methods by which the child overcomes his states of mourning, is, in my view, the testing of reality; this process, however, as Freud stresses, is part of the work of mourning.

In my paper "A Contribution to the Psychogenesis of Manic-Depressive States,"[4] I introduced the conception of the *infantile depressive position,* and showed the connection between the position and manic-depressive states. Now in order to make clear the relation between the infantile depressive position and normal mourning I must first briefly refer to some statements I made in that paper, and shall then enlarge on them. In the course of this exposition I also hope to make a contribution to the further understanding of the connection between normal mourning, on the one hand, and abnormal mourning and manic-depressive states, on the other.

I said there that the baby experiences depressive feelings which reach a climax just before, during and after weaning. This is the state of mind in the baby which I termed the "depressive position," and I suggested that it is a melancholia in *statu nascendi.* The object which is being mourned is the mother's breast and all that the breast and the milk have come to stand for in the infant's mind: namely, love, goodness and security. All these are felt by the baby to be lost, and lost as a result of his own uncontrollable greedy and destructive phantasies and impulses against his mother's breasts. Further distress about impending loss (this time of both parents) arises out of the Oedipus situation, which sets in so early and in such close connection with breast frustrations that in its beginnings it is dominated by oral impulses and fears. The circle of loved objects who are attacked in phantasy and whose loss is therefore feared widens owing to the child's ambivalent relations to his brothers and sisters. The aggression against phantasied brothers and sisters, who are attacked inside the mother's body, also gives rise to feelings of guilt and loss. The sorrow and concern about the feared loss of the "good" objects, that is to say, the depressive position, is, in my experience, the deepest source of the painful conflicts in the Oedipus situation, as well as in the child's relations to people in general. In normal development these feelings of grief and fear are overcome by various methods.

Along with the child's relation, first to his mother and soon to his father and other people, go those processes of internalization on which I have laid so much stress in my work. The baby, having incorporated his parents, feels them to be live people inside his body in the concrete way in which deep unconscious phantasies are experienced—they are, in his mind, "internal" or "inner" objects, as I have termed them. Thus an inner world is being built up in the child's unconscious mind, corresponding to his actual experiences and the impressions he gains from people and the external world, and yet altered by his own phantasies and impulses. If it is a world of people predominantly at peace with each other and with the ego, inner harmony, security and integration ensue.

There is a constant interaction between anxieties relating to the "external" mother—as I will call her here in contrast to the "internal" one—and those relating to the "internal" mother, and the methods used by the ego for dealing with these two sets of anxieties are closely inter-related. In the baby's mind, the "internal" mother is bound up with the "external" one, of whom she is a "double," though one which at once undergoes alterations in his mind through the very process of internalization; that is to say, her image is influenced by his phantasies, and by internal stimuli and internal experiences of all kinds. When external situations which he lives through become internalized—and I hold that they do, from the earliest days onwards—they follow the same pattern: they also become "doubles" of real situations, and are again altered for the same reasons. The fact that by being internalized, people, things, situations and happenings—the whole inner world which is being built up—become inaccessible to the child's accurate observation and judgement, and cannot be verified by the means of perception which are available in connection with the tangible and palpable object-world, has an important bearing on the phantastic nature of this inner world. The ensuing doubts, uncertainty and anxieties act as a continuous incentive to the young child to observe and make sure about the external object-world,[5] from which this inner world springs, and by these means to understand the internal one better. The visible mother thus provides continuous proofs of what the "internal" mother is like, whether she is loving or angry, helpful or revengeful. The extent to which external reality is able to disprove anxieties and sorrow relating to the internal reality varies with each individual, but could be taken as one of the criteria for normality. In children who are so much dominated by their internal world that their anxieties cannot be sufficiently disproved and counteracted even by the pleasant aspects of their relationships with people, severe mental difficulties are unavoidable. On the other hand, a certain amount even of unpleasant experiences is of value in this testing of reality by the child if, through overcoming them, he feels that he can retain his objects as well as their love for him and his love for them, and thus preserve or re-establish internal life and harmony in face of dangers.

All the enjoyments which the baby lives through in relation to his mother are so many proofs to him that the loved object *inside as well as outside* is not injured, is not turned into a vengeful person. The increase of love and trust, and the diminishing of fears through happy experiences, help the baby step by step to overcome his depression and feeling of loss (mourning). They enable him to test his inner reality by means of outer reality. Through being loved and through the enjoyment and comfort he has in relation to people his confidence in his own as well as in other people's goodness becomes strengthened, his hope that his "good" objects and his own ego can be saved and preserved increases, at the same time as his ambivalence and acute fears of internal destruction diminish.

Unpleasant experiences and the lack of enjoyable ones, in the young child, especially lack of happy and close contact with loved people, increase ambivalence, diminish trust and hope and confirm anxieties about inner annihilation and external persecution; moreover they slow down and perhaps permanently check the beneficial processes through which in the long run inner security is achieved.

In the process of acquiring knowledge, every new piece of experience has to be fitted into the patterns provided by the psychic reality which prevails at the time; whilst the psychic reality of the child is gradually influenced by every step in his progressive knowledge of external reality. Every such step goes along with his more and more firmly establishing his inner "good" objects, and is used by the ego as a means of overcoming the depressive position.

In other connections I have expressed the view that every infant experiences anxieties which are psychotic in content,[6] and that the infantile neurosis[7] is the normal means of dealing with and modifying these anxieties. This conclusion I can now state more precisely, as a result of my work on the infantile depressive position, which has led me to believe that it is the central position in the child's development. In the infantile neurosis the early depressive position finds expression, is worked through and gradually overcome; and this is an important part of the process of organization and integration which, together with his sexual development,[8] characterizes the first years of life. Normally the child passes through his infantile neurosis, and among other achievements arrives step by step at a good relation to people and to reality. I hold that this satisfactory relation to people depends upon his having succeeded in his struggles against the chaos inside him (the depressive position) and having securely established his "good" internal objects.

Let us now consider more closely the methods and mechanisms by which this development comes about.

In the baby, processes of introjection and projection, since they are dominated by aggression and anxieties which reinforce each other, lead to fears of persecution by terrifying objects. To such fears are added those of losing his loved objects; that is to say, the depressive position has arisen. When I first introduced the conception of the depressive position I put forward the suggestion that the introjection of the whole loved object gives rise to concern and sorrow lest that object should be destroyed (by the "bad" objects and the id), and that these distressed feelings and fears, in addition to the paranoid set of fears and defences, constitute the depressive position. There are thus two sets of fears, feelings and defences, which, however varied in themselves and however intimately linked together, can in my view, for purposes of theoretical clearness, be isolated from each other. The first set of feelings and phantasies are the persecutory ones, characterized by fears relating to the destruction of the ego by internal persecutors. The defenses against these fears are predominantly the destruction of the persecutors by violent or secretive and cunning methods. With these fears and defences I have dealt in detail in other contexts. The second set of feelings which go to make up the depressive position I formerly described without suggesting a term for them. I now propose to use for these feelings of sorrow and concern for the loved objects, the fears of losing them and the longing to regain them, a simple word derived from everyday language—namely the "pining" for the loved object. In short—persecution (by "bad" objects) and the characteristic defences against it, on the one hand, and pining for the loved ("good") object, on the other, constitute the depressive position.

When the depressive position arises, the ego is forced (in addition to earlier defences) to develop methods of defence which are essentially directed against the "pining" for the loved object. These are fundamental to the whole ego-organization. I formerly termed some of these methods *manic defences,* or the *manic position,* because of their relationship to the manic-depressive illness.[9]

The fluctuations between the depressive and the manic position are an essential part of normal development. The ego is driven by depressive anxieties (anxiety lest the loved objects as well as itself should be destroyed) to

build up omnipotent and violent phantasies, partly for the purpose of controlling and mastering the "bad," dangerous objects, partly in order to save and
restore the loved ones. From the very beginning, these omnipotent phantasies, both the destructive and the reparative ones, stimulate and enter into all
the activities, interests and sublimations of the child. In the infant, the
extreme character both of his sadistic and of his constructive phantasies is in
line with the extreme frightfulness of his persecutors—and, at the other end
of the scale, the extreme perfection of his "good" objects.[10] Idealization is
an essential part of the manic position, namely denial. Without partial and
temporary denial of psychic reality the ego cannot bear the disaster by
which it feels itself threatened when the depressive position is at its height.
Omnipotence, denial and idealization, closely bound up with ambivalence,
enable the early ego to assert itself to a certain degree against its internal
persecutors and against a slavish and perilous dependence upon its loved
objects, and thus to make further advances in development. I will here quote
a passage from my former paper:

In the earliest phase the persecuting and the good objects (breasts) are kept wide
apart in the child's mind. When, along with the introjection of the whole and real
object, they come closer together, the ego has over and over again recourse to that
mechanism—so important for the development of the relations to objects—namely,
a splitting of its imagos into loved and hated, that is to say, into good and dangerous
ones.

One might think that is is actually at this point that ambivalence which, after
all, refers to object-relations—that is to say, to whole and real objects—sets in.
Ambivalence, carried out in a splitting of the imagos, enables the small child to gain
more trust and belief in its real objects and thus in its internalized ones—to love them
more and to carry out in an increasing degree its phantasies of restoration on the loved
object. At the same time the paranoid anxieties and defences are directed towards the
"bad" objects. The support which the ego gets from a real "good" object is
increased by a flight-mechanism, which alternates between its external and internal
good objects. [Idealization.]

It seems that at this stage of development the unification of external and internal,
loved and hated, real and imaginary objects is carried out in such a way that each step
in the unification leads again to a renewed splitting of the imagos. But as the
adaptation to the external world increases, this splitting is carried out on planes which
gradually become increasingly nearer and nearer to reality. This goes on until love for
the real and the internalized objects and trust in them are well established. Then
ambivalence, which is partly a safeguard against one's own hate and against the hated
and terrifying objects, will in normal development again diminish in varying degrees.[11]

As has already been stated, omnipotence prevails in the early phantasies, both the destructive and the reparative ones, and influences sublimations as well as object relations. Omnipotence, however, is so closely bound up in the unconscious with the sadistic impulses with which it was first associated that the child feels again and again that his attempts at reparation have not succeeded, or will not succeed. His sadistic impulses, he feels, may easily get the better of him. The young child, who cannot sufficiently trust his reparative and constructive feelings, as we have seen, resorts to manic omnipotence. For this reason, in an early stage of development the ego has not adequate means at its disposal to deal efficiently with guilt and anxiety. All this leads to the need in the child—and for that matter to some extent in the adult also—to repeat certain actions obsessionally (this, in my view, is part of the repetition compulsion);[12] or—the contrasting method—omnipotence and denial are resorted to. When the defences of a manic nature fail, defences in which dangers from various sources are in an omnipotent way denied or minimized, the ego is driven alternately or simultaneously, to combat the fears of deterioration and disintegration by attempted reparations carried out in obsessional ways. I have described elsewhere[13] my conclusion that the obsessional mechanisms are a defence against paranoid anxieties as well as a means of modifying them, and here I will only show briefly the connection between obsessional mechanisms and manic defences in relation to the depressive position in normal development.

The very fact that manic defences are operating in such close connection with the obsessional ones contributes to the ego's fear that the reparation attempted by obsessional means has also failed. The desire to control the object, the sadistic gratification of overcoming and humiliating it, of getting the better of it, the *triumph* over it, may enter so strongly into the act of reparation (carried out by thoughts, activities or sublimations) that the benign circle started by this act becomes broken. The objects which were to be restored change again into persecutors, and in turn paranoid fears are revived. These fears reinforce the paranoid defence mechanisms (of controlling it or keeping it in suspended animation, and so on). The reparation which was in progress is thus disturbed or even nullified—according to the extent to which these mechanisms are activated. As a result of the failure of the act of reparation, the ego has to resort again and again to obsessional and manic defences.

When in the course of normal development a relative balance between love and hate is attained, and the various aspects of objects are more unified, then also a certain equilibrium between these contrasting and yet closely related methods is reached, and their intensity is diminished. In this connection I wish to stress the importance of *triumph,* closely bound up with contempt and omnipotence, as an element of the manic position. We know the part rivalry plays in the child's burning desire to equal the achievements of the grown-ups. In addition to rivalry, his wish, mingled with fears, to "grow out" of his deficiencies (ultimately to overcome his destructiveness and his bad inner objects and to be able to control them) is an incentive to achievements of all kinds. In my experience, the desire to reverse the child-parent relation, to get power over the parents and to triumph over them, is always to some extent associated with the impulse towards the attainment of success. A time will come, the child phantasies, when he will be strong, tall and grown up, powerful, rich and potent, and father and mother will have changed into helpless children, or again, in other phantasies, will be very old, weak, poor and rejected. The triumph over the parents in such phantasies, through the guilt to which it gives rise, often cripples endeavours of all kinds. Some people are obliged to remain unsuccessful, because success always implies to them the humiliation or even the damage of somebody else, in the first place the triumph over parents, brothers and sisters. The efforts by which they seek to achieve something may be of a highly constructive nature, but the implicit triumph and the ensuing harm and injury done to the object may outweigh these purposes, in the subject's mind, and therefore prevent fulfilment. The effect is that the reparation to the loved objects, which in the depths of the mind are the same as those over which he triumphs, is again thwarted, and therefore guilt remains unrelieved. The subject's triumph over his objects necessarily implies to him their wish to triumph over him, and therefore leads to distrust and feelings of persecution. Depression may follow, or an increase in manic defences and more violent control of his objects, since he has failed to reconcile, restore, or improve them, and therefore feelings of being persecuted by them again have the upper hand. All this has an important bearing on the infantile depressive position and the ego's success or failure in overcoming it. The triumph over his internal objects which the young child's ego controls, humiliates and tortures is a part of the destructive aspect of the manic position which disturbs the reparation and re-creating of his inner world and of internal peace and harmony; and thus triumph impedes the work of early mourning.

To illustrate these developmental processes let us consider some features which can be observed in hypomanic people. It is characteristic of the hypomanic person's attitude towards people, principles and events that he is inclined to exaggerated valuations: over-admiration (idealization) or contempt (devaluation). With this goes his tendency to conceive of everything on a large scale, to think in *large numbers,* all this in accordance with the greatness of his omnipotence, by which he defends himself against his fear of losing the one irreplaceable object, his mother, whom he still mourns at bottom. His tendency to minimize the importance of details and small numbers, and a frequent casualness about details and contempt of conscientiousness contrast sharply with the very meticulous methods, the concentration on the smallest things (Freud), which are part of the obsessional mechanisms.

This contempt, however, is also based to some extent on denial. He must deny his impulse to make extensive and detailed reparation because he has to deny the cause for the reparation, namely the injury to the object and his consequent sorrow and guilt.

Returning to the course of early development, we may say that every step in emotional, intellectual and physical growth is used by the ego as a means of overcoming the depressive position. The child's growing skills, gifts and arts increase his belief in the psychical reality of his constructive tendencies, in his capacity to master and control his hostile impulses as well as his "bad" internal objects. Thus anxieties from various sources are relieved, and this results in a diminution of aggression and, in turn, of his suspicions of "bad" external and internal objects. The strengthened ego, with its greater trust in people, can then make still further steps towards unification of its imagos—external, internal, loved and hated—and towards further mitigation of hatred by means of love, and thus to a general process of integration.

When the child's belief and trust in his capacity to love, in his reparative powers and in the integration and security of his good inner world increases as a result of the constant and manifold proofs and counter-proofs gained by the testing of external reality, manic omnipotence decreases and the obsessional nature of the impulses towards reparation diminishes, which means in general that the infantile neurosis has passed.

We have now to connect the infantile depressive position with normal mourning. The poignancy of the actual loss of a loved person is, in my view, greatly increased by the mourner's unconscious phantasies of having lost his *internal* "good" objects as well. He then feels that his internal "bad" objects predominate and his inner world is in danger of disruption. We know that the loss of a loved person leads to an impulse in the mourner to reinstate the lost loved object in the ego (Freud and Abraham). In my view, however, he not only takes into himself (re-incorporates) the person whom he has just lost, but also reinstates his internalized good objects (ultimately his loved parents), who became part of his inner world from the earliest stages of his development onwards. These too are felt to have gone under, to be destroyed, whenever the loss of a loved person is experienced. Thereupon the early depressive position, and with it anxieties, guilt and feelings of loss and grief derived from the breast situation, the Oedipus situation and all other such sources, are reactivated. Among all these emotions, the fears of being robbed and punished by both dreaded parents—that is to say, feelings of persecution—have also been revived in deep layers of the mind.

If, for instance, a woman loses her child through death, along with sorrow and pain, her early dread of being robbed by a "bad" retaliating mother is reactivated and confirmed. Her own early aggressive phantasies of robbing her mother of babies gave rise to fears and feelings of being punished, which strengthened ambivalence and led to hatred and distrust of others. The reinforcing of feelings of persecution in the state of mourning is all the more painful because, as a result of an increase in ambivalence and distrust, friendly relations with people, which might at that time be so helpful, become impeded.

The pain experienced in the slow process of testing reality in the work of mourning thus seems to be partly due to the necessity, not only to renew the links to the external world and thus continuously to re-experience the loss, but at the same time and by means of this to rebuild with anguish the inner world, which is felt to be in danger of deteriorating and collapsing.[14] Just as the young child passing through the depressive position is struggling, in his unconscious mind, with the task of establishing and integrating his inner world, so the mourner goes through the pain of re-establishing and re-integrating it.

In normal mourning early psychotic anxieties are reactivated; the mourner is in fact ill, but, because this state of mind is so common and seems so natural to us, we do not call mourning an illness. (For similar reasons, until recent years, the infantile neurosis of the normal child was not recognized as such.) To put my conclusions more precisely: I should say that in mourning the subject goes through a modified and transitory manic-depressive state and overcomes it, thus repeating, though in different circumstances and with different manifestations, the process which the child normally goes through in his early development.

The greatest danger for the mourner comes from the turning of his hatred against the lost loved person himself. One of the ways in which hatred expresses itself in the situation of mourning is in feelings of triumph over the dead person. I refer in an earlier part of this paper to triumph as part of the manic position in infantile development. Infantile death wishes against parents, brothers and sisters are actually fulfilled whenever a loved person dies, because he is necessarily to some extent a representative of the earliest important figures, and therefore takes over some of the feelings pertaining to them. Thus his death, however shattering for other reasons, is to some extent also felt as a victory, and gives rise to triumph, and therefore all the more to guilt.

At this point I find that my view differs from that of Freud, who stated: "First, then: in normal grief too the loss of the object is undoubtedly surmounted, and this process too absorbs all the energies of the ego while it lasts. Why then does it not set up the economic condition for a phase of triumph after it has run its course or at least produce some slight indication of such a state? I find it impossible to answer this objection off-hand." [15] In my experience, feelings of triumph are inevitably bound up even with normal mourning, and have the effect of retarding the work of mourning, or rather they contribute much to the difficulties and pain which the mourner experiences. When hatred of the lost loved object in its various manifestations gets the upper hand in the mourner, this not only turns the loved lost person into a persecutor, but shakes the mourner's belief in his good inner objects as well. The shaken belief in the good objects disturbs most painfully the process of idealization, which is an essential intermediate step in mental development. With the young child, the idealized mother is the safeguard against a retaliating or a dead mother and against all bad objects, and therefore represents security and life itself. As we know, the mourner obtains great relief from recalling the lost person's kindness and good qualities, and this is partly due to the reassurance he experiences from keeping his loved object for the time being as an idealized one.

The passing states of elation [16] which occur between sorrow and distress in normal mourning are manic in character and are due to the feeling of possessing the perfect loved object (idealized) inside. At any time, however, when hatred against the lost loved person wells up in the mourner, his belief in him breaks down and the process of idealization is disturbed. (His hatred of the loved person is increased by the fear that by dying the loved one was seeking to inflict punishment and deprivation upon him, just as in the past he felt that his mother, whenever she was away from him and wanted her, had died in order to inflict punishment and deprivation upon him.) Only gradually, by regaining trust in external objects and values of various kinds, is the normal mourner able once more to strengthen his confidence in the lost loved person. Then he can again bear to realize that this object was not perfect, and yet not lose trust and love for him, nor fear his revenge. When this stage is reached, important steps in the work of mourning and towards overcoming it have been made.

To illustrate the ways in which a normal mourner re-established connections with the external world I shall now give an instance. Mrs. A., in the first few days after the shattering loss of her young son, who had died suddenly while at school, took to sorting out letters, keeping his and throwing others away. She was thus unconsciously attempting to restore him and keep him safe inside herself, and throwing out what she felt to be indifferent, or rather hostile—that is to say, the "bad" objects, dangerous excreta and bad feelings.

Some people in mourning tidy the house and re-arrange furniture, actions which spring from an increase of the obsessional mechanisms which are a repetition of one of the defences used to combat the infantile depressive position.

In the first week after the death of her son she did not cry much, and tears did not bring her the relief which they did later on. She felt numbed and closed up, and physically broken. It gave her some relief, however, to see one or two intimate people. At this stage Mrs. A., who usually dreamed every night, had entirely stopped dreaming because of her deep unconscious denial of her actual loss. At the end of the week she had the following dream:

She saw two people, a mother and son. The mother was wearing a black dress. The dreamer knew that this boy had died, or was going to die. No sorrow entered into her feelings, but there was a trace of hostility towards the two people.

The associations brought up an important memory. When Mrs. A. was a little girl, her brother, who had difficulties in his school work, was going to be tutored by a school-fellow of his own age (I will call him B.). B.'s mother had come to see Mrs. A.'s mother to arrange about the coaching, and Mrs. A. remembered this incident with very strong feelings. B.'s mother behaved in a patronizing way, and her own mother appeared to her to be rather dejected. She herself felt that a fearful disgrace had fallen upon her very much admired and beloved brother and the whole family. This brother, a few years older than herself, seemed to her full of knowledge, skill and strength—a paragon of all the virtues, and her ideal was shattered when his deficiencies at school came to light. The strength of her feelings about this incident as being an irreparable misfortune, which persisted in her memory, was, however, due to her unconscious feelings of guilt. She felt it to be the fulfilment of her own harmful wishes. Her brother himself was very much chagrined by the situation, and expressed great dislike and hatred of the other boy. Mrs. A. at the time identified herself strongly with him in these resentful feelings. In the dream, the two people whom Mrs. A. saw were B. and his mother, and the fact that the boy was dead expressed Mrs. A.'s early death wishes against him. At the same time, however, the death wishes against her own brother and the wish to inflict punishment and deprivation upon her mother through the loss of her son—very deeply repressed wishes—were part of her dream thoughts. It now appeared that Mrs. A., with all her admiration and love for her brother, had been jealous of him on various grounds, envying his greater knowledge, his mental and physical superiority, and also his possession of a penis. Her jealousy of her much beloved mother for possessing such a son had contributed towards her death wishes against her brother. One dream thought, therefore, ran: "A mother's son has died, or will die. It is this unpleasant woman's son, who hurt my mother and brother, who should die." But in deeper layers, the death wish against her brother had also been reactivated, and this dream thought ran: "My mother's son died, and not my own." (Both her mother and her brother were in fact already dead.) Here a contrasting feeling came in—sympathy with her mother and sorrow for herself. She felt: "One death of the kind was enough. My mother lost her son; she should not lose her grandson also." When her brother died, besides great sorrow, she unconsciously felt triumph over him, derived from her early jealousy and hatred, and corresponding feelings of guilt. She had carried over some of her feelings for her brother into her relations to her son. In her son, she also loved her brother; but at the same time, some of the ambivalence towards her brother, though modified through her strong motherly feelings, was also transferred on to her son. The mourning for her brother, together with the sorrow, the triumph and the guilt experienced in relation to him, entered into her present grief, and was shown in the dream.

Let us now consider the interplay of defences as they appeared in this material. When the loss occurred, the manic position became reinforced, and denial in particular came especially into play. Unconsciously, Mrs. A.

strongly rejected the fact that her son had died. When she could no longer carry on this denial so strongly, but was not yet able to face the pain and sorrow, triumph, one of the other elements of the manic position, became reinforced. "It is not at all painful," the thought seemed to run, as the associations showed, "if a boy dies. It is even satisfactory. Now I get my revenge against this unpleasant boy who injured my brother." The fact that triumph over her brother had also been revived and strengthened became clear only after hard analytic work. But this triumph was associated with control of the *internalized* mother and brother, and triumph over them. At this stage the *control* over her internal objects was reinforced, the misfortune and grief were *displaced* from herself on to her internalized mother. Here denial again came into play—denial of the psychical reality that she and her internal mother were one and suffered together. Compassion and love for the internal mother were denied, feelings of revenge and triumph over the internalized objects and control of them were reinforced, partly because, through her own revengeful feelings, they had turned into persecuting figures.

In the dream there was only a slight hint of Mrs. A.'s growing unconscious knowledge (indicating that the denial was lessening) that it was she *herself* who lost her son. On the day preceding the dream she was wearing a black dress with a white collar. The woman in the dream had something white round her neck on her black dress.

Two nights after this dream she dreamt again: *She was flying with her son, and he disappeared. She felt that this meant his death—that he was drowned. She felt as if she, too, were to be drowned—but then she made an effort and drew away from the danger, back to life.*

The associations showed that in the dream she had decided that she would not die with her son, but would survive. It appeared that even in the dream she felt that it was good to be alive and bad to be dead. In this dream the unconscious knowledge of her loss is much more accepted than in the one of two days earlier. Sorrow and guilt had drawn closer. The feeling of triumph had apparently gone, but it became clear that it had only diminished. It was still present in her satisfaction about remaining alive—in contrast to her son's being dead. The feelings of guilt which already made themselves felt were partly due to this element of triumph.

I am reminded here of a passage in Freud's "Mourning and Melancholia";[17] "Reality passes its verdict—that the object no longer exists—upon each single one of the memories and hopes through which the libido was attached to the lost object, and the ego, confronted as it were with the decision whether it will share this fate, is persuaded by the sum of its narcissistic satisfactions in being alive to sever its attachment to the non-existent object." In my view, this "narcissistic satisfaction" contains in a milder way the element of triumph which Freud seemed to think does not enter into normal mourning.

In the second week of her mourning Mrs. A. found some comfort in looking at nicely situated houses in the country, and in wishing to have such a house of her own. But this comfort was soon interrupted by bouts of despair and sorrow. She now cried abundantly, and found relief in tears. The solace she found in looking at houses came from her rebuilding her inner world in her phantasy by means of this interest and also getting satisfaction from the knowledge that other people's houses and good objects existed. Ultimately this stood for re-creating her good parents, internally and exter-nally, unifying them and making them happy and creative. In her mind she made reparation to her parents for having, in phantasy, killed their children, and by this she anticipated their wrath. Thus her fear that the death of her son was a punishment inflicted on her by retaliating parents lost in strength, and also the feeling that her son frustrated and punished her by his death was lessened. The diminution of hatred and fear all round allowed the sorrow itself to come out in full strength. Increase of distrust and fears had intensi-fied her feeling of being persecuted and mastered by her internal objects and strengthened her need to master them. All this had expressed itself by a hardening in her internal relationships and feelings—that is to say, in an increase in manic defences. (This was shown in the first dream.) If these again diminish through the strengthening of the subject's belief in good-ness—his own and others'—and fears decrease, the mourner is able to surrender to his own feelings, and to cry out his sorrow about the actual loss.

It seems that the process of projecting and ejecting which are closely connected with giving vent to feelings, are held up in certain stages of grief by an extensive manic control, and can again operate more freely when that control relaxes. Through tears, which in the unconscious mind are equated to excrement, the mourner not only expresses his feelings and thus eases ten-sion, but also expels his "bad" feelings and his "bad" objects, and this adds to the relief obtained through crying. This greater freedom in the inner world implies that the internalized objects, being less controlled by the ego, are also allowed more freedom: that these objects themselves are allowed, in particular, greater freedom of feeling. In the mourner's situation, the feelings of his internalized objects are also sorrowful. In his mind, they share his grief, in the same way as actual kind parents would. The poet tells us that "Nature mourns with the mourner." I believe that "Nature" in this connection represents the internal good mother. This experience of mutual sorrow and sympathy in internal relationships, however, is again bound up with external ones. As I have already stated, Mrs. A.'s greater trust in actual people and things and help received from the external world contributed to a relaxing of the manic control over her inner world. Thus introjection (as well as projection) could operate still more freely, more goodness and love could be taken in from without, and goodness and love increasingly experienced within. Mrs. A., who at an earlier stage of her mourning had to some extent felt that her loss was inflicted on her by revengeful parents, could now in phantasy experience the sympathy of these parents (dead long since), their desire to support and to help her. She felt that they also suffered a severe loss and shared her grief, as they would have done had they lived. In her internal world harshness and suspicion had diminished, and sorrow had increased. The tears which she shed were also to some extent the tears which her internal parents shed, and she also wanted to comfort them as they—in her phantasy—comforted her.

If greater security in the inner world is gradually regained, and feelings and inner objects are therefore allowed to come more to life again, re-creative processes can set in and hope return.

As we have seen, this change is due to certain movements in the two sets of feelings which make up the depressive position: persecution decreases and the pining for the lost loved object is experienced in full force. To put it in other words: hatred has receded and love is freed. It is inherent in the feeling of persecution that it is fed by hatred and at the same time feeds hatred. Furthermore, the feeling of being persecuted and watched by internal "bad" objects, with the consequent necessity for constantly watching them, leads to a kind of dependence which reinforces the manic defences. These defences, in so far as they are used predominantly against persecutory feelings (and not so much against the pining for the loved object), are of a very sadistic and forceful nature. When persecution diminishes, the hostile dependence on the object, together with hatred, also diminishes, and the manic defences relax. The pining for the lost loved object also implies dependence on it, but dependence of a kind which becomes an incentive to reparation and preservation of the object. It is creative because it is dominated by love, while the dependence based on persecution and hatred is sterile and destructive.

Thus, while grief is experienced to the full and despair at its height, the love for the object wells up and the mourner feels more strongly that life inside and outside will go on after all, and that the lost loved object can be preserved within. At this stage in mourning, suffering can become productive. We know that painful experiences of all kinds sometimes stimulate sublimations, or even bring out quite new gifts in some people, who may take to painting, writing or other productive activities under the stress of frustrations and hardships. Others become more productive in a different way—more capable of appreciating people and things, more tolerant in their relation to others—they become wiser. Such enrichment is in my view gained through processes similar to those steps in mourning which we have just investigated. That is to say, any pain caused by unhappy experiences, whatever their nature, has something in common with mourning. It reactivates the infantile depressive position, and encountering and overcoming adversity of any kind entails mental work similar to mourning.

It seems that every advance in the process of mourning results in a deepening in the individual's relation to his inner objects, in the happiness of regaining them after they were felt to be lost. ("Paradise Lost and Regained"), in an increased trust in them and love for them because they proved to be good and helpful after all. This is similar to the ways in which the young child step by step builds up his relations to external objects, for he gains trust not only from pleasant experiences, but also from the ways in which he overcomes frustrations and unpleasant experiences, nevertheless retaining his good objects (externally and internally). The phases in the work of mourning when manic defences relax and a renewal of life inside sets in, with a deepening in internal relationships, are comparable to the steps which in early development lead to greater independence from external as well as internal objects.

To return to Mrs. A. Her relief in looking at pleasant houses was due to the setting in of some hope that she could re-create her son as well as her parents; life started again inside herself and in the outer world. At this time she could dream again and unconsciously begin to face her loss. She now felt a stronger wish to see friends again, but only one at a time and only for a short while. These feelings of greater comfort, however, again alternated with distress. (In mourning as well as in infantile development, inner security comes about not by a straightforward movement but in waves.) After a few weeks of mourning, for instance, Mrs. A. went for a walk with a friend through the familiar streets, in an attempt to re-establish old bonds. She suddenly realized that the number of people in the street seemed overwhelming, the houses strange and the sunshine artificial and unreal. She had to retreat into a quiet restaurant. But there she felt as if the ceiling were coming down, and the people in the place became vague and blurred. Her own house suddenly seemed the only secure place in the world. In analysis it became clear that the frightening indifference of these people was reflected from her internal objects, who in her mind had turned into a multitude of "bad" persecuting objects. The external world was felt to be artificial and unreal, because real trust in inner goodness had gone.

Many mourners can only make slow steps in re-establishing the bonds with the external world because they are struggling against the chaos inside; for similar reasons the baby develops his trust in the object-world first in connection with a few loved people. No doubt other factors as well, e.g. his intellectual immaturity, are partly responsible for this gradual development in the baby's object relations, but I hold that this also is due to the chaotic state of his inner world.

One of the differences between the early depressive position and normal mourning is that when the baby loses the breast or bottle, which has come to represent to him a "good" helpful, protective object inside him, and experiences grief, he does this in spite of his mother being there. With the grown-up person however the grief is brought about by the actual loss of an actual person; yet help comes to him against this overwhelming loss through his having established in his early life his "good" mother inside himself. The young child, however, is at the height of his struggles with fears of losing her internally and externally, for he has not yet succeeded in establishing her securely inside himself. In this struggle, the child's relation to his mother, her actual presence, is of the greatest help. Similarly, if the mourner has people whom he loves and who share his grief, and if he can accept their sympathy, the restoration of the harmony in his inner world is promoted, and his fears and distress are more quickly reduced.

Having described some of the processes which I have observed at work in mourning and in depressive states, I wish now to link up my contribution with the work of Freud and Abraham.

Following Freud's and his own discoveries about the nature of the archaic processes at work in melancholia, Abraham found that such processes also operate in the work of normal mourning. He concluded that in this work the individual succeeds in establishing the lost loved person in his ego, while the melancholic has failed to do so. Abraham also described some of the fundamental factors upon which that success or failure depends.

My experience leads me to conclude that, while it is true that the characteristic feature of normal mourning is the individual's setting up the lost loved object inside himself, he is not doing so for the first time but, through the work of mourning, is reinstating that object as well as all his loved *internal* objects which he feels he has lost. He is therefore *recovering* what he had already attained in childhood.

In the course of his early development, as we know, he establishes his parents within his ego. (It was the understanding of the processes of introjection in melancholia and in normal mourning which, as we know, led Freud to recognize the existence of the super-ego in normal development.) But, as regards the nature of the super-ego and the history of its individual development, my conclusions differ from those of Freud. As I have often pointed out, the processes of introjection and projection from the beginning of life lead to the institution inside ourselves of loved and hated objects, who are felt to be "good" and "bad," and who are interrelated with each other and with the self: that is to say, they constitute an inner world. This assembly of internalized objects becomes organized, together with the organization of the ego, and in the higher strata of the mind it becomes discernible as the super-ego. Thus, the phenomenon which was recognized by Freud, broadly speaking, as the voices and the influence of the actual parents established in the ego is, according to my findings, a complex object-world, which is felt by the individual, in deep layers of the unconscious, to be concretely inside himself, and for which I and some of my colleagues therefore use the term "internalized," or an internal (inner) world. This inner world consists of innumerable objects taken into the ego, corresponding partly to the multitude of varying aspects, good and bad, in which the parents (and other people) appeared to the child's unconscious mind throughout various stages of his development. Further, they also represent all the real people who are continually becoming internalized in a variety of situations provided by the multitude of ever-changing external experiences as well as phantasied ones. In addition, all these objects are in the inner world in an infinitely complex relation both with each other and with the self.

If I now apply this conception of the super-ego organization as compared with Freud's super-ego to the process of mourning, the nature of my contribution to the understanding of this process becomes clear. In normal mourning the individual re-introjects and reinstates, as well as the actual lost person, his loved parents—who are felt to be his "good" inner objects. His inner world, the one which he has built up from his earliest days onwards, in his phantasy was destroyed when the actual loss occurred. The rebuilding of this inner world characterizes the successful work of mourning.

An understanding of this complex inner world enables the analyst to find and resolve a variety of early anxiety-situations which were formerly unknown, and is therefore theoretically and therapeutically of an importance so great that it cannot yet be fully estimated. I believe that the problem of mourning also can only be more fully understood by taking account of these early anxiety situations.

I shall now illustrate in connection with mourning one of these anxiety-situations which I have found to be of crucial importance also in manic-depressive states. I refer to the anxiety about the internalized parents in destructive sexual intercourse; they as well as the self are felt to be in constant danger of violent destruction. In the following material I shall give extracts from a few dreams of a patient, D., a man in his early forties, with strong paranoid and depressive traits. I am not going into details about the case as a whole: but am here concerned only to show the ways in which these particular fears and phantasies were stirred in this patient by the death of his mother. She had been in failing health for some time, and was, at the time to which I refer, more or less unconscious.

One day in analysis, D. spoke of his mother with hatred and bitterness, accusing her of having made his father unhappy. He also referred to a case of suicide and one of madness which had occurred in his mother's family. His mother, he said, had been "muddled" for some time. Twice he applied the term "muddled" to himself and then said: "I know you are going to drive me mad and then lock me up." He spoke about an animal being locked up in a cage. I interpreted that his mad relative and his muddled mother were now felt to be inside himself, and that the fear of being locked up in a cage partly implied his deeper fear of containing these mad people inside himself and thus of going mad himself. He then told me a dream of the previous night: *He saw a bull lying in a farmyard. It was not quite dead, and looked very uncanny and dangerous. He was standing on one side of the bull, his mother on the other. He escaped into a house, feeling that he was leaving his mother behind in danger and that he should not do so; but he vaguely hoped that she would get away.*

To his own astonishment, my patient's first association to the dream was of the blackbirds which had disturbed him very much by waking him up that morning. He then spoke of buffaloes in America, the country where he was born. He had always been interested in them and attracted by them when he saw them. He now said that one could shoot them and use them for food, but that they are dying out and should be preserved. Then he mentioned the story of a man who had been kept lying on the ground, with a bull standing over him for hours, unable to move for fear of being crushed. There was also an association about an actual bull on a friend's farm; he had lately seen this bull, and he said it looked ghastly. This farm had associations for him by which it stood for his own home. He had spent most of his childhood on a large farm his father owned. In between, there were associations about flower seeds spreading from the country and taking root in town gardens. D. saw the owner of this farm again the same evening and urgently advised him to keep the bull under control. (D. had learnt that the bull had recently damaged some buildings on the farm.) Later that evening he received the news of his mother's death.

In the following hour, D. did not at first mention his mother's death, but expressed his hatred of me—my treatment was going to kill him. I then reminded him of the dream of the bull, interpreting that in his mind his mother had become mixed up with the attacking bull father—half dead himself—and had become uncanny and dangerous. I myself and the treatment were at the moment standing for this combined parent-figure. I pointed out that the recent increase of hatred against his mother was a defence against his sorrow and despair about her approaching death. I referred to his aggressive phantasies by which, in his mind, he had changed his father into a dangerous bull which would destroy his mother; hence his feeling of responsibility and guilt about this impending disaster. I also referred to the patient's remark about eating buffaloes, and explained that he had incorporated the combined parent-figure and so felt afraid of being crushed internally by the bull. Former material had shown his fear of being controlled and attacked internally by dangerous beings, fears which had resulted among other things in his taking up at times a very rigid and immobile posture. His story of the man who was in danger of being crushed by the bull, and who was kept immobile and controlled by it, I interpreted as a representation of the dangers by which he felt threatened internally.[18]

I now showed the patient the sexual implications of the bull's attacking his mother, connecting this with his exasperation about the birds waking him that morning (this being his first association to the bull dream). I reminded him that in his association birds often stood for people, and that the noise the birds made—a noise to which he was quite accustomed—represented to him the dangerous sexual intercourse of his parents, and was so unendurable on this particular morning because of the bull dream, and owing to his acute state of anxiety about his dying mother. Thus his mother's death meant to him her being destroyed by the bull inside him, since—the work of mourning having already started—he had internalized her in this most dangerous situation.

I also pointed out some hopeful aspects of the dream. His mother might save herself from the bull. Blackbirds and other birds he is actually fond of. I showed him also the tendencies to reparation and re-creation present in the material. His father (the buffaloes) should be preserved, i.e. protected against his—the patient's—own greed. I reminded him, among other things, of the seeds which he wanted to spread from the country he loved to the town, and which stood for new babies being created by him and by his father as a reparation to his mother—these live babies being also a means of keeping her alive.

It was only after this interpretation that he was actually able to tell me that his mother had died the night before. He then admitted, which was unusual for him, his full understanding of the internalization processes which I had interpreted to him. He said that after he had received the news of his mother's death he felt sick, and that he thought, even at the time, that there could be no physical reason for this. It now seemed to him to confirm my interpretation that he had internalized the whole imagined situation of his fighting and dying parents.

During this hour he had shown great hatred, anxiety and tension, but scarcely any sorrow; towards the end, however, after my interpretation, his feelings softened, some sadness appeared, and he experienced some relief.

The night after his mother's funeral, D. dreamt that X. (a father figure) and another person (who stood for me) were trying to help him, but actually he had to fight for his life against us; as he put it: "Death was claiming me." In this hour he again spoke bitterly about his analysis, as disintegrating him. I interpreted that he felt the helpful external parents to be at the same time the fighting, disintegrating parents, who would attack and destroy him—the half-dead bull and the dying mother inside him—and that I myself and analysis had come to stand for the dangerous people and happenings inside himself. That his father was also internalized by him as dying or dead was confirmed when he told me that at his mother's funeral he had wondered for a moment whether his father also was not dead. (In reality the father was still alive.)

Towards the end of this hour, after a decrease of hatred and anxiety, he again became more co-operative. He mentioned that the day before, looking out of the window of his father's house into the garden and feeling lonely, he disliked a jay he saw on a bush. He thought that this nasty and destructive bird might possibly interfere with another bird's nest with eggs in it. Then he associated that he had seen, some time previously, bunches of wild flowers thrown on the ground—probably picked and thrown away by children. I again interpreted his hatred and bitterness as being in part a defence against sorrow, loneliness and guilt. The destructive bird, the destructive children— as often before—stood for himself, who had, in his mind, destroyed his parents' home and happiness and killed his mother by destroying her babies inside her. In this connection his feelings of guilt related to his *direct* attacks in phantasy on his mother's body; whilst in connection with the bull dream the guilt was derived from his *indirect* attacks on her, when he changed his father into a dangerous bull who was thus carrying into effect his—the patient's—own sadistic wishes.

On the third night after his mother's funeral, D. had another dream:

He saw a 'bus coming towards him in an uncontrolled way—apparently driving itself. It went towards a shed. He could not see what happened to the shed, but knew definitely that the shed "was going to blazes." Then two people, coming from behind him, were opening the roof of the shed and looking into it. D. did not "see the point of their doing this," but they seemed to think it would help.

Besides showing his fear of being castrated by his father through a homosexual act which he at the same time desired, this dream expressed the same internal situation as the bull dream—the death of his mother inside him and his own death. The shed stood for his mother's body, for himself, and also for his mother inside him. The dangerous sexual intercourse represented by the 'bus destroying the shed happened in his mind to his mother as well as to himself; but in addition, and that is where the predominant anxiety lay, to his mother inside him.

His not being able to see what happened in the dream indicated that in his mind the catastrophe was happening internally. He also knew, without seeing it, that the shed was "going to blazes." The 'bus "coming towards him," besides standing for sexual intercourse and castration by his father, also meant "happening inside him." [19]

The two people opening the roof from behind (he had pointed to my chair) were himself and myself, looking into his inside and into his mind (psychoanalysis). The two people also meant myself as the "bad" combined parent-figure, myself containing the dangerous father—hence his doubts whether looking into the shed (analysis) could help him. The uncontrolled 'bus represented also himself in dangerous sexual intercourse with his mother, and expressed his fears and guilt about the badness of his own genitals. Before his mother's death, at a time when her fatal illness had already begun, he accidentally ran his car into a post—without serious consequences. It appeared that this was an unconscious suicidal attempt, meant to destroy the internal "bad" parents. This accident also represented his parents in dangerous sexual intercourse inside him, and was thus an acting out as well as an externalization of an internal disaster.

The phantasy of the parents combined in "bad" intercourse—or rather, the accumulation of emotions of various kinds, desires, fears and guilt, which go with it—had very much disturbed his relation to both parents, and had played an important part not only in his illness but in his whole development. Through the analysis of these emotions referring to the actual parents in sexual intercourse, and particularly through the analysis of these internalized situations, the patient became able to experience real mourning for his mother. All his life, however, he had warded off the depression and sorrow about losing her, which were derived from his infantile depressive feelings, and had denied his very great love for her. In his mind he had reinforced his hatred and feelings of persecution, because he could not bear the fear of losing his loved mother. When his anxieties about his own destructiveness decreased and confidence in his power to restore and preserve her became strengthened, persecution lessened and love for her came gradually to the fore. But together with this he increasingly experienced the grief and longing for her which he had repressed and denied from his early days onward. While he was going through this mourning with sorrow and despair, his deeply buried love for his mother came more and more into the open, and his relation to both parents altered. On one occasion he spoke of them, in connection with a pleasant childhood memory, as "my dear old parents"— a new departure in him.

I have described here and in my former paper the deeper reasons for the individual's incapacity to overcome successfully the infantile depressive position. Failure to do so may result in depressive illness, mania or paranoia. I pointed out (*op. cit.*) one or two other methods by which the ego attempts to escape from the sufferings connected with the depressive position, namely either the flight to internal good objects (which may lead to severe psychosis) or the flight to external good objects (with the possible outcome of neurosis). There are, however, many ways, based on obsessional, manic and paranoid defences, varying from individual to individual in their relative proportion, which in my experience all serve the same purpose, that is, to enable the individual to escape from the sufferings connected with the depressive position. (All these methods, as I have pointed out, have a part in normal development also.) This can be clearly observed in the analyses of people who fail to experience mourning. Feeling incapable of saving and securely reinstating their loved objects inside themselves, they must turn away from them more than hitherto and therefore deny their love for them. This may mean that their emotions in general become more inhibited; in other cases it is mainly feelings of love which become stifled and hatred is increased. At the same time, the ego uses various ways of dealing with paranoid fears (which will be the stronger the more hatred is reinforced). For instance, the internal ''bad'' objects are manically subjugated, immobilized and at the same time denied, as well as strongly projected into the external world. Some people who fail to experience mourning may escape from an outbreak of manic-depressive illness or paranoia only by a severe restriction of their emotional life which impoverishes their whole personality.

Whether some measure of mental balance can be maintained in people of this type often depends on the ways in which these various methods interact, and on their capacity to keep alive in other directions some of the love which they deny to their lost objects. Relations to people who do not in their minds come too close to the lost object, and interest in things and activities, may absorb some of this love which belonged to the lost object. Though these relations and sublimations will have some manic and paranoid qualities, they may nevertheless offer some reassurance and relief from guilt, for through them the lost loved object which has been rejected and thus again destroyed is to some extent restored and retained in the unconscious mind.

If, in our patients, analysis diminishes the anxieties of destructive and persecuting internal parents, it follows that hate and thus in turn anxieties decrease, and the patients are enabled to revise their relation to their parents—whether they be dead or alive—and to rehabilitate them to some extent even if they have grounds for actual grievances. This greater tolerance makes it possible for them to set up ''good'' parent-figures more securely in their minds, alongside the ''bad'' internal objects, or rather to mitigate the fear of these "bad" objects by the trust in "good" objects. This means enabling them to experience emotions—sorrow, guilt and grief, as well as love and trust—to go through mourning, but to overcome it, and ultimately to overcome the infantile depressive position, which they have failed to do in childhood.

To conclude. In normal mourning, as well in abnormal mourning and in manic-depressive states, the infantile depressive position is reactivated. The complex feelings, phantasies and anxieties included under this term are of a nature which justifies my contention that the child in his early development goes through a transitory manic-depressive state as well as a state of mourning, which become modified by the infantile neurosis. With the passing of the infantile neurosis, the infantile depressive position is overcome.

The fundamental difference between normal mourning, on the one hand, and abnormal mourning and manic-depressive states, on the other, is this. The manic-depressive and the person who fails in the work of mourning, though their defences may differ widely from each other have this in common, that they have been unable in early childhood to establish their internal "good" objects and to feel secure in their inner world. They have never really overcome the infantile depressive position. In normal mourning, however, the early depressive position, which had become revived through the loss of the loved object, becomes modified again, and is overcome by methods similar to those used by the ego in childhood. The individual is reinstating his actually lost loved object; but he is also at the same time re-establishing inside himself his first loved objects—ultimately the "good" parents—whom, when the actual loss occurred, he felt in danger of losing as well. It is by reinstating inside himself the "good" parents as well as the recently lost person, and by rebuilding his inner world, which was disintegrated and in danger, that he overcomes his grief, regains security, and achieves true harmony and peace.

NOTES

1. *Collected Papers*, Vol. IV, p. 163.
2. *Ibid.*, p. 154.
3. *Ibid.*, p. 166.
4. *International Journal of Psycho-Analysis*, Vol. XVI, 1935. The present paper is a continuation of that paper, and much of what I have now to say will of necessity assume the conclusions I arrived at there.

5. Here I can only refer in passing to the great impetus which these anxieties afford to the development of interests and sublimations of all kinds. If these anxieties are over-strong, they may interfere with or even check intellectual development. (*Cf.* Klein, "A Contribution to the Theory of Intellectual Inhibition," *International Journal of Psycho-Analysis,* Vol. XII, 1931.)

6. *The Psycho-Analysis of Children,* 1932; in particular, Chapter VIII.

7. In the same book (p. 149), referring to my view that every child passes through a neurosis differing only in degree from one individual to another, I added: "This view, which I have maintained for a number of years now, has lately received valuable support. In his book, *Die Frage der Laienanalyse* (1926), Freud writes: 'Since we have learnt to see more clearly we are almost inclined to say that the occurrence of a neurosis in childhood is not the exception but the rule. It seems as though it is a thing that cannot be avoided in the course of development from the infantile disposition to the social life of the adult.' (S. 61)."

8. At every juncture the child's feelings, fears and defenses are linked up with his libidinal wishes and fixations, and the outcome of his sexual development in childhood is always interdependent with the processes I am describing in this paper. I think that new light will be thrown on the child's libidinal development if we consider it in connection with the depressive position and the defences used against that position. It is, however, a subject of such importance that it needs to be dealt with fully, and is therefore beyond the scope of this paper.

9. "A Contribution to the Psychogenesis of Manic-Depressive States," *International Journal of Psycho-Analysis,* Vol. XVI, 1935.

10. I have pointed out in various connections (first of all in "The Early Stages of the Oedipus Complex," *International Journal of Psycho-Analysis,* Vol. IX, 1928) that the fear of phantastically "bad" persecutors and the belief in phantastically "good" objects are bound up with each other. Idealization is an essential process in the young child's mind, since he cannot yet cope in any other way with his fears of persecution (a result of his own hatred). Not until early anxieties have been sufficiently relieved owing to experiences which increase love and trust, is it possible to establish the all-important process of bringing together more closely the various aspects of objects (external, internal, "good" and "bad," loved and hated), and thus for hatred to become actually mitigated by love—which means a decrease of ambivalence. While the separation of these contrasting *aspects*—felt in the unconscious as contrasting *objects*—operates strongly, feelings of hatred and love are also so much divorced from each other that love cannot mitigate hatred.

   The flight to the internalized "good" object, which Melitta Schmideberg (in "Psychotic Mechanisms in Cultural Development," *International Journal of Psycho-Analysis,* Vol. XI, 1930) has found to be a fundamental mechanism in schizophrenia, thus also enters into the process of idealization which the young child normally resorts to in his depressive anxieties. Schmideberg has also repeatedly drawn attention to the connections between idealization and distrust of the object.

11. "A Contribution to the Psychogenesis of Manic-Depressive States," pp. 172–3.

12. *The Psycho-Analysis of Children,* pp. 170 and 278.

13. *Ibid.,* Chapter IX.

14. These facts I think go some way towards answering Freud's question which I have quoted at the beginning of this paper: "Why this process of carrying out the behest of reality bit by bit, which is in the nature of a compromise, should be so extraordinarily painful is not at all easy to explain in terms of mental economics. It is worth noting that this pain seems natural to us."

15. "Mourning and Melancholia," *Collected Papers,* Vol. IV, p. 166.

16. Abraham writes of a situation of this kind: 'We have only to reverse [Freud's] statement that 'the shadow of the lost love-object falls upon the ego' and say that in this case it was not the shadow but the bright radiance of his loved mother which was shed upon her son.'' (*Selected Papers*, p. 442.)

17. *Collected Papers*, Vol. IV, p. 166.

18. I have often found that processes which the patient unconsciously feels are going on inside him are represented as something happening on top of or closely round him. By means of the well-known principle of representation by the contrary, an external happening can stand for an internal one. Whether the emphasis lies on the internal or the external situation becomes clear from the whole context—from the details of associations and the nature and intensity of affects. For instance, certain manifestations of very acute anxiety and the specific defence mechanisms against this anxiety (particularly an increase in denial of psychic reality) indicate that an internal situation predominates at the time.

19. An attack on the outside of the body often stands for one which is felt to happen internally. I have already pointed out that something represented as being on top of or tightly round the body often covers the deeper meaning of being inside.

Introductory Notes to Chapter 10

Rita V. Frankiel

In this important paper, Loewald explores the relation between separation, loss, and the development of psychic structure. Internalization is his focus, and he illuminates the way that love objects lost through separation and death and those from whom disengagement must be effected (as in the transformation of passionate oedipal attachments into elements in the superego) are ultimately represented in some significant form in either the ego or the superego. Following Freud, he views the superego as a product of internalization, which is set in motion by separation and loss and the normal mourning that can follow when events are favorable. A parallel is drawn between processes set in motion during the planned termination of analysis and other losses that lead to mourning with internalization as a consequence. Loewald relates his thinking to Freud's not fully developed thoughts on internalization; in his view, transference analysis fosters the patient's seeking for improved substitutes for lost infantile love objects; it aims the patient toward resolutions based on finally relinquishing infantile loves and the unending search for them in adult life. The complexity of termination of analysis in this context is considered. He makes the point that emancipation must be distinguished from rebellion as a means of separation from external objects since rebellion maintains the external tie to the object while emancipation maintains the tie via a relation to an internal object.

This paper supplies a link between the literature on processes of mourning and the literature on termination of psychoanalysis, in which it should have a significant place. (See Parkin [1981] in this connection.)

10. Internalization, Separation, Mourning, and the Superego

Hans W. Loewald

In this paper I shall speak of the superego as a product of internalization, and of internalization in its relations to separation, loss, and mourning. A brief consideration of some aspects of the termination of an analysis will be presented in this context. I shall describe some of the differences and similarities between ego identifications and superego identifications and shall introduce the concept of degrees of internalization, suggesting that the introjects constituting the superego are more on the periphery of the ego system but are capable of mobility within this system and may thus merge into the ego proper and lose their superego character. The proposition will be presented that the superego, an enduring structure whose elements may change, has important relations to the internal representation of the temporal mode future.

As an introduction to the subject it may be useful to recall that for Freud the superego is the heir of the oedipus complex. Introjections and identifications preceding the oedipal phase and preparing the way for its development go into the formation of the ego proper. The origins of the superego are to be found also, according to Freud, in those early identifications which he calls immediate and direct and which are not the outcome of relinquished object cathexes. But the identifications which constitute the superego proper are the outcome of a relinquishment of oedipal objects; they are relinquished as external objects, even as fantasy objects, and are set up in the ego, by which process they become internal objects cathected by the id— a narcissistic cathexis. This is a process of desexualization in which an internal relationship is substituted for an external one.

Thus we can distinguish two types or stages of identification: those that precede, and are the basis for, object cathexes and those that are the outcome of object cathexes formed in the oedipal phase. The latter constitute the

Reprinted by permission of the author and *The Psychoanalytic Quarterly* 31 (1962):483–504.

precipitate in the ego which Freud calls the superego; the former constitute the forerunners, the origins of the superego, but are, considered in themselves, constituent elements of the ego proper. I think it is correct to say that the early (''ego-'') identifications take place during stages of development when inside and outside—ego and objects—are not clearly differentiated, which is to say that the stage where ''objects'' can be ''cathected'' is not yet reached or that a temporary regression from this stage has taken place. The later type of identifications with differentiated objects of libidinal and aggressive cathexis—objects which themselves cathect in such way. The later identifications thus can be based on the relinquishment of these objects. In actuality, of course, there is a continuum of stages between these two types and much overlapping and intermingling of them.

I

The relinquishment of external objects and their internalization involves a process of separation, of loss and restitution in many ways similar to mourning. During analysis, problems of separation and mourning come to the fore in a specific way at times of interruption and most particularly in the terminal phases of treatment. In fact, the end-phase of an analysis may be described as a long-drawn-out leave-taking—too long-drawn-out, it often seems, from the point of view of ordinary life. In everyday life, many of us tend to cut short a farewell, perhaps in order to diminish the embarrassment, the ambiguity, and pain, even though we may be torn between the grief of separation and the eager anticipation of the future awaiting us. Others seem to wish to prolong the farewell; yet it is not the farewell they want too prolong but the presence of the beloved person so as to postpone the leave-taking as long as possible. In both cases an attempt is made to deny loss: either we try to deny that the other person still exists or did exist, or we try to deny that we have to leave the beloved person and must venture out on our own. Either the past or the future is denied. At the death of a beloved person, either form of denial may occur internally as there is no possibility of realizing the denial by external action with the other person. In true mourning, the loss of the beloved person is perhaps temporarily denied but gradually is accepted and worked out by way of a complex inner process.

Analysis is not and should not be like ordinary life although it is a replica of it in certain essential features while it is fundamentally different in other respects. Compared with everyday life, the leave-taking of the end-phase of analysis is too long-drawn-out; compared with the leave-taking involved in the resolution of the oedipus complex, the terminal phase of an analysis is likely to be a considerably shortened and condensed leave-taking. One of the differences between analysis and ordinary life is that experiences purposefully and often painfully made explicit in analysis usually remain implicit in ordinary life; they are lifted onto a level and quality of awareness which they do not usually possess in ordinary life. To gain such awareness, inner distance and perspective are needed, and to acquire them time is needed which is not often available or used in such ways in the urgency of immediate life experiences.

If the experience of parting, of ending the relationship with another person (here the analyst) is felt explicitly, consciously, and in the hypercathected mode that is characteristic of analysis and is prompted by the analytic interpretation, then neither the existence of the person from whom we part nor the anticipated life without him can be denied. In the explicit experience of parting, the person from whom we take leave is becoming part of the past, and at the same time we move into the future which is to be without him. Neither past nor future are denied but are recognized and taken hold of in the present. The extended leave-taking of the end-phase of analysis is a replica of the process of mourning. The analyst who during the analysis has stood at times for mother, father, and other loved and hated figures of the patient's past is to be left. The internal relationships the patient had established with these loved and hated figures of the past have become partially external again during analysis. The internalizations by which the patient's character structure became established in earlier years have been partially undone in the analytic process and have been replaced by relationships with an external object—the analyst standing for various objects at different times. In other words, internalizations have been, to a degree, reversed; internal relationships constituting elements of the ego structure have been re-externalized.

Analysis, understood as the working out of the transference neurosis, changes the inner relationships which had constituted the patient's character by promoting the partial externalization of these internal relationships, thus making them available for recognition, exploration, and reintegration. By partial externalization, psychic structures in their inner organization are projected onto a plane of reality where they become three-dimensional, as it were. However, the analyst, as was the case with the original parental figures, is only a temporary external object in important respects. The relationship with the analyst, like that with parental figures in earlier ego development, has to become partially internalized—a process which to varying degrees goes on during all but the initial stages of analysis, but which is to come to its fruition and more definitive realization during the terminal phase. The pressure of the impending separation helps to accelerate this renewed internalization, although the process of internalization will continue and come to relative completion only after termination of the analysis.

The death of a love object, or the more or less permanent separation from a love object, is the occasion for mourning and for internalization. The unconscious and conscious experiences of threats to one's own existence as an individual, heightened by the increasing awareness of one's own eventual death, is, I believe, intimately connected with the phenomenon of internalization. It seems significant that with the advent of Christianity, initiating the greatest intensification of internalization in Western civilization, the death of God as incarnated in Christ moves into the center of religious experience. Christ is not only the ultimate love object which the believer loses as an external object and regains by identification with Him as an ego ideal, He is, in His passion and sacrificial death, the exemplification of complete internalization and sublimation of all earthly relationships and needs. But to pursue these thoughts would lead us far afield into unexplored psychological country.

Loss of a love object does not necessarily lead to mourning and internalization. The object lost by separation or death may not be mourned, but either the existence or the loss of the object may be denied. Such denial is the opposite of mourning. Instead of internalizing the relationship, external substitutions may be sought. One patient, for instance, used all available figures in the environment as substitutes for the lost parents, clinging forever to relatives and friends of his parents and from his own childhood, appealing to them, often successfully, for care and love. But he was unable to establish lasting new relationships and lasting and effective sublimations; his capacity for productive work was severely limited; his superego development was rudimentary. Both the ability to form lasting new external relationships and the capacity for stable sublimations appear to be based on, among other things, firmly established internalizations.

Another patient appeared to be the victim of his father's denial of the death of the father's beloved brother. The patient became the substitute for the brother and the father now clung to him with all the force of this never-relinquished attachment. The patient had great difficulty in emancipating himself from his father because of the guilt involved in severing this tie. Of course this was only one aspect of the patient's neurotic attachment to his father. For many complex reasons, a third patient denied the existence of his sister with whom he had had an early overt sexual relationship. This sister, now married, remained strongly attached to the patient while he denied the early relationship as well as any present feeling for her by complete condemnation of her and refusing to have anything to do with her. In the analysis he kept "forgetting" her existence, as well as the significance of the childhood relationship in his current life, despite its prominent evidence. For this patient the process of mourning was something to be avoided; for instance, even a temporary separation had to be abrupt and he would not let friends or relatives accompany him to the station if he were going away on a trip. When we began to think of termination of the analysis, he had a strong impulse to terminate practically from one day to the next, and insisted that after the analysis we would never meet again.

An analysis is itself a prime example of seeking a substitute for the lost love objects, and the analyst in the transference promotes such substitution. The goal, however, is to resolve the transference neurosis, a revival of the infantile neurosis. The failure to resolve the oedipus complex can be understood as a failure to achieve stable internalizations based on true relinquishment of the infantile incestuous object relations, leading to faulty superego formation. The resolution of the transference neurosis is thus intimately related to the achievement of true mourning by which relationships with external objects are set up in the ego system as internal relationships in a process of further ego differentiation. This is the reason why it is so important to work through the separation involved in the termination of analysis.

Ideally termination should culminate in or lead into a genuine relinquishment of the external object (the analyst) as an incestuous love object and, in the transformation of the external relationship, into an internal relationship within the ego-superego system. Such internalization does not necessarily imply that a relationship, once it becomes internal, cannot further develop as an internal relationship. To avoid misunderstanding I should like to stress again that a sharp distinction must be maintained between a relationship to fantasy objects and an internal relationship that is a constituent of ego structure.

II

It is time to consider more closely the problem of internalization and its relation to separation and mourning. I use the term "internalization" here as a general term for certain processes of transformation by which relationships and interactions between the individual psychic apparatus and its environment are changed into inner relationships and interactions within the psychic apparatus. Thus an inner world is constituted and it in turn entertains relationships and interactions with the outer world. The term "internalization" therefore covers such "mechanisms" as incorporation, introjection, and identification, or those referred to by the terms "internal object" and "internalized object," as well as such "vicissitudes of instincts" as the "turning inward" of libidinal and aggressive drives. The word "incorporation" most often seems to emphasize zonal, particularly oral, aspects of internalization processes. "Introjection" probably is the term that is most ambiguous. There are reasons to assume that internalization per se is only one element of at least certain kinds of identification and that projection plays an important part in them. The term "identification," in accordance with general psychoanalytic parlance, is used here in a somewhat loose fashion so as not to prejudge what might be implied in the concept.

The significance of separation has been of concern to psychoanalysis since its beginnings, and in many different contexts and ramifications. To name some at random: separation anxiety, castration fear, birth trauma, loss of the love object, loss of love, the implications of the oedipal situation (relinquishment of the libidinal object, incest barrier) mourning, depression, ego boundaries and early ego development (detachment from the environment), superego origins, oral aggression, frustration, and others beside. If one asks how human beings deal with the anxieties and frustrations of separation and loss, the answer may be either by external action designed to reduce or abolish the sense of separation and loss, or by an internal process meant to achieve the same end. Yet separation may be experienced not as deprivation and loss but as liberation and a sign of mastery. Separation from a love-hate object may be brought about by oneself in an attempt to effect emancipation from such objects, or it may be facilitated by others, even the love objects themselves; if it is not facilitated, or if it is prevented by others, the lack of separation may be experienced as deprivation. However, it seems that emancipation as a process of separation from external objects—to be distinguished from rebellion which maintains the external relationship—goes hand in hand with the work of internalization which reduces or abolishes the sense of external deprivation and loss. Whether separation from a love object is experienced as deprivation and loss or as emancipation and mastery will depend, in part, on the achievement of the work of internalization. Speaking in terms of affect, the road leads from depression through mourning to elation.

In the event of aggression and overwhelming intrusion and invasion from the outside, the need for separation may become imperative. Such a need may be satisfied by removal of the aggressor or of oneself. On the other hand, under such circumstances the need for union may become imperative ("identification with the aggressor"); through such union aggression is removed by a different means. As we explore these various modes of separation and union, it becomes more and more apparent that the ambivalence of love-hate and of aggression-submission (sadism-masochism) enters into all of them and that neither separation nor union can ever be entirely unambivalent. The deepest root of the ambivalence that appears to pervade all relationships, external as well as internal, seems to be the polarity inherent in individual existence of individualism and "primary narcissistic" union—a polarity which Freud attempted to conceptualize by various approaches but which he recognized and insisted upon from beginning to end by his dualistic conception of instincts, of human nature, and of life itself.

The relinquishment of oedipal love objects and the concomitant identifications are generally seen as being enforced by these very objects (castration threat, threat of loss of love, incest taboo). But if this development be a necessary evil, it is the kind of evil that is turned into a virtue in the course of human evolution. It is an example of the "change of function" which led Hartmann to the concept of the secondary autonomy of the ego.[1] As pointed out before, separation from love objects, while in one sense something to be overcome and undone through internalization, is, in so far as it means individuation and emancipation, a positive achievement brought about by the relinquishment and internalization of the love objects. The change of function taking place here is that a means of defense against the pain and anxiety of separation and loss becomes a goal in itself.

But can we be satisfied with the description of these internalizations as originating in defensive needs even though we grant that they are important elements in oedipal identifications? The oedipal identifications, constituting the elements of the superego, are new versions—promoted by new experiences of deprivation and loss—of identifications which precede the oedipal situation. The narcissistic cathexis, replacing object cathexis in internalization, is secondary and is founded on an older, "primary" narcissism of which it is a new version. The same appears to hold true not only for the libidinal but for the aggressive aspects of oedipal identifications. If we accept Freud's views on primary aggression, behind aggression turned inward, as manifested in phenomena of guilt and masochism, lies what Freud called "primary masochism" which, in terms of the aggressive drives, corresponds to primary narcissism. Without going into further details here, the conception is that in ontogenetic development a primitive stage of primary narcissism and primary aggression (death instinct) is followed by some process of externalization. Once such externalizations have occurred, reinternalizations may take place and sexual and aggressive drives may be turned inward. Yet they are not quite the same drives as they were before externalization; they have been qualified and differentiated by externalization, that is, by having become object-cathected. (Freud wrote: "The shadow of the object fell upon the ego.") Figuratively speaking, in the process of internalization the drives take aspects of the object with them into the ego. Neither drive nor object is the same as before, and the ego itself becomes further differentiated in the process. Internalization is structure building.

But we must go one step further. It has been recognized recently that we have to understand the stage of primary narcissism and primary aggression not as a stage where libido and aggression are still cathected in a primitive ego rather than in objects, but as a stage where inside and outside, an ego and an object-world, are as yet not distinguishable one from the other. To quote from a recent summary of views on early ego development, "no difference exists between the 'I' and the 'non-I' in the first weeks of life. The first traces of such distinction begin in the second month. This lack of boundaries is a prerequisite for both projection and introjection." [2] To ask whether externalization preceded internalization or vice versa becomes, in the light of this insight, meaningless. There are primary externalizations and internalizations, and there are secondary externalizations and internalizations. In the secondary externalization something that was internal becomes external, and in secondary internalization something that was external becomes internal. The meaning of the terms externalization and internalization, when we speak of the primary forms, is different: primary externalization signifies that *externality is being established;* primary internalization signifies that *internality is being constituted.* On this level, then, we cannot speak of externalization ("projection") and internalization as defenses (against inner conflict or external deprivation); we must speak of them as boundary-creating processes and as processes of differentiation of an undifferentiated state. It is true, nevertheless, that defenses against inner conflict and against outer deprivation promote and color such differentiation.

Hence the relinquishment and internalization of oedipal objects, while "enforced" by these objects in the oedipal situation, must at the same time be seen as a resumption on a new level of boundary-creating processes. Ego, objects, and boundaries of and between them—at first nonexistent, later still indistinct and fluid—gradually become more distinct and fixed, although by no means in an absolute or definitive fashion. Side by side with object relations, processes of identification persist and re-enter the picture in new transformations representing resumptions of boundary-setting, differentiating processes, notwithstanding their prominent aspects as defenses against loss of love objects.

Earlier I referred to the end-phase of an analysis as an extended leave-taking and as a replica of the process of mourning. Mourning involves not only the gradual, piecemeal relinquishment of the lost object, but also the internalization, the appropriation of aspects of this object—or rather, of aspects of the relationship between the ego and the lost object which are "set up in the ego" and become a relationship within the ego system. This process is similar to the relinquishment of the oedipal objects that leads to the formation of the superego. A relationship with an external libidinal-aggressive object is replaced by an internal relationship. In the work of mourning— a lost relationship, lost by death or actual separation—this change from object cathexis to narcissistic cathexis is a repetition, within certain limits, of the previous experience of the relinquishment of oedipal object relations and of their being set up in the ego. There is, of course, an important difference between the resolution of the oedipus complex and mourning in later life: in the oedipal situation the external objects not only remain present during the resolution of the conflict, but the fact that they remain present actively promotes the process of internalization. The parents remain present during this period but change their attitude; they promote a partial detachment, a decathexis of libidinal-aggressive drives from themselves as external objects so that an amount of such drive energy is freed for narcissistic recathexis. Moreover, some drive energy becomes available for eventual recathexis in nonincestuous external relationships: parents promote emancipation. Deca-thexis of drive energy from the incestuous object relations promotes, in varying proportions, both a narcissistic recathexis (internalization) and recathexis in external object relations, the new external object relations remain incestuous in character; without further differentiation of the inner world no further differentiation of the object world takes place. The latency period exemplifies, in its essentials, such a silent phase of internalization.

The promotion by the parents of partial decathexis from themselves as libidinal-aggressive objects, and of narcissistic recathexis (omitting in this context the recathexis in new object relations), is not merely in the interest of the child's development but represents a developmental change in the parents: they themselves achieve a partial decathexis of libidinal-aggressive drive energy from the child as *their* external object, leading to further internalizing processes in themselves and modifications of their own ego structures.[3] Such mutuality, to use Erikson's term, is essential for normal resolution of the oedipus complex and development of the superego.

If the resolution of the oedipus complex is a prototype of mourning, it is this prototype, achieved through the interaction between the objects involved in the oedipal situation, that enables the individual to mourn external objects in later life without the object's interacting help. The analytic situation re-embodies this interaction and the termination of analysis leads, if things go well, to a healthier resolution of the oedipus complex than the patient had been able to achieve before, and to a more stable superego. Patients at the termination of treatment frequently express a feeling of mutual abandonment which, if analyzed, becomes the pathway to the relinquishment of the analyst as an external object and to the internalization of the relationship. This is similar to the experience of emancipation in adolescence, which repeats the oedipal struggle on a higher level.

Internal and external relationships, of course, continue to supplement and influence each other in various ways during adult life; there are more or less continuous shifts and exchanges between internal and external relationships. Freud first alluded to them in his paper "On Narcissism."

III

"Ideal ego" and "ego ideal" were the first names Freud gave to the "differentiating grade in the ego" which he later called the superego. The ideal ego, by identification with the parental figures—perceived as omnipotent—represents, in Freud's view, a recapturing of the original, primary narcissistic, omnipotent perfection of the child himself. It represents an attempt to return to the early infantile feeling of narcissistic sufficiency, so rudely disillusioned by the inevitable frustrations and deprivations inherent in the conditions of extrauterine existence. This presumed omnipotent sufficiency appears to be maintained, for a time, by the close "symbiotic" relationship with the mother, and is gradually replaced by reliance on the seeming parental omnipotence. The ideal ego, in contrast to the child's frequent experience of an impotent, helpless ego, is then a return, in fantasy, to the original state; it is an ego replenished, restored to the wholeness of the undifferentiated state of primary narcissistic union and identity with the environment, by identification with the all-powerful parents. The process could be described—naively yet perhaps quite aptly—as one whereby the child reaches out to take back from the environment what has been removed from him in an ever-increasing degree since his birth: identification that attempts to re-establish an original identity with the environment. This identity of the past, at first "hallucinated" by the child in the manner of hallucinatory wish fulfilment, gradually becomes something to be reached for, wished for in the future. Representatives of such a future state of being are parents, perhaps siblings, and later other "ideals."

If the ideal ego represents something like a hallucinated or fantasied state of perfection, the term "ego ideal" indicates more clearly that this state of narcissistic perfection is something to be reached for. In so far as this wholeness is the original state of the infant in his psychic identity with the environment, and in so far as (from the point of view of the disillusioned observer) the parental environment is far from such a state of omnipotent wholeness and perfection, we must describe the identifications just mentioned as containing an element of projection. Undoubtedly such infantile projections evoke responses in the parent which in turn help to shape the child's developing conception of ideals, just as in general the parents' responses to his needs, demands, and expectations contribute to the character of his idealizations. But the child's ideals are also shaped by the parents' own projections, by *their* idealizations of the child, and by their demands, expectations, and needs in respect to the child. In a sense, both the child and the parents can be said to have fantasies—some would say illusions—about the other's state of perfection and wholeness, or at least about the other's perfectibility.

But let us not scoff at such fantasies. The demands and expectations engendered by them are essential for the development and maintenance of a sound superego in the object of such expectations—provided that the expectations are allowed to be continuously shaped and tempered by an increasing realistic appraisal of the stage of maturity and of the potentialities of the object. The inevitable elements of disillusionment are no less important for superego development in the one so disillusioned, for it is such disillusionment that under reasonably favorable circumstances (if frustration is not overwhelming) contributes to the internalization of expectations and demands. Regarding the child, then, parental projective fantasies of the child's narcissistic perfection and wholeness, as well as infantile projective fantasies of the parent's omnipotent perfection, have an important bearing on the development of his superego. Such fantasies, based on old longings in all concerned, in normal development are gradually being cleared and modified in accordance with a more realistic comprehension of the potentialities and limitations of the object relation involved. The parents are to be the guides in this process of clearing and resolving which leads to a more rational mutual relationship externally, as well as to a reasonably balanced internal relationship within the ego-superego system in so far as the internalized demands lose their archaic insistence on narcissistic perfection.

The term "superego"—in accordance with Freud's view that the superego is the heir of the oedipus complex—is used after the distinction between ego and objects, and the distinction between heterosexual and homosexual objects, is relatively firmly established, and after boundaries of and between ego and objects, and limitations of the oedipal object relations, are acknowledged. (In the particular context of this paper, I can only allude to the paramount importance of the sexual differentiation of objects and of self for the superego problem and must leave further consideration of this issue for another occasion.) It is only then that an external and an internal world can be said to exist in the experience of the child and that ideals and demands are more definitely sorted out into external and internal. There are now external and internal authorities, with their demands, their love and hate, their images of what should be, their rewards and punishments. The superego is constituted of those authorities that are clearly internal and have become a "differentiating grade in the ego," thus being clearly differentiated from external love-hate authorities and ideal images.

Demands, expectations, hopes, and ideals change in the course of development. Some are reached and fulfilled and are no longer beckonings from a future; others are not. Some are given up, others remain as ideals and demands though never reached and fulfilled. New demands and ideals arise. Some are realized for a time but then are lost or become remote again. Clinical evidence, particularly clear in some psychotic and borderline states because of the fragility and transparency of the ego structure, indicates a mobility of so-called introjected objects within the ego system, suggesting shifting degrees of internalization and externalization which bring the introjects more or less close to the ego core. If we think in such terms as "degrees of internalization," of greater or lesser "distance from an ego core," it is of great importance to keep in mind that the modification of external material for introjection, brought about by internalization, varies with the degree of internalization. A comparison with physiological assimilation is suggested whereby organic compounds are ingested and subjected to catabolic and anabolic changes in the course of assimilation into the body substance. Underlying the concept of the superego as a differentiating grade in the ego is the idea of a distance from an ego core. Unless there is a degree of tension between this ego core and the superego, they are not distinguishable.

Let me give a simple example of progressive internalization and re-externalization, taken from precursory stages of superego development. Ferenczi spoke of sphincter morality, and there can be no doubt that the expectation of sphincter control becomes increasingly internalized as an expectation. But a point is reached where such control is established and no longer an external or internal demand which may or may not be realized; it becomes an automatic control which now can be said to be a rather primitive ego function. Since maturation must have advanced to a state where such expectations become feasible, it is obvious that a correspondence between external and internalized expectation, on the one hand, and internal potentiality, on the other hand, is very important. Sphincter control, under certain conditions of stress, may be lost temporarily, at which time it regains the quality of a demand. Or it may retain this quality unconsciously from early times; for instance, if the original parental expectation of it was not in tune with the maturational stage of the child—a lack of empathic interaction which interferes with internalization.

A second example is taken from the experience of mourning. The outcome of mourning can show something like a new intake of objects into the superego structure in so far as elements of the lost object, through the mourning process, become introjected in the form of ego-ideal elements and inner demands and punishments. Such internalization of aspects of a lost love object, if observed over long periods of time (we must think in terms of years in adults) may be found to be progressive, so that eventually what was an ego-ideal or superego element becomes an element of the ego proper and is realized as an ego trait rather than an internal demand. We see this, for instance, in a son who increasingly becomes like his father after the father's death. It is as though only then can he appropriate into his ego core given elements of his father's character. It would lead too far to give clinical examples from psychotic conditions, although shifts in degrees of internalization and externalization, because of the instability of the ego structure, are often particularly impressive here.[4]

The foregoing discussion leads to a conception of the superego as a structure, and enduring as a structure whose constituent elements may change.[5] Elements of it may become elements of the ego proper and may, under conditions of ego disorganization and reorganization, return, as it were, into the superego and even be further externalized.

During analysis we can observe the projection or externalization of superego elements onto the analyst. During the periods of psychic growth—in childhood as well as in adult life—the change of superego elements into ego elements is a continuing process, it seems. The superego itself, in its turn, receives new elements through interaction with the object world. The changing of superego elements into ego elements involves a further desexualization and deaggressivization; it involves a return, as in a spiral, to the type of identifications characterized as ego or primary identification—regaining a measure of narcissistic wholeness which inevitably, as in childhood, leads again to loss of such self-sufficiency by further involvement with others. The progressive differentiation and enrichment of the ego during life, to the extent to which it occurs, is a return in a new dimension to an identity of ego and objects, on the basis of which new reaches of the object world become accessible. The ripening of the personality in adult life, whether through analysis or other significant life experiences, is based on the widening and deepening relations that the enriched and more differentiated ego entertains with external reality, understood and penetrated in new dimensions.

Inner ideals, expectations, hopes, demands, and, equally, inner doubts, fears, guilt, despair concerning oneself—all this is reaching toward or feeling defeated by a future. The voice of conscience tells us what we should do or should have done, speaking from a future which we ask ourselves to reach or tell ourselves we are failing to reach—perhaps a future which should bring back a lost past, but certainly a future whose image in the course of development becomes imbued with all that is still alive from the hopes, expectations, demands, promises, ideals, aspirations, self-doubt, guilt, and despair of past ages, ancestors, parents, teachers, prophets, priests, gods, and heroes. Maturation and development, which are movements into a future, are promoted, defined, and channeled, or hindered and inhibited, by the hopes and expectations, fears, doubts, and demands, by the guidance and positive and negative examples given by parents and other authorities, depending on whether or not they are commensurate with the stage and speed of development and with the potentialities of the child, and depending on the superego development of the authorities themselves. Seen from the other side, parental expectations, fears, and hopes, the guidance and example-giving of authorities, their standards, prohibitions, and punishments for the child are promoted and channeled, or inhibited and frustrated, by the child's maturation and development which bring some new potentialities into the parents' view and limit and exclude others. The superego, inasmuch as it is the internal representative of parental and cultural standards, expectations, fears, and hopes, is the intrapsychic representation of the future. Only in so far as we are ahead of ourselves, in so far as we recognize potentialities in ourselves which represent *more* than we are at present, can we be said to have a conscience. The voice of conscience speaks to us as the mouthpiece of the superego, from the point of view of the inner future which we envision. One might say that in the voice of conscience the superego speaks to the ego as being capable or incapable of encompassing the superego as the inner future toward which to move.

As an aspect of the inner future of the ego becomes an inner actuality, this superego element merges into the ego as an element no longer differentiated from the ego. Guilt in respect to this element vanishes, as guilt is a form of tension between ego and superego. We have a sense of guilt concerning past or present thoughts, feelings, and deeds, but only inasmuch as they represent a nonfulfilment of the inner image of ourselves, of the internal ideal we have not reached, of the future in us that we have failed.

The greater or lesser distances from the ego core—the degrees of internalization of which I spoke—perhaps are best understood as temporal in nature, as relations between an inner present and an inner future. Such structuralization obviously is not spatial. Physical structures are in space and organized by spatial relations. It may be that we can advance our understanding of what we mean when we speak of psychic structures if we consider the possibility of their mode of organization as a temporal one, even though we do not as yet understand the nature of such organization. It might well be useful to explore further not only the superego in its relations to the temporal mode future, but also the time dimensions of id and ego and their relations to the temporal modes past and present.

SUMMARY

The formation of the superego, as the "heir of the oedipus complex," is considered in its relation to the phenomena of separating and mourning. Separation is described in its aspect as the occasion for processes of internalization, especially as it is related to mourning. The work of mourning is not confined to a gradual relinquishment of the lost object but also encompasses processes of internalizing elements of the relationship with the object to be relinquished. Such internalizations, in so far as they occur as part of the resolution of the oedipus complex, lead to further differentiation of the ego of which the superego is a "differentiating grade." Some illustrations of the psychological processes involved in separation are given and there is a brief discussion of the termination of analysis from this point of view.

Separation from love objects constitutes a loss and may be experienced as deprivation. But separation, in certain crucial events in human life, also has the significance of emancipation and lack of separation may be experienced as deprivation. It is suggested that the emancipation involved in the normal resolution of the oedipus complex, as well as in subsequent separations in which successful mourning takes place, can be understood in two ways: first, as an internal substitution for an externally severed object relationship (internal "restitution of the lost object"), and second, as as resumption of early boundary-setting processes by which a further differentiation and integration of the ego and of the object world on higher levels of development takes place. In other words, so-called superego identifications represent an undoing, so to speak, of separation in so far as object loss is concerned and they also represent the achievement of separation in so far as boundary-setting and further ego and object differentiation is concerned. The differences and similarities between so-called primary and secondary identifications, as well as between primary and secondary aggression, are briefly discussed from this point of view. It is pointed out that both internality and externality, an inner world and an outer world, are constituted by the primary forms of these processes and that their secondary forms, notwithstanding their defensive functions, continue to contribute to the further organization of an inner and an outer world.

Some concrete aspects of superego formation through the interaction between child and parents are briefly cited, and the duality or polarity of individuation and primary narcissistic identity with the environment is emphasized as a basic phenomenon of human development underlying the ambivalent significances of separation and of internalization.

The concept of degrees of internalization is advanced. This implies shifting distances of internalized "material" from the ego core and shifting distances within the ego-superego system, as well as transformations in the character of the introjects according to the respective degrees of internalization. The superego is conceived as an enduring structure pattern whose elements may change and move either in the direction of the ego core or in an outer direction toward object representation. Thus elements of the superego may lose their superego character and become ego elements, or take on the character of object representations (externalization). It is postulated that the superego has the temporal character of futurity inasmuch as the superego-ego ideal may be understood as the envisioned inner future of the ego. Conscience, as the voice of the superego, speaks to the ego from the point of view of the inner future toward which the ego reaches or which the ego has failed. It is suggested that the degrees of internalization, the distances from the ego-core, are temporal in nature, representing relations between an inner present and an inner future, although we but vaguely grasp the nature of such temporal structuralization.

NOTES

1. Hartmann, Heinz: *Ego Psychology and the Problem of Adaptation.* New York: International Universities Press, Inc., 1958, pp. 25–26. Certain aspects of internalization and of the all-important phenomenon of change of function in biology and mental life were seen clearly by Nietzsche. He used the term "internalization." *Cf.* his *The Genealogy of Morals* (1887). Garden City, New York: Doubleday Anchor Books, 1956.
2. Panel on *"Some Theoretical Aspects of Early Psychic Functioning,"* reported by David L. Rubinfine. *J. Amer. Psa. Assn.,* VII, 1959, p. 569.
3. Compare Benedek, Therese: *"Parenthood as a Developmental Phase." I. Amer. Psa. Assn.,* VII, 1959, pp. 389–417, and pertinent formulations in many of Erik Erikson's writings.
4. Cameron, Norman: *"Introjection, Reprojection, and Hallucination in the Interaction between Schizophrenic Patient and Therapist." Int. J. Psa.,* XLII, Parts 1–2, 1961.
5. See also Novey, Samuel: *"The Role of the Superego and Ego Ideal in Character Formation." Int. J. Psa.,* XXXVI, 1955. Here he speaks of the superego as a "functional pattern of introjection rather than as a fixed institution."

Introductory Notes to Chapter 11

Rita V. Frankiel

Pollock's numerous publications on mourning have spanned a thirty-year period. His recently published two-volume book on the subject (1989) reprints his most important contributions to this literature. There is hardly an aspect of the dynamics and symptomatology of object loss, mourning, and its potentially creative sequelae that Pollock has not written about. These contributions include numerous papers on clinical phenomena associated with grief and mourning—anniversary reactions in their vast diversity and meaning (1971), trauma as it relates to potential for recovery from bereavement (1970), homicide and suicide related to pathological mourning (1975a, 1975b), the lasting effects of the death of siblings and children (1962, 1978a, 1982). He has been especially interested in the way that phenomena of mourning are also present in times of transition—intrapsychic, interpersonal, and transcultural (1989).

In the paper included here, Pollock conceives the mourning process to be a response to an alteration in the outer world, the loss of a significant object. The mourning process is seen as an operation designed to restore ego equilibrium by adapting to the fact that the loss has actually occurred. Two phases are postulated—acute and chronic. Mammals and birds seem to go through a reaction similar to the acute phase in humans. In the course of developing his ideas and describing the course that mourning can take, Pollock describes anniversary reactions, the way that mourning can be perpetuated through a variety of enactments occurring on a timetable set by the unconscious of the mourner.

Pollock's work in applied analysis on creative products as the outcome of the resolution of a process of mourning in their creators is described in the section on creativity below.

11. Mourning and Adaptation

George H. Pollock

I. ADAPTATION

Claude Bernard (1813–1878), the French physiologist, was the first to advance the concept that animals exist in two environments: an external milieu in which the organism is actually situated, and an internal milieu in which the tissue elements are present. Although Bernard was concerned mainly with the physiological and biochemical aspects of the organism, he concluded that the "primary condition for freedom and independence of existence" was the constancy and stability of the internal milieu and the mechanisms that allowed this state to continue. Bernard felt that the organism had to be "so perfect that it can continually compensate for and counterbalance external variations." The equilibrium had to be constantly maintained and all vital mechanisms had "only one object: that of preserving constant the conditions of life in the milieu intérieur."

I am taking the liberty of extending Bernard's ideas to the psychological environment. Here too we find an external and an internal milieu. In both we find definite regulatory devices designed to deal with various alterations that may occur. Freud extensively studied the internal psychological milieu and advanced various theoretical constructs which allowed a conceptual framework to be formulated. As early as 1892, Freud alone and with Breuer proposed the idea of the constancy of excitation. When the nervous system had difficulty in dealing with increases in excitation through associative thinking or motor discharge, Freud and Breuer suggested that a "psychical trauma" occurred. In 1911, Freud advanced his understanding of psychological processes with his "Formulations on the Two Principles of Mental Functioning." Here he introduced two modes of constancy adaptations—the immediate energetic discharge or avoidance of the pleasure-pain principle,

Reprinted by permission of the author and *The International Journal of Psycho-Analysis* 42 (1961):341–61. Copyright © Institute of Psycho-Analysis.

and the capacity, oriented to external reality, for discharge delay of the reality principle. This later type of adaptation used mechanisms involving consciousness, attention, notation, and memory storage as well as decision-making with action to alter external reality and thought, as means of coping with new and potentially disrupting situations. In *Beyond the Pleasure Principle,* Freud once more emphasized the principle of constancy and its relationship to the mental apparatus. We can see that Freud's idea of the psychological constancy of the internal milieu paralleled Bernard's model of the physico-biochemical stability. In both the internal milieu was optimally maintained within a certain range. Less variation could occur here in contrast to the external milieu, and various defence mechanisms were necessary to maintain this constancy of the inside.

Walter Cannon (1871–1945) extended and elaborated this concept of stability by his principle of homeostasis, which emphasized the various biological processes tending to re-establish steady states of equilibrium and constancy when disturbing elements upset the state of balance. As biologists have continued their investigations, various optimal ranges for particular body processes have been discovered. With disease interferences, these ranges vary in accordance with the degree of impairment imposed upon the organism, as well as with the restitutive capacity operative within the organism.

Cannon envisioned the extension of his homeostasis idea to include "some general principles for the establishment, regulation, and control of steady states" which could be applicable to social and industrial organizations. He wrote that "perhaps a comparative study would show that every complex organization must have more or less effective self-righting adjustments in order to prevent a check on its functions or a rapid disintegration of its parts when it is subjected to stress."

Although Freud was aware of defensive manoeuvres utilized in psychological adaptation early in his work, it was in 1923 that he first presented us with the structural organization of the mental apparatus in *The Ego and the Id.* The ego's integrative role was elaborated and its relationship to the external millieu (reality) as well as to the psychic internal milieu explained. In 1936, Anna Freud (17) developed in further detail the protective and sustaining aspects of the ego's function. In 1937, Hartmann's classic essay on *Ego Psychology and the Problem of Adaptation* first appeared. These last two contributions focused the direction of later psycho-analytic developments and investigations upon ego activities.

It was Cannon who noted that "the perfection of the process of holding a stable state in spite of extensive shifts of outer circumstances is not a special gift bestowed upon the highest organisms but is the consequence of a gradual evolution."

Charles Darwin (1809–1882), in *The Origin of Species*, suggested that, by a process of natural selection, less well adapted forms of life would have on the average a heavier death-rate and a lower multiplication-rate. Again dealing with physical characteristics, he postulated his idea of the "survival of the fittest." Undoubtedly the homeostatic stabilizing mechanisms came into being through a process of gradual evolution and natural selection. These included both psychological and physiological processes for reintegrating and re-establishing the self-regulating internal equilibrium. It was Bernard who wrote that "the phenomena of living beings must be considered as a harmonious whole."

We can thus see that a fundamental property of every living organism, at every stage of its existence, is the capacity for adaptive response to its external environment which allows for a state of balance in its internal milieu. Natural selection seems to have favoured those individuals and species that possess the greatest power of responsive plasticity of the individual within the optimal range of adaptation. Both the theory of evolution and that of the dynamic steady state or homeostatic adaptation are necessary to the understanding of human responses to psychological and physiological stresses both external and internal. We must have adaptation to the environment now, and the capacity for it in future, if smooth functioning is to be secured.

Adaptation involves a series of processes that are goal-directed and designed to facilitate the establishment of a state of equilibrium between the organism and its environment. In some instances the optimal level of equilibrium is fixed and various mechanisms attempt to adjust to this constancy. In other situations, devices are utilized to allow for a state as close to the optimal as possible. In any event the adaptational process is a dynamic one, having its roots in the biological structure and constantly attempting to balance intersystemic and intrasystemic tensions by way of the ego (Hartmann, 23).

Phylogenetic evolution has been directed towards allowing the organism increased independence of its environment, but this freedom is operative only within a certain range. As biological evolution has proceeded there has been a concomitant internalization of vital structures and functions. This applies to essential physiological, anatomical, and psychological process and structures. We may view the appearance of intra-psychic structures along this continuum of evolving internalization. The simplest unicellular organism operates on the uncomplicated stimulus-response level. Man also may in some instances do this, but he can perceive many stimuli which can be internally understood and stored without any immediate external response. Hartmann suggests that animals may have some kind of ego, though it is not comparable to that which we think is present in man. He feels that, in lower animals, reality relationships provide the patterns for the aims and means of pleasure-gain to a greater extent than they do in adult man. In view of Freud's "Formulations on the Two Principles of Mental Functioning," this statement can be elaborated to indicate that certain infra-human species, as well as the egos of very young children, operate primarily on the basis of the pleasure principle, whereas more mature and integrated human egos function in accordance with the reality principle and utilize secondary process thinking which includes intra-psychic representations of external objects and memory. Pleasure-principle operations view the object mainly in terms of the function it performs for the individual being, namely that of the reduction of tension. Only with greater maturation and development does the object become differentiated as an individual entity with distinct personal characteristics of its own in addition to those that are overtly functional. We see that psychological adaptation may occur at levels which have phylogenetic significance as well as ontogenetic importance.

Hartmann differentiates the state of adaptedness from the adaptive process which brings this state about. In this adaptive process, various defensive techniques are utilized. But "adaptation achievements may turn into adaptation disturbances," when reality situations are altered. Thus when an object relationship is interrupted by the death of one of the significant participants, a new ego-adaptive process has to be instituted in order to deal with the altered internal-external psychological situation. Where there is a possibility of substitution with little difficulty, the adaptive task may be easily accomplished, as is the case with certain animals and very young infants. But when the lost object has taken on psychic significance in addition to functional fulfilment, the adaptive process involves in part an undoing of the previous adaptational equilibrium established with that object, and the gradual reestablishment of new relationships with reality-present figures. The complex adaptive process instituted in such a situation is called mourning.

A process may come about in one of two ways. There may be the stepwise series of consecutively followed specific stages, or the situation where many stages exist simultaneously and concomitantly. Even in this latter type of process, where varying intermediate phases are present at the same time, there are quantitative differences between the varying stages, but definite starting and end points may be ascertained. In the intermediate phases of the process, reactions and interactions may have inhibitory, facilitatory, or neutralizing effects.

It is only by carefully studying each component part that we can gain an approximate appreciation of the complex relationship of the entire process. For the sake of simplicity, this second type of process may be described as if it occurred in seemingly isolated consecutive steps, although this may not be so in fact.

The mourning process consists of a series of operations and stages whose appearance seems to follow a sequential pattern. In line with the above, however, it is necessary to indicate that although certain aspects of the process are more apparent at particular times; the succession of one stage by another does not necessarily indicate that a former stage may not be present later in time, or that a later one was not in evidence earlier.

II. THE MOURNING PROCESS IN MAN

Psychological lesions result when there is a disruption of the state of equilibrium that is established to allow for optimal functioning. As indicated above, reactions evoked by the upset in adaptation give rise to a process designed to re-establish an intra-psychic homeostatic steady state. Characteristically, mourning refers to the response following the death of a meaningful figure. As will be postulated below, this mourning reaction is an ego-adaptive process which includes the reaction to the loss of the object, as well as the readjustment to an external environment wherein this object no longer exists in reality. The mourning process is not species-specific, and is obviously intrapsychic, as the external loss cannot be undone. Usually we assume that mourning and the reaction to permanent loss without death are equivalent. This equation, though not rejected, requires further demonstration. Differences may be present which allow for more precise description.

The ante-mortem nature of the relationship between the bereaved and the deceased will be an important factor in the resultant mourning process. The type of ego development, maturation, and the level of integration and organization, however, will be the crucial variables in determining the course and extent of the mourning process. Thus an ego that has developed to the point where reality is correctly perceived, and objects distinctly and uniquely differentiated, will mourn differently from an ego that is poorly integrated and immature.

A. Historical Considerations

In a discussion attached to the case history of Fraulein Elisabeth von R, which appeared in the *Studies on Hysteria* (1893), Freud described

a highly-gifted lady who suffers from slight nervous states and whose whole character bears evidence of hysteria, though she has never had to seek medical help or been unable to carry on her duties. She has already nursed to the end three of four of those whom she loved. Each time she reached a state of complete exhaustion; but she did not fall ill after these tragic efforts. Shortly after her patient's death, however, there would begin in her a work of reproduction which once more brought up before her eyes the scenes of the illness and death. Every day she would go through each impression once more, would weep over it and console herself—at her leisure, one might say. This process of dealing with her impressions was dovetailed into her everyday tasks without the two activities interfering with each other. The whole thing would pass through her mind in chronological sequence. I cannot say whether the work of recollection corresponded day by day with the past.

An editorial comment in the Standard Edition at this point indicates that this account of the "work of recollection" anticipated Freud's later concept of the "work of mourning."

Freud goes on to say that "In addition to these outbursts of weeping with which she made up arrears and which followed close upon the fatal termination of the illness, this lady celebrated annual festivals of remembrance at the period of her various catastrophes, and on these occasions her vivid visual reproduction and expressions of feeling kept to the date precisely." Freud gives a specific instance of her husband's death which had occurred three years earlier.

This careful clinical description not only presented Freud's precursory ideas referable to the mourning work, but also was the first conceptualization of what we now call anniversary reactions. This type of reaction, more currently rediscovered and elaborated upon, is clearly a variation and an incomplete form of the mourning process. In the patient described by Freud, these observations are made only in passing, but in retrospect they already predict some of his later significant contributions.

In 1895 in Draft G, on Melancholia, Freud related depression and melancholia to mourning and grief. He spoke of a "longing for something that is lost," and "a loss in the subject's instinctual life." Again anticipating his later formulations, he also commented that "the uncoupling of associations is always painful." In Draft N, written on 31 May 1897, Freud not only gave us the first hint of the oedipus complex, but also connected mourning with melancholia. This comparison he further commented on in his 1910 discussion of suicide, where he referred to the "affect of mourning."

Freud described mourning as a normal emotional process in his *Five Lectures on Psycho-Analysis* (1909), and in the same year in his "Notes upon a Case of Obsessional Neurosis," he states that "I told him, a normal period of mourning would last from one to two years." The essays on *Totem and Taboo* (1912–13) further develop Freud's ideas on the mourning process. He writes that "Mourning has a quite specific psychical task to perform: its function is to detach the survivors' memories and hopes from the dead. When this has been achieved, the pain grows less and with it the remorse and self-reproach" (p. 65). In the same work Freud points out that after a death both affection and hostility to the deceased exist. The mourning relates to the positive feelings, while satisfaction is the reaction of triumph related to the hostile feelings. The hostility, however, is repressed and becomes unconscious, because the mourning process which derives from an intensification of the loving feelings does not allow of any satisfaction. But this hostility may be dealt with by projection onto the dead object, and this gives rise to the fear of the dead. This phenomenon also is related to the feelings of anger which will be discussed below.

In January 1914, Freud spoke to Jones about his paper on mourning and melancholia, and in December of that year he presented his ideas to the Vienna Psychoanalytical Society. He wrote his first draft in February 1915, and the manuscript was finished in May 1915. In March and April 1915, Freud wrote his paper "Thoughts for the Times on War and Death." In November 1915, Freud's "On Transience" was written, and published the following year.

In attempting a correlation of events in Freud's life with the appearance of these papers, we note that Freud's father died on 23 October 1896. In July 1897 Freud began his self-analysis, and on 15 October 1897 in a letter to Fliess announced his discovery of the oedipus complex. Draft N, it seems, was written at a time when Freud himself was in the midst of working out his own mourning for his dead father. In 1910 the difficulties with Adler were increasing, and in 1911 the break with him actually occurred. In 1913 the dissension with Jung was very painful to Freud, and in 1914 came Jung's resignation from psycho-analytic associations. The distress these oppositions caused to Freud is well known. Although it is speculative, his more formal conceptualization of mourning may have been related to his grief over the loss of Jung and what Jung represented to him. The 1913 Congress was an unpleasant experience for Freud, and in 1914 Jung's formal separation occurred. In November 1914, Freud's beloved brother Emmanuel died in a railway accident. Jones states "he was eighty-one years old, the same as their father when he died." About this same time, "there was also the loss of the famous raider, the *Emden,* to be mourned; Freud said he had got quite attached to her." In December 1914, "Freud's spirits were very low, and he begged Abraham to come and cheer him up." It was in the same month that Freud spoke to the Vienna Society on mourning and melancholia in a discussion of a paper by Tausk on melancholia.

In 1915 Freud's two sons were actively involved in the war and he was quite concerned over them. Jones notes that "Freud had several dreams about calamities to his sons, which he interpreted as envy of their youth." Many of his close associates (Abraham, Ferenczi, Rank, Sachs) were also on army service during this period. It was in 1915 that the three major works above referred to were written. We may infer that all the losses, disappointments, and threats undoubtedly influenced Freud, so that his introspective activities yielded insights on mourning that were reflected in his papers on this theme.

In his essay "On Transience," Freud notes that individuals "recoil from anything that is painful," and so there is "a revolt in their minds against mourning." Thus thoughts about the transience of an object involve "a foretaste of mourning over its decease" with resultant avoidance of thoughts on this theme. Until recent months surprisingly few investigations have been made of the mourning process *per se* by psychoanalysts and others involved in psychological research. Perhaps Freud's statements quoted above are in part an explanation of the apparent lack of study of this normal and omnipresent phenomenon.

In "Mourning and Melancholia" Freud states that "mourning is regularly the reaction to the loss of a loved person, or to the loss of some abstraction which has taken the place of one, such as fatherland, liberty, an ideal, and so on." He indicates that a mourning process as such can occur after varying losses. The loss of the abstraction, however, is reacted to as if it were the intra-psychic object that is lost. In this investigation, the loss following the death of a significant figure will be the major source of clinical data, and the major definition of the mourning process. In the various clinical and theoretical reports appearing on this subject some terminological differences seem to confuse aspects of the mourning process. Thus grief is an affect that may follow on a multitude of situations. It is seen in the mourning process, but grief as such may be seen in situations where there is no such process. Transitory object loss in time and in space may give rise to various reactions that are components of the mourning process, but this again must be differentiated from the permanent loss in time and space of a significant object.

In *The Ego and the Id,* Freud states that the "character of the ego is a precipitate of abandoned object-cathexes" as well as the recording of "past object-choices." Thus all prior frustrations and renunciations were seemingly followed by mourning processes. When viewed in this broad way, the mourning process becomes very significant, as it is apparently one of the more universal forms of adaptation and growth through structuralization available to man. Not all aspects of this process necessarily occur with every loss. In studying the responses to the death of meaningful figures, various facets not usually seen in other types of frustration and loss may be described and delineated. Mourning may result when there is rejection by an object not by death, but the important focus here is on the resulting process and not necessarily on the precipitating event. We mourn something that is lost but previously had been strongly cathected, and through this process the ego is built.

Klein has commented on the close connexion between the testing of reality in normal mourning and the early mental processes. It is her contention that the early mourning characteristic of the child's reactions to frustrations is revived and re-experienced whenever grief occurs in later life. Just as Freud has stressed the importance of reality testing as the most important part of the adult mourning work, so Klein emphasizes this ego activity in overcoming a mourning-like process seen in young children where in external reality no death has occurred.

In this paper an attempt will be made mainly to delineate and discuss more specifically the various stages of the mourning process as it customarily occurs in man after the death of an object. These findings will then in the last section be related to observations made on infra-human responses to death. More deviant types of mourning reactions will be briefly mentioned, to be more fully elaborated in a later paper.

B. Stages of the Mourning Process

Approximately five years ago, while intimately involved in a mourning adaptation of his own, the author had occasion to experience and observe more closely the changing aspects of the mourning process in himself and also in family members of various ages and developmental levels. As the mourning continued it became apparent that different aspects of the process could be distinguished. These stages consisted of a series of reactions occurring in a temporal sequence, having distinct degrees of acuteness and chronicity, and seemingly divided into component parts. Stimulated by these observations, a more systematic study of the mourning process was undertaken, and the following conclusions were arrived at.

When a death occurs, the first response is that of shock. This results from the sudden upset in ego equilibrium, and is related to the initial awareness that the object no longer exists in space, time, or person. The particular emotional orientation to this being is disrupted, and initially there is excessive stimulation due to this initial awareness that cannot be integrated. The overwhelming task may unsuccessfully be dealt with and result in a panic response, which includes shrieking, wailing, or moaning, or may be manifested by a complete collapse with paralysis and motor retardation. The behaviour in this shock stage indicates acute regression to a much earlier ego-organizational level. The narcissistic loss, related to the resulting shock, is connected with the suddenness of the event. The phenomenon of narcissistic mortification is applicable to this shock state. There is "a sudden loss of control over external and internal reality, or both, by virtue of which the emotion of terror is produced, along with the damming up of narcissistic libido or destrudo" (12). The shock phase results when the ego is narcissistically immobilized by the suddenness and massiveness of the task that confronts it.

The response noted in this initial stage varies in intensity according to the suddenness of the death and the degree of preparation the ego underwent prior to the death. Thus death following chronic and prolonged serious illness is reacted to differently from the acute unexpected demise of a close object. Nonetheless, a shock response will be present in both situations, although the intensity will vary. Previous shocks of a similar kind may suddenly be catapulted into this most recent one and can result in a total regressive immobilization. In susceptible individuals this shock can be of such magnitude as to precipitate a serious somatic dysfunction such as thyrotoxicosis (1). In instances where death is anticipated as a result of a long-standing debilitation, acute mourning reactions may occur prior to the actual death. In several patients, whose parents were dying of malignant conditions, the shock response came when the patients first heard of the hopeless malignant diagnosis, and only very slightly when the actual death occurred. In these persons, the ego was able to react to the upset in present reality more gradually, so that when death supervened much preparation had already been done.

It is the sudden impingement of reality on the unprepared ego that results in an overwhelming of the stimulus barrier and the integrative capacity of the organism. Massive regression with panic can ensue until further restitutive activities take over. The duration of this shock phase is usually short, although the immobilization may persist owing to faulty later reparative reactions. It may be that the degree of shock ranges through a spectrum of responses depending upon the type of ego stimuli barriers that have previously been integrated.

The second stage in the mourning process, very closely following the shock response, is the grief reaction. Darwin describes the physical aspects of this response in his *Expression of the Emotions in Man and Animals*. He indicates that early grief is characterized by much muscular hyperactivity such as hand wringing, aimless wild walking, hair and clothes pulling. Darwin interprets this behaviour as indicative of the impotence the bereaved feels to undo the death that has just occurred. This frantic movement changes when it is realized that nothing can be done. Then deep despair and sorrow take over, and the sufferer becomes very quiet, sits motionless or gently rocks to and fro, sighs deeply and becomes muscularly flaccid. All the facial features are lengthened and the characteristic grief appearance results. Darwin specially calls attention to the grief muscles, whose innervation results in the typical obliquity of the eyebrow and the depression of the corners of the mouth. As grief lessens, the change may be detected in muscular alterations even before feelings are altered. Lindemann has described the feelings of fatigue, exhaustion, and anorexia seen in this acute grief phase. The energy impoverishment seen in grief has been related to the mourning process by Freud in his *Inhibitions, Symptoms, and Anxiety*.

As the shock stage merges into the grief phase a subjective feeling of intense psychic pain is felt. The suffering ache is initially of much greater intensity than what subsequently follows in the later chronic grief phase. Accompanying this psychic pain may be the sudden screaming, yelling, and other non-verbal but vocal manifestations of this grief reaction. This acute initial response later becomes the more characteristic depression. The spasmodic crying changes to tearful lamentations, and gradually verbal communications become more frequent, though still accompanied by much sobbing.

What explanations can we seek for the phenomena described in this phase? Initially we must consider the "Formulations on the Two Principles of Mental Functioning" of Freud. The pleasure ego, operating under the pleasure-pain principle, strives for the release of tension and excitement. In the very young child this is completely related to the external object. Thus when there is an increase in excitation without release because the object is absent, pain results. With the death of the object, there is temporary ego disruption with regression to an ego state where the pleasure-pain principle is the chief axis of mental functioning. Since reality principle functioning is temporarily abrogated, the capacity to wait for discharge and the ability to seek alternative ways of handling the increase in tension is very much diminished.

Thus the external reality loss so overwhelms the ego that immobilization and shock occur with regression to the earlier pleasure-pain principle operation. This pain may result from the heightened non-discharged "energic cathexis" due to the absence of the object. As greater ego integration occurs, reality-principle functioning and secondary process thinking return with the resulting amelioration of the psychic pain. Freud has noted the feeling of pain that occurs in mourning is his "Mourning and Melancholia." In this paper, however, Freud initially refers to the pain as *Schmerz* and not *Unlust*, the "mental antithesis of pleasure," also translated as "pain." Later he calls the pain that is present *Schmerz-Unlust*. It is my contention that this pain is both *Schmerz* and *Unlust*, and represents the regression to the earlier phase of mental functioning. The idea that the lost object can no longer hopefully fulfil the needs of the mourner seems to be the key point. This reality awareness, however, is more characteristic of the later chronic mourning process. This early intense pain is seemingly more closely tied to the reaction to frustration at not having the object there.

In his paper "On Narcissism," Freud notes that as libidinal interest and investment is withdrawn from a love object into the ego, there is a damming-up of libido in the ego. With this increase in tension, pain is experienced.

This conceptualization allows us to view this aspect of the mourning process as analogous to the model of the actual neuroses. When the libido is discharged, the pain diminishes.

The pain phenomenon may alternatively be approached from the point of view of Federn. Thus the object is gone and temporarily libido may be avulsed along with it. This can result in an ego impoverishment and an inability to bind stimuli so that withdrawal is the emergency adaptation to conserve libido by avoiding stimuli that additionally tax the ego. Regression to an earlier ego state requires less expenditure of ego cathexis. Utilizing this concept of ego depletion in mourning may assist in differentiating the reaction after the death of an object from that on the loss of an object not through death but through growth. Thus in analysis mourning-like reactions occur when childhood objects are given up. The grief involved in losing all retained relationships revived in the transference neurosis is not due to impoverishment. This latter is a living process leading to a particular goal of detachment. This process is different from the mourning following the actual death of a significant being. I cannot say whether the avulsion hypothesis or the "swelling" hypothesis causes the pain. Either phenomenon can result in this reaction, and further study is necessary to find specifically which is more significant.

Convergent evidence for the presence of pain is to be found in understanding the rather "animal-like" crying seen in the earlier phase of mourning. The cry is an alarm signal that is vocalized very early in life. In addition it expresses unpleasurable feelings and emotions. The cry in not only a proclamation of pain or some other non-pleasurable state, but is also the earliest form of vocal communication and command. It seems to announce that something undesired is present, and it usually arouses the simple and appropriate response on the part of those who hear it. Thus as "pain" occurs, it is accompanied initially by the primitive crying that is indicative of this pain. As the local communications become more verbal, the crying also seems to be less primitive and less wail-like, and the needs are expressed in more advanced ways.

With separation we get crying. This is commonly seen when a young child is spatially and temporally removed from its mother. It is also seen in adults on various occasions of parting. French has postulated that underlying the crying is the wish for reconciliation. In certain of the anthropoids this seems to be the case; initially, however, it is the cry of distress that accompanies separation from the mother. When the child becomes aware of the mother's response to the crying, it may then become the signal for reconciliation in addition to its earlier significance.

In "Mourning and Melancholia," Freud states that mourning work involves the testing of reality that shows that the loved object no longer exists and requires "that all the libido shall be withdrawn from its attachment to this object." Thus when reality-principle operation takes over, there is a consciousness of the external world without the departed object. This absence is not only perceived but is confirmed by repeated confrontations of the external world, and is finally noted and remembered. There may be a partial repression of the pain involved in the loss. This pain will be re-experienced periodically throughout the mourning process and the experience integrated in the later stage of mourning work. As the ego passes judgement on the truth and permanence of the loss, action and thought processes are utilized to facilitate appropriated alterations of reality with subsequent adaptation.

Fantasy-making and day-dreaming, however, not being dependent upon real objects and reality testing, still remain subordinated to the pleasure-principle alone, and so repression remains as the all-powerful defense. Thus fantasies and day-dreams concerning the deceased object can interfere with the mourning work, and in instances where the death of the object is not realistically appreciated, the object may continue to exist as an unassimilated introject with whom internal conversations can be carried on. This phenomenon has been observed in several patients who lost their parents in childhood. The use of fantasy defensively in ignoring reality is commonly seen in various clinical pictures. But the fantasied monologue and interior dialogue is quite frequently found in this phase of the mourning process.

In the "Formulation on the Two Principles of Mental Functioning," Freud relates a repetitive dream of a man whose father died after a long illness, the dream occurring months after the death. In it the father was alive again and the patient talked to him as of old. "But as he did so he felt it exceedingly painful that his father was nevertheless dead, only not aware of the fact." Freud in 1911, involved in working out problems of id psychology, related the pain to the dreamer's death wishes towards the father when he was alive. This pain, however, may have resulted from the awareness of the death as it had been described above, and in the dream we can see how the reality of the father's death is avoided by portraying him as alive, and yet the dreamer is simultaneously aware of the fact that he is dead. In other words, this dream represents the mourning work involved in partially accepting the father's death, yet at the same time avoiding this recognition.

In his paper "Fetishism" (1927), Freud discusses two male analysands who lost their fathers at the age of two and ten respectively. He mentions that each patient had refused to acknowledge his father's death, yet neither of them had developed a psychosis. On further investigation, Freud found that "only one current of their mental processes" had not accepted the father's death. "There was another which was fully aware of the fact; the one which was consistent with reality stood alongside the one which accorded with a wish." One of these cases was a severe obsessional and "in every situation in life he oscillated between two assumptions—on the one his father was sill alive and hindered him from action, on the other his father was dead and he had a right to regard himself as his successor." We can infer here that the patient's mourning process was such that he still could not accept the reality of the father's death. Freud (21) points out that in certain states of conflict the synthetic function of the ego is abrogated and both reality and instinct may be satisfied at great cost. This type of non-synthetic ego functioning related to isolation may be the adaptive technique utilized by this patient.

In the chronic mourning stage, pain may continue to be felt. It is however less intense, less generalized, and less continuous, related to specific recollections or perceptions, and gradually extinguished. In the acute mourning phase the pain does not have these buffering characteristics.

In instances of chronic illness, these painful grief responses may antedate the actual death, as we have said above for the shock responses. The reaction here is that the loved person is already lost in the internal milieu, even though death has not yet occurred in reality. An individual speaking of a close relative who had recently been diagnosed as having a fatal illness, referred to the ill person in the past tense throughout the conversation. Spontaneously the speaker remarked, "You know he is dead for me already." This indicated that the internal loss and mourning process was already in motion. Mourning work is still required, however, after the actual death has occurred. If there is no evidence of it, it may represent a defensive short-circuiting of the process to avoid pain, and hence does not allow for full resolution and integration.

To be sure, any previous ambivalent feelings, conflicts, or hostilities with death wishes can play an important part in the mourning process. The magical belief in the causality of the death with great guilt may be the major contributor to subsequent serious psycho-pathology. Freud discussed this point in his paper on "Dostoevsky and Parricide" (1928). There he clearly related the pre-death wish for the object's demise to the actual death of the object followed by a transient period of triumph and joy. This, however, quickly gave rise to guilt, and the self-punishing attitude persisted. In his biography, Jones mentions that when Freud was nineteen months old, his next younger sibling, a brother, died aged eight months. "In a letter to Fliess (1897) he (Freud) admits the evil wishes he had against his rival and adds that their fulfilment in his death had aroused self-reproaches, a tendency to which had remained ever since." These self-reproaches can in susceptible persons result in abnormal mourning reactions, which may include melancholia and psychosis. In this paper, these pathological conditions, though considered, are not specifically focused upon.

The third phase of the acute mourning process is that of the separation reaction. This may manifest itself in various ways, and will be more intense in individuals with earlier unresolved conflicts in this sphere. The reality of the loss intensifies this reaction, and initially recognition of the traumatic event may be avoided. Thus the absence of grief described by Deutsch may be involved in this inability to recognize that the object's absence is not temporary but permanent, and that the object is dead.

A patient talking of her inability to face the idea of her mother's death reported in an analytic session that to face it was "too difficult." Not only had she become aware of her grief and pain, but she was attempting to defend herself against what she described as feelings of "nothingness and emptiness." She gradually recognized that to mourn was to acknowledge the nothingness of her mother, and this meant emptiness inside her. Defensively she kept her mother alive in heaven and used "religion" as an aid to her ego in avoiding the "total nothingness of death."

The ego-adaptive task in this aspect of the mourning process requires a reorientation in the perceptual sphere involving both self and object. In order to master that part of the early anxiety experience related to separation, a total internalization is required, or a greater dependence on previously internalized and integrated relationships in the ego of object representations. Anna Freud (17) has described this as object constancy. Where internal object representations are not well integrated, where tensions exist in the form of ambivalences unsolved and with non-neutralized aggression, the energy balance is seriously disturbed. The integrative task becomes greater at reconciling external reality with internal structures where the prior developmental pattern was defective or distorted.

The representation of the lost object is re-cathected because the instinctual energies that would have been discharged in actual relationship to the object, being now undischarged, recathect the internalized object image. Where there is poor differentiation between self and not-self, where there is poor ego integration, the hypercathected internal object may be projected and hallucinated as an external figure. The hallucinatory process in this instance is a manifestation of what happens when instinctual tension is not discharged because the real object is lost, and we have a primitive type of ego organization. Separation is not accepted and the lost object is halluncinatively retained.

Introjection and identification in terms of psychic structural formation relate to this point. Both, however, are internalization operations. If we view introjection as a process, mode, or technique, and identification as the end-result of the process in which introjection is initially present, the confusion between these two terms may be clarified and may shed light on subsequent mourning processes.

In a healthy object relationship, where there has been total assimilation or identification, the mourning process is comparatively short-lived, and comes to a spontaneous end. It may reflect whatever unresolved components of incorporation without identification are still present, but a comparatively healthy ego integration allows reality to be perceived, accepted, and dealt with appropriately without lasting ego immobilization. Grief is present, but is of such intensity and duration that it is not considered pathological. When an object has been introjected without identification, it exists as an encapsulated image in the ego as the result of the lack of assimilation. This introjected object retains characteristics of the original object, in many ways intensified as a result of the ambivalent feelings connected with the object. When the external object dies, an abnormal mourning process ensues. This may be reflected in the inability to accept the actual death of the object, and the retention of the introjected image with responses indicative of the fact that this introjected object still exists. Because of the lack of completeness of identification and ego integration, the ambivalences directed towards this object enhance the mourning process, if it occurs, with the formation of severe symptoms of melancholia or self-destruction, or both. When the actual death of the external object is totally denied with the absence of grief, what is found is a retention of the introjected object as an entity of the relationship, and this object is perpetuated externally by means of secret internal "communications" with this object. An example of this phenomenon has been observed in three adult patients, one of whom has been briefly discussed above.

In all the cases a parent had died prior to the patient's sixth birthday. Throughout the years there had been a retention of the deceased parent in the form of a fantasied figure who was in heaven; to whom the patient could talk and tell whatever he or she wished; who never verbally or actively responded to the patient; and who was always all-seeing and omnipresent. The fantasies about these retained figures came out with great caution and difficulty lest the patients be shamed for retaining these images. In all three instances the patients denied ever visiting the cemetery where the deceased parent was buried, and there was a period of amnesia that extended from the moment when the patient was told of the parent's death until many months later.

In one of these cases, the man's father died when he was a very young child, and his mother died when he was an adult. The process described above was observed in connexion with his father's decease. In the case of his mother, however, he was able to accept her death, but continued to visit her grave regularly and to speak to her. He still envisioned her as alive, but not able to answer him.

This retention of the object as a figure that can be spoken to and envisioned, and the denial of its demise, interferes with mourning. When there has been incomplete identification, i.e. when the identification process had not come about or has been arrested at a preliminary stage owing to immaturity or arrest of development, there is either a melancholic depressive response, or a denial of the death of the deceased with ego arrestation, distortion, or defect.

Patients report that following particular analytic hours they continue to talk to the analyst even though they have left his office. In these reports the analyst rarely answers, and as the analytic process proceeds, this "talking to the analyst as analyst" gradually diminishes and finally ceases with the integrated assumption of a "communication with self." It is maintained that in these instances a process occurs similar to that mentioned above, namely initial introjection of the analyst as an object with later identification and assimilation. He is retained in a somewhat encapsulated form with whom internal communication proceeds. When identification is complete, the introject is assimilated and the presence of the separate imago disappears.

In "Group Psychology and the Analysis of the Ego," Freud discusses the relationship of identifications to object cathexes and object relations. Object cathexis implies an object that is outside and energized. Identification is the process and end result wherein changes occur in the ego and actions take place without reference to the assimilated object. "Identification with an object that is renounced or lost as a substitute for that object'' occurs through the ''introjection of it into the ego.'' We assume that ''identification is the earliest and original form of emotional tie with an object.'' Thus ''in a regressive way it becomes a substitute for a libidinal object-tie'' by introjection. In identification with an object, the result is being like the object; in choosing the person as an object, the result is having the object. Identification may appear regressively and defensively in lieu of ''object-choice.'' In mourning this defensive wholesale identification with the lost object can be used to avoid the painful resolution of mourning work.

In Freud's monumental *Inhibitions, Symptoms, and Anxiety*, (1926), the last seven pages are directed to a discussion of anxiety, pain, and mourning. In this section, Freud differentiates mourning from anxiety, in that the former results from the loss of an object, while the latter is ''a reaction to the danger of losing the object.'' In both responses there is pain, although it may be more clearly identified in the mourning reaction of the adult. Freud, citing the infant's response to the loss of the mother, even on a temporary basis, states that ''the first determinant of anxiety which the ego itself introduces is loss of perception of the object (which is equated with loss of the object itself).'' This antedates the fear of loss of love which has not as yet appeared. It is regression to this early stage of separation and its defences that characterizes this phase of the mourning process.

The response to recognizing the separation and its permanence gives rise to anxiety and also to anger. Both these affects are experienced in the acute mourning stage. Defences to deal with these threatening affects may quickly come into existence. Freud states the pain is ''the actual reaction to the loss of the object, and anxiety is the reaction to the danger which that loss entails, and in its further displacement a reaction to the danger of the loss of the object itself.'' This differentiation, though valid, need not be mutually exclusive. The object is dead and is no longer externally present. This results in pain, but also in anxiety. The ego cannot completely accept the reality and finality of the separation in time and space, and so anxiety about the loss is experienced. That part of the ego which regresses to pleasure-principle operation does feel the pain owing to the absence of the object. The later chronic mourning work is not characterized by excessive anxiety, as the object is more and more accepted as permanently gone. Instead pain continues ''in view of the high degree and insatiable nature of the cathexis of longing which is concentrated on the object by the bereaved person during the reproduction

of the situations in which he must undo the ties that attach him to it.''
(Freud 1926).

The anger at being left and frustrated is also characteristically part of the
acute separation reaction. Typically it comes out in an undisguised fashion in
children. They are frustrated and enraged. In adults, however, this anger may
be displaced onto others, as hostility to the dead is not easily tolerated by the
mourning ego. Thus physicians, hospital personnel, undertakers, become the
focus of displaced hostility. There may be accusations against close relatives,
or even self-accusations about what the mourner could or should have done.
This anger is usually unrealistic and unwarranted, and in the adult may not
be present in identifiable form. It may fuse with the grief, and in the chronic
mourning work be indicated by feelings of depression or through various
guilt-expiating rituals.

When there is anger about the loss, it is indicative that the separation is
recognized and acknowledged. In this sense anger is restitutive, as cathexis
can be discharged through the affective experience of anger. Thus the anger
is in the service of mastery of the shock, panic, and grief. As to the reasons
for the anger, we must recognize that the rage is a narcissistic rage. It is as if
the child is screaming ''It happens to me and I have no control over it. It is
the parents' fault and they should have prevented it.'' When the rage is
discharged diffusely, frustration at being left is avoided, as is the feeling
of helplessness.

Clinically the frustration consequent on the death of a parent or spouse is
due not only to the factors mentioned above, but also to the increased demand
made upon the bereaved by the other survivors. Thus the child who loses a
parent and is expected to fulfil the needs of the bereaved surviving parent
suffers a double loss and is angry at this. The handling of the bereavement
by the various mourners as well as by the social mores and religious customs
can aid or reinforce various expressive and inhibitory activities involved in
the mourning process. This latter point will be discussed elsewhere.

Separation anxiety may manifest itself in various ways. There may be a
reluctance to be separated from the corpse. Thus one may look longingly and
fixedly at it, at the coffin, or at the grave. There may be the false perception
that the dead is still breathing or moving. Afterwards there may be an
inability to accept that the lost object is permanently gone. Thus Queen
Victoria ordered that her husband's study must not be disturbed in a single
detail after his death. It almost seemed as though the reality of permanent

separation could be avoided by keeping the room ready for occupation. Variations of this denial of separation may be manifested by displacement of cathexis from the object onto auxiliaries which are reminders of the departed. Thus old letters, keepsakes, portraits, eyeglasses, bits of hair, clothing, and other intimate possessions are treated as if they have to be constant reminders of the existence of the object. In some instances this reflects the inability to let the object die, be buried and let life go on. In "Mourning and Melancholia," Freud notes that the struggle involved in abandoning a libido position previously occupied by a loved object could be so intense that "a turning away from reality" can result and the object "clung to through the medium of an hallucinatory wish-psychosis." Eventually, however, in the normal individual reality gains the day.

In mourning, libido detachment or object decathexis occurs topographically in the system Unconscious. The process then proceeds through the Preconscious into the Conscious. It is here that reality perception can occur. When this path is blocked owing to ambivalence, as Freud pointed out in "Mourning and Melancholia," repression continues to operate and pathological mourning results.

The task of mourning consists of internal object decathexis with the freeing of energy for later recathectic activities. As Freud pointed out, this process may be stopped at the level of a hallucinatory wish-psychosis which denies the death of the object, or it may go on to completion wherein the ego becomes free and uninhibited when the mourning work is finished. The mourning process end result may stop at various intermediate steps short of completion. Thus one may get total or partial undifferentiated identification with the object, as was seen in the clinical data cited above, or on the side of completion of mourning, partially unneutralized cathexis that is only moderately changed though still bound and ego-inhibiting.

To recapitulate briefly, the acute stage of the mourning process refers to the immediate phases following the loss of the object. These phases consist of the shock, grief, pain, reaction to separation, and the beginning internal object decathexis with the recognition of the loss. The reaction to separation brings with it anxiety as the perception of the loss in time and space is integrated, as well as the anger reaction.

As the acute stage of the mourning process progresses, the chronic stage gradually takes over. Here we find various manifestations of adaptive mechanisms attempting to integrate the experience of the loss with reality so that life activities can go on. Adaptation in the chronic stage of mourning involves the further integration of newer reality demands which include newer functional need gratifications and demands. The ego is able to withstand the more immediate effects of the loss of the object, and to begin the reparative aspect of the more lasting adaptation. Freud has described this chronic stage of the mourning process as the mourning work. This work is a continuation of the process that began more acutely immediately following the loss.

The sequential dreams occurring during the mourning process are indicators of this work of the ego. Changes occurring in the perception of the lost object in the dream reveal the gradual withdrawal of cathexis from the object and its associations. Thus in one instance, initial dreams of the departed object immediately after the death still kept the object alive, functioning and communicating. Gradually the object disappeared from the dreams *per se,* and in late phases of the chronic mourning process, a dream was reported wherein an individual spoke of a funeral and burial that had occurred several months previously. Associations to the dream dealt with "finally accepting" that the figure was dead, buried although still remembered. Here the acceptance of the reality of the loss came about, and secondary process reality-principle-oriented behaviour utilizing memory was in evidence.

Another patient reported that as he accepted the reality of the death of his father, his dreams began to lose colour. Grey was the predominant shade, until one day a grey dream was reported as having a "sprig of green" in it. His associations dealt with "something coming to life again." It was as though the freed energy heralded "the arrival of spring, when things began to grow again after a long cold grey winter."

In analysis the mourning work can be followed by noting the varying restitutive ego activities. One of the patients mentioned above was unable to mourn, as it was indicative of the acceptance of the death. If the death was not accepted, then mourning was not going to occur. This patient at times even wondered if she had ever had a real mother. As the analysis proceeded, her great guilt toward her mother came out. The mother had died when the patient was four and a half. The multi-ambivalences overwhemed the patient with excessive guilt and anxiety. This was strongly reinforced by the strong oedipal feelings towards the father. As the analysis continued, the mourning process gradually began and proceeded in the fashion described above. The transference neurosis provided this woman with objects that rekindled her repressed conflicts. Various shades of her mixed feelings emerged, and her dreams began to deal with meaningful figures. In a similar way to the dreams mentioned above, her early dreams dealt with the deceased object as being alive. This woman actually retained her mother in heaven as a live figure. Each night she spoke to her, and the patient "knew that mother" heard her. As the analyst was cathected, he became the replacement for the mother, and thus it was with him that conversations took place by night. With energizing of the introject of the analyst, the mother was allowed to die, and the patient began to grieve, feel anxious, cry, and dream of meaningful figures who had died. This long and interesting analysis clearly indicated that the degree of ambivalence toward the dead object before the death occurred was related to the stage of psychic development achieved at the time of the loss. This ego distortion in part determined the length of the mourning work as well as the type of mourning reaction. In instances where melancholia or absent mourning occurs, we must look for the pathological interferences with the mourning process. It is not within the scope of this paper to discuss the effect of therapy on the mourning process. This problem has been dealt with by Fleming and Altschul (15), and also by the present author elsewhere.

Any death in childhood, especially that of a parent, interferes with the growth and developmental processes of the gradual detachment of libido from infantile images of the object. These parental internalizations are important in the integration and structuralization of the ego and superego.

In considering the mourning process, it is important to note that similarities can be observed in all such adaptational activities. But there are significant differences also. Firstly, the type of loss suffered must be considered. A permanent loss through death may be quite different from a temporary separation that is time-limited and not absolute. A sudden unexpected death results in a more acute response than a chronic loss due to institutionalization or even death. Secondly, we must recognize the significance of who or what is lost. The death of a parent in childhood differs from the death of a parent in adulthood. The death of the mother during the oedipal stage of a girl may have a different effect from what it has for an oedipal boy. The death of a sibling in childhood differs from the death of one's own child. The death of a spouse may be more significant than the loss of a political election in which there may be great involvement. It is difficult to generalize in this field, but further precision and delineation are necessary in our study of different types of losses and of the different objects that can be lost.

We must also recognize that the degree of maturity of the psychic apparatus of the mourner will be another important variable to investigate in the mourning process. Ego defects, distortions, or arrests cannot result in healthy mourning processes. The function of the lost object to the mourner is closely related to object replacement after the mourning process has ended.

In all probability the purest form of the mourning process occurs in mature adults. Even here, however, the loss of a child can never be fully integrated and totally accepted by the mother or the father. In an exchange of letters with Ludwig Binswanger (3), Freud wrote on the anniversary of his dead daughter's thirty-sixth birthday, "We know that the acute grief we feel after a loss will come to an end, but that we will remain inconsolable, and will never find a substitute. Everything that comes to take the place of the lost object, even if it fills it completely, nevertheless remains something different." In a later note, Freud recalls that he cannot forget the younger child of his deceased daughter, who also had died several years earlier. About this child Freud wrote, "to me this child had taken the place of all of my children and other grandchildren, and since then, since Heinele's death, I don't care for my grandchildren any more, but find no joy in life either. This is also the secret of my indifference—it was called courage—towards the danger to my own life."

Freud touches on the possible different mourning reactions that may occur in later life and senescence. Energies may not be so freely available as internal objects may not be so easily decathected. What one can do with theses liberated energies in older age differs from what may result earlier in life. Personal observations made on this point reveal that external objects may not be invested with the decathected libido, if it is available, by older people. More frequently, economic investments of less object-directed activities are made, and more narcissistic withdrawal occurs. Where there is an inability to make such shifts, too much ego depletion results and death may occur. It is not infrequently observed that shortly after the death of a long-standing marital partner, the survivor also succumbs. In these instances adaptation to life without the object is not possible.

The acute mourning reactions gradually become less intense and more distanced. As the ego is able to perceive reality correctly, various discharge techniques become more apparent. Little episodes that are suddenly recalled may serve as poignant reminders of the past. They may rekindle the dying fire of grief and tears for a short time. The response, however, is short-lived. There may be gradual acceptance of the fact that someone is not in a particular place at a specific time. Slips in conversation may indicate that the death of the object is still partially unaccepted. With the disposal of the dead figure's possessions, and having to deal with the alterations in practical reality, the ego begins to cathect new activities. True, the need to give up a house, a social group, or the like as a result of the separation may serve to institute new mourning processes and increase the integrative task of the ego, but these also are gradually worked through.

As personal possessions are dispersed, living arrangements altered, decisions made without reference to the lost object, the ego recognizes that narcissistic supply can be had elsewhere. Newer external objects become the focus of "give and take." These newer objects are seen not as exact substitutes for the lost objects, but as figures which permit reality relations that are mutually satisfactory. The loss of the dead object is assimilated, accepted, and the bereavement can come to an end.

Intra-psychically the object that is lost becomes part of the ego through identification. This may be manifested by activity such as a woman showed after the death and mourning for her husband. When confronted with a problem one day she said, "I deliberately looked at this in a way that my husband might have done had he been alive. I was surprised that I could honestly face it and deal with it in a way I never could have previously." This identification with facets of the lost object is frequently seen after the death of a close relative. In part it may be due to an increased cathexis of the internalized object to overcome the effects of the external loss, and thus take over some of the functional activities that the dead object previously provided.

Identification with the analyst after the termination of analysis allows the process of self-analysis to continue. The observing ego of the patient becomes sufficiently expanded and integrated for observation, interpretation, and experiencing to occur autonomously and non-volitionally. This healthy development is the end product following termination of a successful analysis. The mechanism is similar to though not the same as that following the successful completion of a mourning process. The ego is enriched and different, and can take over functions that were previously handled by the strongly cathected external object.

In the essay "On Transience," Freud notes that mourning comes to a spontaneous end "when it has renounced everything that has been lost, then it has consumed itself, and one's libido is once more free (in so far as we are still young and active) to replace the lost objects by fresh ones equally or still more precious." The lost object is not forgotten, nor is the new object identical with the lost if the mourner's ego is capable of differentiation. The end of mourning occurs with a resultant identification in the form of a consciously decathected memory trace.

Sporadic episodes of mourning may still occur in connexion with specific events or items, but these become fewer and less time-concentrated. New mourning experiences can serve to revive past mourning reactions that may still have bits of unresolved work present. In the instance of the loss of a very significant object, the total mourning process may never be completed.

Various religious rituals, when divested of their theological implications, emphasize the cultural evolution of mores and folkways which can defensively assist the ego in the adaptation involved in the mourning process. These will be discussed in another paper.

Mourning as a process of adaptation to a significant loss occurs in the attempt to maintain the constancy of the internal psychic equilibrium. The process consists of an acute and chronic stage. Various phases of these stages as well as their characteristic defensive operations have been presented. The ego's ability to perceive the reality of the loss; to appreciate the temporal and spatial permanence of the loss; to acknowledge the significance of the loss; to be able to deal with the acute sudden disruption following the loss with attendant fears of weakness, helplessness, frustration, rage, pain, and anger; to be able effectively to reinvest new objects or ideals with energy, and so re-establish different but satisfactory relationships, are the key factors in this process. The process has certain phenomena, utilizes certain mechanisms, and has a definite end-point. Pathological interferences with it result in maladaptations with resultant psychopathology.

III. INFRA-HUMAN RESPONSES TO DEATH

As mentioned in the first section of this presentation, the evolution of adaptive mechanisms and processes is related to survival of the species. When attempting to find information dealing with the phylogenetic roots of the mourning process, we quickly realize that little has been reported about the response in infra-human animals to death. When accounts have appeared, they have usually been either anecdotal or detailed observational reports and inferences by field workers. Systematic investigations of this problem have not been made. In the examples cited below, the reported data will be presented and comparisons will be made to note any similarities with various component phases of the human mourning process.

Death is a universal biological phenomenon from which no individual animal other than certain protozoa escapes. Although a biological event, with the evolution of familial organization, and psychological internalizations and structuralizations, it has taken on psycho-social significance. Involved in this is the need to differentiate the mourning response for a meaningful deceased object from the significance of death as an event that may involve the survivor himself. It is not my intention here to deal with the latter area except as it relates to the mourning response. Nature had seemingly evolved a homeostatic process to cope with the event of separation through death in the form of the mourning process in man. Investigating the responses of certain animals to the death of meaningful figures, I feel that the mourning process is an adaptation that has evolved phylogenetically. Although we cannot equate the responses observed in infra-human animals to the events of the mourning process as it is characteristically seen in man, the strikingly parallel reactions in non-human animals to certain phases of the mourning process in man seems to indicate phylogenetic evolutionary anlage for the human mourning process.

Systematic observations and investigations of animals' responses to the death of a previously meaningful object have not been carried out. Reports of such events are found with great difficulty, and these are mainly behaviouristic observations. Dr Schneirla, of the American Museum of Natural History, informed the author that behaviour described as depression, occurring after the removal of a meaningful figure, has been observed in certain mammals and birds, but not in reptiles, amphibians, or fish. This would seemingly set a phylogenetic base for the development of this adaptational process. In this paper, only the mammalian references will be cited.

It is common knowledge that dogs attached to their owners go through various grief and "mourning" responses when separations occur. A recent description of such an event, quoted from the newspaper account, stated that:

Corky, a small, forlorn fox terrier, ran away three times to sit in front of Our Lady of the Angels School, waiting for his mistress, Angelene. Angelene, 14, had died in the fire-scarred building. But Corky could not comprehend this. Three times the runaway dog was brought home to Angelene's mother, Mrs Julia Lechnik. Finally, she locked Corky inside the house. Mournfully the dog wandered to Angelene's room and crawled under her bed. Corky did not come out for four days. He neither ate nor slept. Towards Christmas, Corky at last began to perk up. "He'd still go to the front door in the afternoon, looking for Angie," Mrs Lechnik said. "But at least he began eating again."

Another report concerned a Japanese dog named Hachi:

> Born on 20 November, 1923, Hachi was sold a month later to a professor at Tokyo University. Hachi soon formed the habit of going to the railroad station with his master each morning, and waiting there until he returned from the university on the afternoon train.
>
> When the professor died in 1925, his family moved to another part of Tokyo. Hachi, however, returned to the railroad station each day to await the master who would never return. He set out for the station in the morning and remained there until evening. Hachi made his daily trip to the station for ten years, until he died on 8 March, 1935.

Interestingly a statue of Hachi was erected in front of the Tokyo railroad station with the inscription "The Faithful Dog, Hachi." In 1953, Japan issued a stamp in his honour.

Lorenz (28,29), has also reported his own experiences of the faithful devotion shown him by his lupus-derived dogs. His pet, Stasi, refused to return to her young puppies when it interfered with her being with Lorenz. Lorenz has noted that a lupus dog (wolf-derived) who has once sworn his allegiance to a certain man, is forever a one-man dog. No stranger can take the master's place, and if the master leaves, the animal becomes "literally unbalanced," obeying no one and acting like "an ownerless cur." Lorenz has observed that lupus bitches seem to have a monogamous type of fidelity to a particular dog, and in chows especially the oath of fidelity is seemingly irrevocable. Lorenz has advanced a theory that explains the difference in this fixed type of object relationship characteristic of wolf-derived dogs as contrasted with other canine varieties. It would carry us far afield to elaborate his hypothetical premises here. Instead it is interesting to note that the behaviour described as grief, denial, and time-limited anorexia following the death of Angelene seems similar to what we see in man during acute phases of the mourning process. Corky seems to have been able eventually to accept his mistress's absence, but Hachi (wolf-derived no doubt) presumably could not adapt to the change in his life.

Jones (25) has described the behaviour of a ewe when her lamb has died. The ewe does not wish to leave her dead lamb, and if she loses sight of it she "will race around and bleat in demented searching." In order to effect the adoption of another lamb by the "bereaved ewe," the farmer

> quickly ties a length of twine to the lamb's neck and then, when the ewe is near, gives it a little tug. The ewe sees movement, fancies her lamb is alive, and makes to follow. The lamb is kept moving with little tugs of the string until the ewe is

following it into the barn, where it is quickly whisked out of sight round the corner and as rapidly as possible a live lamb is presented to the questing mother.

We can infer from this report that the anxiety attendant on the separation of the dead lamb from its mother is short-lived when a viable substitute is carefully introduced as a new object. Movement as an indicator of life is quite important in sheep. When a viable moving lamb could be substituted for the dead one, the ewe presumably did not know the difference provided no delay occurred. The primitiveness of this response is one that is akin to the functional substitution that is possible for the human neonate in the early months of life. The association of life with bodily movement is also not limited to sheep. We know it is frequently used as evidence of life or death by man as well. Dr Schneirla described the behaviour of a cat, reared with a rat, when the two were separated. The cat yowled, cried, ate very little, and lost weight. Similar accounts for various birds have been recorded by Lorenz and others. The reports of the dogs, unlike that of the ewe, seem to indicate a reaction that includes greater specificity and differentiation of the object.

Spitz (31) writes that substitution of the mother or absence from the mother prior to the sixth month does not give rise to anaclitic depression. If the mother was a "good" object, removal after the sixth month for an unbroken period of three months gave rise to anaclitic depression, whereas if the mother had been a "bad" one, the incidence of depression was markedly reduced, as was its severity when it occurred. Spitz relates these findings to the ego organization in the second half of the first year. The ego then can coordinate "elementary perception and apperception," can co-ordinate elementary volitional motility, and has a capacity for elementary differentiation of affect as is involved in the capacity to produce distinctly discernible positive or negative affective reactions on appropriate stimulation." Before six months, the infant has achieved no locomotion and so is quite passive in its social demands from the environment. The adult initiates all activity. In the sheep, the response seemingly is that of the young child before the sixth month of age. In both, substitution and equivalence are possible without difficulty.

The reports of simian responses to death are more impressive in connexion with an evolutionary concept of the mourning process. Professor Washburn has sent me the following direct account of his observations of baboons:

I witnessed one case of the relations of a mother to a dead baby baboon. One day I heard a tremendous scream of a kind I had not heard before. When I located the troop of baboons (a troop which I had seen repeatedly and knew well) I saw that one of the larger babies was dead. A baby of this size jumps on its mother's back when the troop moves and takes care of itself pretty well. The mother walked away from the baby, but the largest male of the troop refused to leave it and set up a terrific noise of screaming and barking until the mother came back. She then picked up the baby and carried it while walking on three legs. This process was repeated at least four or five times until the troop finally reached their sleeping trees.

I believe this case is unique in that it was the leader of the troop who urged the mother back to the baby after she had left it. Small babies who die are carried by the mother without the urging of other baboons. I never saw this, but it has been observed many times.

The need to deny death and effect separation is inferred from this first-hand report. Zuckerman (35) also in studying baboons has found similar behaviour indicative of the denial of death. Thus young animals would cling to the carcasses of their dead mothers, or mothers would cling to their dead young, and in the London Zoological Gardens baboons as well as apes tried to prevent the removal of a dead animal as if it were the abduction of a live one. Even in the sexual sphere, "when a female baboon dies in a 'sexual fight' on Monkey Hill, the males continue to quarrel over her dead body, which they also use as a sexual object until it is forcibly removed by the keepers." This retention of the dead and attempt to treat it as still living is characteristic only for the higher anthropoids and man. Other species may show some response to the death of the object, but deal with the actual dead body as dead and having no functional appeal. Zuckerman concludes that "monkeys and apes . . . react to their dead companions as if the latter are alive but passive." This may be the manifestation of the primitive denial of death mechanisms relating to separation anxiety that is seen in early stages of mourning in man. Eissler, however, feels that only the human species knows of death and that the apes are ignorant of it. This may be so; animals, however, can discern things that are not alive, so that responding to non-living animals as if they were alive seems rather to involve a denial-like mechanism.

Chimpanzees seem to show even more dramatic responses to death. Brown in his paper "Grief in the Chimpanzee" (1879), writing about the behaviour of the surviving chimpanzee after his partner died, states:

With the chimpanzee, the evidences of a certain degree of genuine grief were well marked. The two animals had lived together for many months, and were much attached to each other; they were seldom apart and generally had their arms about each other's neck; they never quarrelled, even over a pretended display of partiality by their keeper in feeding them, and if occasion required one to be handled with any degree of force, the other was always prepared to do battle in its behalf on the first cry of fright. After the death of the female, which took place early in the morning, the remaining one made many attempts to rouse her, and when he found this to be impossible his rage and grief were painful to witness. Tearing the hair, or rather snatching at the short hair on his head, was always one of his common expressions of extreme anger, and was now largely indulged in, but the ordinary yell of rage which he set up at first, finally changed to a cry which the keeper of the animals assures me he had never heard before, and which would be most nearly represented by hah-ah-ah-ah-ah, uttered somewhat under the breath, and with a plaintive sound like a moan. With this he made repeated efforts to arouse her, lifting up her head and hands, pushing her violently and rolling her over. After her body was removed from the cage—a proceeding which he violently opposed—he became more quiet, and remained so as long as his keeper was with him, but catching sight of the body once when the door was opened and again when it was carried past the front of the cage, he became violent, and cried for the rest of the day. The day following, he sat still most of the time and moaned continuously—this gradually passed away, however, and from that time he has only manifested a sense of a change in his surroundings by a more devoted attachment to his keeper, and a longer fit of anger when he leaves him. On these occasions it is curious to observe that the plaintive cry first heard when the female died is frequently, though not always, made use of, and when present, is heard towards the close of the fit of anger. It may well be that this sound having been specialized as a note of grief, and in this case never having been previously called into use by the occurrence of its proper emotion, now finds expression on the return of even the lesser degree of the same feeling given rise to by the absence of his keeper, and follows the first outbreak of rage in the same manner as the sobbing of a child in the natural sequence of a passionate fit of crying. It may be noted too, that as his attachment to his keeper is evidently stronger than when there was another to divide with him the attention which they received, the grief now caused by the man's absence would naturally be much stronger and a more exact representation of the gestures of grief would be made.

Notwithstanding the intensity of his sorrow at first, it seems sufficiently evident that now a vivid recollection of the nature of the past association is not present. To test this a mirror was placed before him, with the expectation that on seeing a figure so exactly like his lost mate, some of the customary signs of recognition would take place, but even by caressing and pretending to feed the figure in the glass, not a trace of the expected feeling could be excited. In fact, the only visible indication of a change of circumstances is that while the two of them were accustomed to sleep at night in each other's arms on a blanket on the floor, which they moved from place to place to suit their convenience, since the death of the one, the other has invariably slept on a cross-beam at the top of the cage, returning to inherited habit and showing, probably, that the apprehension of unseen dangers has been heightened by his sense of loneliness.

On looking over the field of animal emotion it seems evident that any high degree of permanence in grief of this nature belongs only to man; slight indications of its persistence in memory are visible in some of the higher animals and domesticated races, but in most of them the feeling appears to be excited only by the failure of the inanimate body, while present to the sight, to perform the accustomed actions.

The foundation of the sentiment of grief is probably in a perception of loss sustained in being deprived of services which had been of use. An unrestrained indulgence in an emotion so powerful as this has become in its higher forms, would undoubtedly prevent due attention to the bodily necessities of the animal subjected to it; in man, its prostrating effects are mainly counteracted by an intelligent recognition of the desirability of repairing the injury suffered, and in him, therefore, the feeling may exist without serious detriment to his welfare, but among the lower animals it would seem probable that any tendency to its development would be checked by its own destructive effects—the feeling, for instance, would most frequently occur on the death of a mate—a deep and lasting grief would then tend to prevent a new association of like nature and would thus impede the performance of the first function of animal in its relation to its kind—that of reproduction.

We can see illustrated here the shock, grief, and separation anxiety stages characteristic of the acute mourning responses of man. The sustained mourning work seemed, however, to be absent. This phase of the mourning process seems to be uniquely human. Brown suggests this is because of memory differences. The difference in type of object relationships with intra-psychic representation of specific objects and structuralizations would be the more precise explanation. The apparent anger of the chimpanzee at his inability to rouse his dead companion is seemingly connected with the impotent grief activity described above for man. To be sure, we might postulate that this could be reflective of anger at being left or frustrated, but this would be only a speculative interpretation of these data. In our patients this anger response is often found, though concealed by the depression that is present.

Garner (22) has also reported extensively on the history and observations made on a particular chimpanzee, Aaron, which he studied extensively from his capture in the jungle until his death in captivity. I shall quote parts of his report, as they pertain to our present interest.

At the time of his capture his mother was killed in the act of defending him from the cruel hunters. When she fell to the earth, mortally wounded, this brave little fellow stood by her trembling body defending it against her slayers, until he was overcome by superior force, seized by his captors, bound with strips of bark, and carried away into captivity.

After he was captured, Aaron was placed with another chimpanzee, Moses. In time Moses fell ill, and the following reaction was reported:

At night, when they were put to rest, they lay cuddled up in each other's arms, and in the morning they were always found in the same close embrace.

But on the morning Moses died the conduct of Aaron was unlike anything I had observed before. When I approached their snug little house and drew aside the curtain, I found him sitting in one corner of the cage. His face wore a look of concern, as if he were aware that something awful had occurred. When I opened the door he neither moved nor uttered any sound. I do not know whether or not apes have any name for death, but they surely know what it is.

Moses was dead. His cold body lay in its usual place; but it was entirely covered over with the piece of canvas kept in the cage for bed-clothing. I do not know whether or not Aaron had covered him up, but he seemed to realize the situation. I took him by the hand and lifted him out of the cage, but he was reluctant. I had the body removed and placed on a bench about thirty feet away, in order to dissect it and prepare the skin and the skeleton for preservation. When I proceeded to do this, I had Aaron confined to the cage, lest he should annoy and hinder me at the work; but he cried and fretted until he was released. It is not meant that he shed tears over the loss of his companion, for the lachrymal glands and ducts are not developed in these apes; but they manifest concern and regret, which are motives of the passion of sorrow. But being left alone was the cause of Aaron's sorrow. When released he came and took his seat near the dead body, where he sat the whole day long and watched the operation.

After this Aaron was never quiet for a moment if he could see or hear me, until I secured another of his kind as companion for him; then his interest in me abated in a measure, but his affection for me remained intact. . . .

The new companion, Elisheba, a female, became ill, and once more the opportunity to observe Aaron's reactions presented itself. Hour after hour Aaron sat holding her locked in his arms. He was not posing for a picture, nor was he aware how deeply his manners touched the human heart. Even the brawny men who work about the place paused to watch him in his tender offices to her, and his staid keeper was moved to pity by his kindness and his patience. For days she lingered on the verge of death. She became too feeble to sit up; but as she lay on her bed of straw, he sat by her side, resting his folded arms upon her and refusing to allow any one to touch her. His look of deep concern showed that he felt the gravity of her case in a degree that bordered on grief. He was grave and silent, as if he foresaw the sad end that was near at hand. My frequent visits were a source of comfort to him, and he evinced a pleasure in my coming.

On the morning of her decease I found him sitting by her as usual. At my approach he quietly rose to his feet and advanced to the front of the cage. Opening the door, I put my arm in and caressed him. He looked into my face and then at the prostrate form of his mate. The last dim sparks of life were not yet gone out, as the slight motion of the breast betrayed; but the limbs were cold and limp. While I leaned over to examine more closely, he crouched down by her side and watched with deep concern to see the result. I laid my hand upon her heart to ascertain if the last hope was gone; he looked at me, and then placed his own hand by the side of mine, and held it there as if he knew the purport of the act.

At length the breast grew still, and the feeble beating of the heart ceased. The lips were parted, and the dim eyes were half-way closed; but he sat by as if she were asleep. The sturdy keeper came to remove the body from the cage; but Aaron clung to it and refused to allow him to touch it. I took the little mourner in my arms, but he watched the keeper jealously and did not want him to remove or disturb the body. It was laid on a bunch of straw in front of the cage, and he was returned to his place; but he clung to me so firmly that it was difficult to release his hold. He cried in a piteous tone and fretted and worried, as if he fully realized the worst. The body was then removed from view, but poor little Aaron was not consoled.

After this he grew more attached to me than ever. When I went to visit him he was happy and cheerful in my presence; but the keeper said that while I was away he was often gloomy and morose. As long as he could see me or hear my voice, he would fret and cry for me to come to him. When I had left him, he would scream as long as he had any hope of inducing me to return.

A few days after the death of Elisheba the keeper put a young monkey in the cage with him, for company. This gave him some relief from the monotony of his own society, but never quite filled the place of the lost one. With this little friend, however, he amused himself in many ways. He nursed it so zealously and hugged it so tightly that the poor little monkey was often glad to escape from him in order to have a rest. Both the task of catching it again afforded him almost as much pleasure as he found in nursing it.

Shortly after Elisheba's death, Aaron himself died. Not having been present during his short illness or at the time of this death, I cannot relate any of the scenes accompanying them; but the kind old keeper who attended him declares that he never became reconciled to the death of Elisheba, and that his loneliness preyed upon him almost as much as the disease.

The description of Aaron's reactions, though coloured by the sentimental terms used by Garner, could seemingly be a behaviouristic account of the acute mourning phase in man. Again we have no evidence of mourning work *per se*, but we have ample evidence of grief-like reactions following what seems to have been some form of meaningful object relationship. The possible utilization of Garner as a new object after Moses' death bears some similarity to the recathectic phase following the completion of the mourning work.

Yerkes (33) has described the screaming responses of survivors in gorillas and monkeys, as well as in chimpanzees. In other reports (34), surviving animals insisted on following the body of the deceased companion when it was removed, and on being prevented from doing this, cried for a while, and then became listless and spiritless for several days. They further state "that depression, grief, and sorrow are occasionally manifested by the chimpanzee is beyond dispute. Definitely established also is the fact that weeping in the human sense does not occur. The typical approach to it is whining, moaning, or crying in the manner of a person in distress. Tears we have never observed.''

This tearless moan has been reported to the author by two patients. In one instance when the patient first saw the corpse of his mother, he cried and screamed in what was described as ''an inhuman howl.'' He had no tears. In the second case, the patient on hearing of the death of her mother screamed and shrieked ''like an animal'' but without tears. In both instances the tears occurred after the shock period passed and the grief phase came into focus. This crying response, unlike the tears accompanying grief and depression, is very rarely recovered in any but the original stimulation situation. It is transitory, but undoubtedly is a most primitive means of communication of the unpleasant affect accompanying the first awareness of the death of the object. This initial human reaction, though infrequently reported in man, seems to be more common in anthropoids.

The cry heard in the howling monkeys when there is an acute separation from the mother has been described by Carpenter. It serves initially to indicate distress in the young animal and can signal retrieving activity. Concomitantly, the mother wails and groans until recovery of the infant occurs. The cries of the infant serve as cues which localize it for the other animals that might retrieve it, while the mother's wails not only express her distress, but focus the activities of the clan on recovery of the infant, while also producing stimulation to which the infant may orient and move. Carpenter has been able to distinguish and categorize these cries so that they can be identified.

Carpenter, studying gibbons, has also identified the separation cry of the infant. In gibbons, the family groupings are monogamous, and are inferred to be relatively stable. Thus the tie between infant and mother may more clearly approximate to that of the human infant. Carpenter has reported an interesting observation on the mother-dead child interaction. He states, ''I have observed two rhesus mothers which carried dead babies until only the skins and skeletons remained. They guarded these remains persistently for over three days and seemed confused by the lack of normal responses on the part of the dead infants.'' He reported no crying on the part of the mothers, but Garner has noted that monkeys do not talk when alone, so perhaps the auditory signals between the mothers were sufficient stimuli and this more distressed response was not evoked.

On the basis of the above data and discussion, the hypothesis is advanced that infra-human mammals do show responses to the death of significant figures in their environment. The anthropoids and chimpanzees particularly seem to react in a fashion similar to those of the acute mourning stages as seen in man. No data or evidence exist that true mourning work occurs after the acute reactions. The level of ego functioning in these animals would be comparable to that of a very young pleasure-seeking child. Further investigations of mourning responses in children of various developmental levels of integration are needed to complete our ontogenetic picture of this process of adaptation. It is to be hoped that anthropologists and psychologists may also assist in providing us with additional facts that can confirm or refute the propositions presented in this section.

IV. SUMMARY

The mourning process as an adaptational adjustment of the internal psychic milieu to an altered external milieu has been discussed. This process involves the series of responses to the loss of the object as well as the later reparative aspects of the process. Adaptation must include the capacity to adjust to the failure of a prior adaptation, as well as the capacity to make the initial adaptation. One example of this situation is seen in the response to the death of a significant object. In man, the object relationships that existed prior to death can become anti-adaptational after that object is no longer existent. In order to re-establish ego equilibrium, a mourning process begins. This process consists of an acute and a chronic stage. The first stage may seemingly be seen in mammalia and birds, especially in chimpanzees and baboons. The chronic mourning stage, consisting mainly of the mourning work of object decathexis, is predicated on a qualitatively different type of psychic organization characteristic of the more mature human ego (intra-psychic differentiation and object representation, memory, reality-principle secondary process thinking). Apparently phylogenetic evolution has allowed, through natural selection, for additional adaptation with new object ties after reality has interfered with a prior object relationship. In man object replacement after death depends upon the instinctual needs of the mourner, the degree of energy liberation or replenishment resulting from the mourning process, and the maturity of the ego and the superego. The cathexis of new objects is not part of the mourning process *per se.* but an indicator of its degree of resolution. The objects newly chosen may be substitutes or replacements, but are rarely exact equivalents for the lost object.

REFERENCES

The individual papers and works of Sigmund Freud are referred to specifically in the body of the paper. Wherever possible Standard Edition has been utilized, in other instances the Collected Papers is cited. These latter references are specifically noted below.

1. Alexander, F., Ham, G., and Carmichael, H. (1951). "A Psychosomatic Theory of Thyrotoxicosis." *Psychosom, Med.,* 13, 18–35.
2. Bernard, C. (1865). *An Introduction to the Study of Experimental Medicine,* p. 226. (New York: Dover Publications, 1957.)
3. Binswanger, L. *Sigmund Freud: Reminiscences of a Friendship,* p. 106. (New York: Grune and Stratton. 1957.)
4. Brown, A. E. (1879). "Grief in the Chimpanzee," *American Naturalist,* 13, 173–175.
5. Cannon, W. B. *The Wisdon of the Body,* p. 333. (New York: Norton, 1939.)
6. Carpenter, C. R. (1934). "A Field Study of the Behavior and Social Relations of Howling Monkeys." *Comp. Psychol. Monograph,* 10, 1–168.
7. ———(1940). "A Field Study in Siam of the Behaviour and Social Relations of the Gibbon." *Comp. Psychol. Monograph,* 16, 1–212.
8. ———(1942). "Societies of Monkeys and Apes." *Biological Symposia,* 8, 177–204.
9. Darwin, C. *Origin of Species by Means of Natural Selection* (1859), and *The Descent of Man and Selection in Relation to Sex* (1871) p. 1000. (New York: Modern Library.)
10. ———. *The Expression of the Emotions in Man and Animals.* (London: Murray, 1872.)
11. Deutsch, H. (1937). "Absence of Grief." *Psychoanal. Quart.,* 6, 12–22.
12. Eidelberg, L. (1959). "The Concept of Narcissistic Mortification." *Int. J. Psycho-Anal.,* 40, 164–168.
13. Eissler, K.R. *The Psychiatrist and the Dying Patient,* p. 338. (New York: Int. Univ. Press, 1955.)
14. Federn, P. *Ego Psychology and the Psychoses,* p. 375. (New York: Basic Books, 1952.)
15. Fleming, J. and Altschul, S. (1959). "Activation of Mourning and Growth by Psychoanalysis." *Bull. Philadelphia Assoc. for Psychoanal.,* 9, 37–38.
16. French, T. M. Personal Communication.
17. Freud, A. *The Ego and the Mechanisms of Defence.* (London; Hogarth, 1936.)
18. Freud, S. (1892). Letter to Joseph Breuer (June 29, 1892). *C.P.,* 5, 25–26.
19. Freud, S., and Breuer, J. (1892). "On the Theory of Hysterical Attacks." *C.P.,* 5, 27–30.
20. Freud, S. *The Origins of Psycho-Analysis: Letters, Drafts and Notes: 1887–1902,* p. 486. (New York: Basic Books, 1954.)
21. ———(1938). "Splitting of the Ego in the Defensive Process." *C.P.* 5, 372–375.
22. Garner, R. L. *Apes and Monkeys: Their Life and Language.* (Boston: Ginn, 1900.)
23. Hartmann, H. (1939). *Ego Psychology and the Problem of Adaptation.* (New York: Int. Univ. Press, 1958.)
24. Jones, E. *Sigmund Freud: Life and Work.* (London: Hogarth, 1953–7. 3 vols.)
25. Jones, J. L. (1958). "Animal Psychology on the Farm." *Country Life,* 1512–1513.
26. Klein, M. (1938). "Mourning and Its Relation to Manic-Depressive States." In: *Contributions to Psychoanalysis,* pp. 311–338. (London: Hogarth, 1948.)
27. Lindemann, E. (1944). "Symptomatology and Management of Acute Grief." *Amer. J. Psychiat.,* 101, 141–149.

28. Lorenz, K. *King Solomon's Ring*, p. 202. (London: Methuen, 1952.)

29. ———. *Man Meets Dog*. (London: Methuen, 1954.)

30. Schneirla, T. C. Personal Communication.

31. Spitz, R. A. (1946). "Anaclitic Depression." *Psychoanal. Study Child*, 2, 313–342.

32. Washburn, S. L. Personal Communication.

33. Yerkes, R. M. *Almost Human*, p. 278. (New York: Century, 1925.)

34. Yerkes, R. M. and Yerkes, A. W. *The Great Apes*, p. 652. (New Haven: Yale Univ. Press, 1929.)

35. Zuckerman, S. *The Social Life of Monkeys and Apes*, p. 357. (London: Kegan Paul, 1932.)

PART III

CHARACTERISTICS OF PATHOLOGICAL MOURNING

Introductory Notes to Chapter 12

Rita V. Frankiel

Bowlby began his major work in this area with a monograph for the World Health Organization on deprivation of maternal care (1951). In this work, he amassed statistics on the devastating effects of maternal deprivation, demonstrating that early loss of the mother without adequate substitute care-givers was associated with delinquency and criminality in later life and with severe and long-lasting psychiatric illness.

The paper included in this volume is the fifth in a series exploring the meaning and consequences of object loss in early childhood. His twofold thesis in this entire body of work is, first, that once the tie to a mother figure is formed, separation anxiety and grief result when that tie is ruptured, initiating processes of mourning; and, second, that in early life, these mourn-ing processes often take a pathological turn and predispose the child to later psychiatric illness. The first part of his thesis, that even very young children mourn, stirred a major controversy in the psychoanalytic literature (see especially Bowlby [1960] and responses by Anna Freud, Spitz, and Schur in the same journal). This disagreement will be summarized in section 5, which addresses the question, "Do children mourn?"

In "Processes of Mourning" (1961), Bowlby's view of the stages of the mourning process in adults and children is set forth. The first stage is characterized by perseveration of thought, feeling, and behavior oriented toward the lost partner, weeping, and aggressive thought and action. These have as their function the recovery of the object. When this is not successful and the object does not appear, in normal mourning these behaviors gradually disappear over time. In the next phase, despair and disorganization come to the fore, succeeded finally by reorganization and hope. In pathological mourning the searching, perseveration, and aggression persist, often in dis-guised forms. The bereaved person remains preoccupied with the lost object, organizing his or her life as though the object were still recoverable.

In the paper reprinted here, Bowlby further develops his argument that adults and children have similar patterns of mourning. What is characteristic of pathological mourning is the inability to acknowledge and express yearning for and angry striving for the return of the lost object. Instead, the striving is repressed and unconscious, and, thus insulated from change, it persists. Bowlby describes four patterns of pathological mourning—unconscious yearning to recover the object; persistent anger and reproach; vicarious caring for someone else who is bereaved; and denial that the object is permanently lost. Following Engel (see chapter 1), Bowlby makes an analogy between recovering from loss and the process of healing from a wound or a burn. If the processes of mourning take a favorable course, eventually there will be a renewal of the capacity to make and maintain loving attachments; if they become pathological, this function remains impaired to some extent. Bowlby takes issue with the insistent focus by psychoanalytic writers since Freud on identification as central in the resolution of mourning. He also disagrees with Melanie Klein, feeling that her emphasis on guilt and reparation draws attention away from processes of mourning, particularly searching for the lost object and experiencing and expressing the need to reclaim the lost object. These disagreements with the major psychoanalytic figures of this era have probably contributed greatly to the lack of attention to Bowlby's less controversial but vastly significant contributions to understanding the events in external reality that can lead to a pathological mourning process.

12. Pathological Mourning and Childhood Mourning

John Bowlby

This is the fifth in a series of papers in which I am exploring the theoretical implications of the behavior to be observed when young children are removed from the mother figures to whom they are attached and are placed with strangers. The thesis I am advancing is twofold: "first, that once the child has formed a tie to a mother-figure, which ordinarily occurred by the middle of the first year, its rupture leads to separation anxiety and grief and sets in train processes of mourning; secondly, that in the early years of life these mourning processes not infrequently take a course unfavourable to future personality development and thereby predispose to psychiatric illness." Since in earlier papers I have discussed the theory of separation anxiety and mourning, it is to the second part of the thesis that this and later papers are directed.

In the preceding paper, "Processes of Mourning" (5), reasons were given for dividing healthy mourning, whether it occurs in human infants or adults or in lower species, into three main phases. Particular attention was given to the first phase, during which the instinctual response systems binding the bereaved to the lost object remain focused on the object, because during this phase yearning and an angry effort to recover the lost object seem to be the rule. The hypothesis was advanced that, so far from being pathological, an open expression of such angry striving to recover the object is a sign of health and that it enables the bereaved gradually to relinquish the object. What seems to characterize much pathological mourning is an inability to accept and express this striving; instead, it becomes repressed and unconscious and so, insulated from change, persists.

If grief itself is to be regarded as a disease, as Engel (11) has persuasively

Reprinted by permission of the author's estate and International Universities Press, Inc. from JAPA 11 (1963):500–41.

argued, how, it may be asked, are the terms "healthy" and "pathological" best applied? Engel's own analogies are useful. If the experience of loss is likened to the experience of being wounded or being burned, the processes of mourning that follow loss can be likened to the processes of healing that follow a wound or burn. Such healing processes, we know, may take a course which in time leads to full, or nearly full, function being restored; or they may, on the contrary, take one of many courses each of which has as its outcome an impairment of function of greater or less degree. In the same way, processes of mourning may take a favorable course that leads in time to restoration of function, namely, to a renewal of the capacity to make and maintain love relationships, or they may take a course that leaves this function impaired in greater or less degree. Just as the terms healthy and pathological are applicable to the different courses taken by healing processes, so may they be applied to the different courses run by mourning processes.

Four main variants of pathological response that are shown by bereaved adults will be considered. I shall begin with those clinical conditions, often suffused with anxiety and depression, in which a persistent and unconscious yearning to recover the lost object is most evident. A main reason for starting here is that an unconscious urge to recover the lost object is a dynamic that probably is present or at least latent in all the other pathological variants of mourning but, because more deeply repressed, is more difficult to see. Moreover, little attention hitherto seems to have been directed to it, and much in my thesis rests on a clear understanding of its role.

The second variant to be considered is intense and persistent anger and reproach expressed toward various objects, including the self. Although such aggressive thought and action, concerned as they often are with events of the past, seem pointless enough to the outsider, I believe their function, of which the subject is not usually fully conscious, is always to achieve reunion with the lost object.[1] And this I believe to be the case even where feelings of revenge and hatred for the lost object seem to be the chief underlying motives, and even, too, where these are directed not toward the lost object but toward the self.

The third variant is the way in which, instead of grieving, some bereaved people become absorbed in caring for someone else who has also been bereaved, an absorption that seems at times to amount to a compulsion.

The fourth variant, denial that the object is permanently lost, is a way of responding very different from the first three. In each of these variants the bereaved acknowledges the reality of loss; the pathology lies in the repression of certain of the instinctual response systems evoked by it. Where, on the other hand, reality of the loss itself is denied such response systems are not evoked: instead a main part of the pathology is at a cognitive level. Such denials, however, rarely represent the complete picture. Probably always they coexist with some awareness of the object's loss. As a result there comes into being a split in the ego of the kind Freud was interested in from the beginning to the end of his professional life (e.g., *Studies on Hysteria* [7] and "Splitting of the Ego in the Defensive Process" [23]).

Although it is convenient to discuss each of these four main variants of pathological mourning separately, it will be evident that they are not mutually exclusive. On the contrary, they exist together in a multitude of combinations and give rise to clinical conditions of protean variety: anxiety and depressive illness, fetishism, and hysterical and psychopathic behavior appear to be among the commoner. Here, however, my concern is with pathological process, not with clinical syndrome. For this reason, instead of attempting to elucidate all the features of any one clinical picture, which is the task most analytic authors set themselves, my interest is to trace the manifold ways in which processes of mourning can affect the lives of individuals. Once this has been well done, it seems likely, the pathology of each of the many clinical syndromes will be easier to decipher.

One very important variant of pathological mourning is a distortion of the process of identification with the object. Since it is this variant that has been the center of theoretical attention in the psychoanalytic literature, its omission requires explanation. One reason is that the problems raised by identification, healthy and pathological, are so complex that together they require a series of papers to themselves. Another is that the primary data on which we are drawing—the responses of young children to separation—do not lend themselves readily to the study of identificatory processes and their deviations. Above all, as just explained, the task I set myself is different from that of most analytic authors who have discussed mourning and its pathology. The reason that Freud (19) became interested in identification with the lost object is because he was grappling with the problem of how it is that reproach, originally directed against the lost object, comes in melancholic patients to be directed instead against the self. Although my discussion will touch on this problem, it does not seek to solve it. Instead, its concern is with the origin and function of the reproach itself.

In describing the four main variants of pathological mourning, illustrations drawn from a number of case reports will be presented. In several of them, it will be noted, the loss that gave rise to the mourning from which the patient is still suffering is the loss of a parent that occurred in the patient's childhood. That this should be so is no accident. Apart from any bias I may have to select such cases, there is much evidence, statistical and clinical, that many though by no means all cases of pathological mourning in adults have originated following a loss in childhood. This evidence, which is of much consequence to my thesis, is reviewed in part elsewhere.

In this paper the main aim is, having first delineated certain pathological patterns of mourning, to compare these pathological patterns with patterns of response that are known to be typical of infants and young children following loss. The result is a conclusion of great significance. This is that the two sets of patterns are substantially the same: in other words, the mourning responses that are commonly seen in infancy and early childhood bear many of the features which are the hallmarks of pathological mourning in the adult.

This discussion will throw into relief the problem of defense. The mourning responses of infancy and early childhood, it will be seen, can no more be understood without reference to defense than can the pathological variants of mourning in adults. Processes of repression, splitting, and denial are all at work. Because, however, the issues raised by them and by their relation to mourning are large and controversial, there is no room to do them justice in this paper.

When describing the four patterns of pathological response that are shown by bereaved adults I shall frequently draw on case material reported by other analysts. The discussion of literature dealing with theory, however, will be postponed till the end. There are three main features of pathological mourning to which I am drawing attention. They are: (1) the role of an unconscious urge to recover the lost object; (2) the tendency for defensive processes to come into action after a bereavement; and (3) the frequency with which individuals prone to pathological mourning have experienced loss of a parent in childhood. Only the literature dealing with the first will be discussed here.

PATHOLOGICAL VARIANTS OF MOURNING

Unconscious Yearning for Lost Object

When in the previous paper I described the first phase of the normal mourning process I emphasized, in addition to perseveration of thought, feeling, and behavior oriented toward the lost partner, two main features: the first is weeping, and the second aggressive thought and action. Both it seemed had as their function the recovery of the object. When in fact the object is only temporarily lost responses of these kinds are useful and this, it was suggested, accounts in large part for their being so regularly the initial reaction to loss. When, however, the object proves to be permanently lost they are no longer useful; in due course, therefore, they may be expected to diminish and disappear. In healthy mourning this is what occurs, and the second and third phases of mourning duly follow: despair and disorganization are succeeded by reorganization and hope. In pathological mourning, on the other hand (or at least in some of its commonest forms), they persist, albeit in disguised forms. The bereaved person remains preoccupied in thought and action with the lost object, not only organizing his life as though it were still recoverable but continuing to weep for it and commonly also to display dissatisfaction and ill temper with his friends and himself.

Consideration of these kinds led to the hypothesis being advanced that an open expression of protest and of demand for the object's return is a necessary condition for a healthy outcome. Such an outcome, it seems, requires the expression both of the yearning for the lost object, accompanied by sadness and crying, and also of the anger and reproach that are felt toward the object for its desertion. That the open expression of *both* these components of ambivalence in healthy mourning is common is well illustrated by the case of Mrs. B. which was chosen by Edith Jacobson (26) as a contrast to her cases of pathological mourning.

Mrs. B. was a middle-aged woman in a state of profound mourning following the loss of her husband. On the one hand, there was evident a deep yearning for him: "She would weep copiously when alone dwelling on her memories of the beloved partner. She would feel the need again and again to visit the same places in the mountains whose beauty they had enjoyed together. . . . A beautiful view . . . now evoked outbursts of weeping in association with her memories of the delight she has shared with her husband." On the other, was hostility directed against him "of which she apparently had been and was fully aware," and also some hostility directed against herself in the shape of remorse for some of her behavior toward him. Incompatible both with each other and with reality though these responses appear, and in some respects indeed are, it is my hypothesis that if mourning is to run a healthy course, it is necessary that they be experienced and expressed. When they are not, it is suggested, reality testing is more likely to fail and the unrealistic demand for the object's return to live on at an unconscious level. Certainly this is characteristic of many cases of pathological mourning.

A case of neurosis in an adolescent girl reported by Root (39) has many features which appear to be fairly typical. The condition, he believed, stemmed from unsatisfactory mourning following the death in an accident of the patient's mother when the patient herself was aged ten. The main symptoms were those of anxiety and depression, with inhibition, indecision, nausea and sickness. "In the analysis," it is reported, "she could not at first comprehend, even intellectually, that she missed her mother." In her dreams and fantasies, on the other hand, mother constantly appeared. In some of them there was a happy reunion with her mother; in others the picture of her mother in a sanatorium, or a frightening scene of her mother "with the gory signs of head and face injuries." From such evidence we may conclude that, unknown to herself, this girl was still in the first phase of mourning and still unconsciously striving for reunion with her lost mother. This view is supported by a remark she made when well on in the analysis: "she spoke of grieving as 'letting her mother die.' " Only after she could accomplish the task of mourning her mother's death, Root reports, did improvement in her condition develop.

There are two points in this girl's history which are of interest. In the first place her initial reaction to her mother's death appears to have been one of incredulity and denial, and there had been no expression of grief. At the same time there was much concern for vicarious figures: "she could shed tears for an orphaned beggar girl," and, during the analysis, "often displaced her sadness onto something else or felt sad for someone else"; moreover, her marriage at seventeen had been to a man who, like herself, had lost his mother when he was aged ten.

The second point refers to the patient's early childhood. Her mother had continued working and the patient had been looked after by maids. How many is not stated, but when one to whom she had been attached left when she was seven, there seems to have been a "tearful parting" which in the analysis "was easily recalled with much emotion and weeping." The question therefore arises whether perhaps this patient had had experiences in the earlier years that had predisposed her to respond to her mother's death with a pathological form of mourning, amounting to an "absence of grief." This is what my theoretical position leads me to predict.

Two of the three cases reported by Joan Fleming et al. (13) show many resemblances to this case of Root's. The first is of a woman of thirty complaining of anxiety and depression precipitated by failure in an examination and disappointment in a love affair. At fifteen years she had left Germany as a refugee and three years later had heard of her father's death; the fate of her mother remained uncertain. Although she insisted that she "never mourned them and never seemed to miss them," in her dreams "she cried as she rushed to meet them." Because she was tearful when reminded of her parents, "she fought against this response by becoming angry and condemning of the grief responses of others." Although in analysis she protested her ability to cope without help, later she admitted: "Time stopped for me at fifteen." The second patient, a man of twenty-three, showed many of the same features.

In both these patients the repression of yearning for the lost object is clear enough, and in neither does the analyst seem to have had too great a difficulty in enabling the patient once more to experience it and thereby to get over it. In other cases the unconscious yearning is more deeply repressed and therefore less evident. Thus Helene Deutsch (10) reports the case of a man whose personality had developed in such a way that, but for a fantasy about a dog, it would be very difficult to convince a skeptic that unconscious yearning was really present.

Helene Deutsch's patient was in his early thirties when, without apparent neurotic difficulties, he came into analysis for nontherapeutic reasons. The clinical picture was one of a wooden and affectionless character. She describes how "he showed complete blocking of affect without the slightest insight. In his limitless narcissism he viewed his lack of emotion as 'extraordinary control.' He had no love-relationship, no friendships, no real interests of any sort. To all kinds of experiences he showed the same dull and apathetic reaction. There was no endeavor and no disappointment. . . . There were no reactions of grief at the loss of individuals near to him, no unfriendly feelings, and no aggressive impulses."

As regards history, we learn that his mother had died when he was five years old and that he had reacted to her death without feeling. Later he had repressed not only the memory of his mother but also everything else preceding her death.

"From the meager childhood material brought out in the slow, difficult analytic work," Helene Deutsch continues, "one could discover only negative and aggressive attitudes towards his mother, especially during the forgotten period, which were obviously related to the birth of a younger brother.

The only reaction of longing for his dead mother betrayed itself in a fantasy, which persisted through several years of his childhood. In the fantasy he left his bedroom door open in the hope that a large dog would come to him, be very kind to him, and fulfill all his wishes. Associated with this fantasy was a vivid childhood memory of a bitch which had left her puppies alone and helpless, because she had died shortly after their birth.''

In each of the cases reported by Helene Deutsch, and especially this one, the bereaved person adopted a hostile, aggressive attitude in place of yearning for the loved figure that is missed. This common tendency has been commented upon by a number of analysts, for example Lindemann (33) and Melanie Klein (28). Edith Jacobson (26), referring to the same thing, notes that ''during treatment severely depressed patients . . . may even consciously realize that, could they only be sad and weep, they would 'feel for the world' again,'' and that when in fact they are able to yearn for what is lost ''a relieving 'sweet sadness' may break through.'' It is my hypothesis that the yearning which these patients are initially unable to experience is the muted expression of a demand for the object's return and of an urge to recover it which is active at an unconscious level. To some extent their anger, even if conscious, is to be understood in the same light. Although in part it seems to represent a wish that the lost and therefore pain-arousing object should be removed or destroyed, in part it is the distorted expression of an angry desire that the object return.

Unconscious Reproach against Object: Self-Reproach

Ever since Freud published ''Mourning and Melancholia'' there has been awareness among analysts of the immense importance that anger with the lost object plays in pathological mourning. Indeed, Freud himself and many others have been so struck by it that its presence has often been thought to be diagnostic of pathological mourning. I believe this to be a mistake, and that anger with the lost object, with others, and with the self is extremely common even in healthy mourning. In fact, only by clear recognition of its presence and function in healthy mourning, I believe, are we able to understand its place in pathological mourning.

In addition to its very existence, there are a number of other features of the anger following loss that have proved puzzling. Among them are its bitterness, its persistence, and its frequent selection of inappropriate targets, including its tendency to turn against the self. The difficulty in understanding these features has given birth to many complexities of psychoanalytic theory. In the theoretical schema advanced here I hope it may be possible to explain them more simply.

The cardinal feature of my hypothesis is that loss of object almost always results in an effort to recover it, and this effort is often the more successful when infused with a dash of aggression. Furthermore, at reunion after temporary loss, reproaches leveled against the object may be expected to insure that the object becomes less prone to go away again. For example, there is many a mother who has vowed never again to leave her young child in strange surroundings after she has been exposed to the reproaches he levels against her following his return home. Such reproaches, more or less bitter, and an angry clinging to her are, we now know, the rule following temporary loss in childhood. In most cases, it is clear, they perform a useful function; they are part and parcel of the effort to undo the loss, to recover the lost object and to insure that it never deserts again. Their appearance after bereavement in a way that seems to be maladaptive is due, I have suggested, to irretrievable loss of object being statistically so rare that it has not been taken into account in the design of our biological equipment.

Such then is the function of anger and reproach. The targets to which they may be directed in a way that is more or less appropriate include the lost object, third parties, and the self. When directed at third parties they are apt to take quasi-paranoid forms;[2] doctors or others connected with the loss are accused, often unjustly. When directed against the self they give rise to self-reproach. I wish to emphasize that each of these targets may be legitimate. Sometimes the loss has been caused or at least facilitated by third parties; sometimes by acts of omission or commission the bereaved has himself contributed to the loss. Even when in reality this is not so, it may not be altogether unreasonable to suppose it to be so. In all such cases, although the reproaches may be powerless to reverse the loss in question, they cannot be regarded as unrealistic.

It is a main characteristic of pathological reproaches, on the other hand, toward whatever target they are directed, that they are inappropriate to the person reproached. It was their inapplicability to the self in cases of melancholia that struck Freud so forcibly and led him to his famous hypothesis regarding the origin of pathological self-reproaches. "If one listens patiently to a melancholic's many and various self-accusations," he writes, "one cannot in the end avoid the impression that often the most violent of them are hardly at all applicable to the patient himself, but that with insignificant modifications they do fit someone else, someone whom the patient loves or has loved or should love. . . . So we find the key to the clinical picture: we perceive that the self-reproaches are reproaches against a loved object which have been shifted away from it on to the patient's own ego'' (19, p. 248). As a result the anger and reproach felt toward the loved object cease to be conscious and instead persist unconsciously.

Although this hypothesis regarding the origin of pathological self-reproach has been widely accepted by analysts, there are some who have attenuated or even at times reversed it; for example, Melanie Klein and her colleagues and also Weiss (44) have emphasized instead the degree to which reproach against the self is appropriate and reproach against the object not so. The position I am adopting is near to Freud's; it expands his hypothesis by putting it into a more generalized form.

As we have seen, depending on the circumstances of each case and the degree of understanding of the bereaved, blame for loss of object may reasonably be attributed by him to one or more of several persons: the object, the self, and third parties. This being so, in principle reproach directed toward any one person may be shifted away from that person toward any other. In practice, of course, such shifts tend to be of particular kinds and are usually designed to spare either the self or the object. The commonest are away from the self and toward third parties, and away from the object and toward the self. When the self is spared blame, the clinical picture is paranoid; when the object is spared it is depressive. In each case, it is held, the pathology lies not in the existence of anger and reproach but in their displacement away from an appropriate object toward an inappropriate one. As a result angry and reproachful feelings toward the original object become unconscious.

This leads to a consideration of the place of guilt. Within the context sketched, guilt over loss is seen to be generated in at least three different ways. First, there is guilt that springs from a more or less realistic appraisal of the part the bereaved himself has played in the loss, and may be large or small according to circumstances. This was clearly recognized by Freud: there are, he remarks in discussing the self-reproaches of melancholics, "a few genuine self-reproaches . . . scattered among those that have been transposed back'' (19, p. 248). Secondly, there is the rather less realistic guilt that arises from the bereaved knowing consciously or unconsciously that, even if he is not in reality responsible for the loss, he has often wished the lost object away. Much neurotic guilt over loss appears to be of this character. Finally, there is the wholly irrational guilt that arises from the turning toward the self of reproaches initially and more or less appropriately aimed at the object. It was one of Freud's great discoveries to recognize that psychotic guilt is to be accounted for by a shift of this kind.

This picture of guilt and its role in mourning, it will be noted, distinguishes it sharply from grief. In some formulations, especially Melanie Klein's, grief is so closely identified with guilt that the two are almost indistinguishable. In this formulation, on the other hand, whereas grief is conceived as an "amalgam of anxiety, anger and despair following the experience of irretrievable loss" (5), guilt is conceived as resulting from those components of angry reproach which happen, whether appropriately or inappropriately, to be directed toward the self. These different formulations, it will be evident, lead to substantial differences in the content of interpretations that are given to patients suffering from pathological mourning.

It seems probable that it is the turning of anger and reproach away from an appropriate object and toward an inappropriate one, so that one of their main components becomes unconscious, that accounts for their tendency in cases of pathological mourning to persist long beyond the normal period. Experience suggests that, if from the first they are openly expressed toward their appropriate object, both yearning for the lost object and angry reproach against it or others (including the self) tend gradually to fade. In so far as there is hope of recovery they have performed their function: in so far as there is no hope this has been demonstrated beyond peradventure. It is when yearning and reproach are not openly expressed toward their appropriate object that they persist. It is as though secretly and unconsciously hope remains that strenuous enough effort to recover the lost object may still succeed and bitter enough reproach against it for deserting may still prevent repetition. Until the effort is made and the reproach expressed these possibilities remain: and so displaced and unconscious yearning and also angry reproach rumble on over the years causing misery to everyone in their orbit.

Large part though displacement seems to play in accounting for the persistence of angry reproach, another factor probably enters also. It is not only when displaced and unconscious that reproach remains ineffectively expressed. Inevitably when loss is prolonged or permanent it remains so. This fact seems also to contribute to its becoming so bitter. This is best seen by contrasting the psychological situations of subjects exposed to short and to prolonged (or permanent) separations respectively.

When separation is only temporary opportunity soon comes for the expression of the angry reproach felt toward the lost object. Once expressed the affectionate components of the relationship can become active once more and, although anger and reproach may persist, they are constantly corrected and modified by the presence of the object and the positive feelings it arouses. In a situation of prolonged or permanent loss on the other hand, not only is opportunity to express anger and reproach missing but the affectionate components of the relationship inevitably wane. As a result the anger and reproach, never directly expressed, fester.

Thus it is seen that, our biological equipment being what it is, a loss of any kind that is permanent carries with it a special risk that anger and reproach, always evoked by loss, will persist instead of fading. Nonetheless this does not occur in all cases of mourning. As Melanie Klein, Edith Jacobson, and others have pointed out, in the healthy mourning of adults loving memories of the lost object are strong enough to hold these angry reproaches in check, to permit their limited expression, and so to enable the bereaved to get over the loss. Evidently in cases of pathological mourning special conditions are present which lead this process to miscarry. One of them, it is well known, is the existence in the previous attitude of the bereaved of unduly strong tendencies toward both possessiveness and anger for the object. Although this is a point repeatedly made by analysts who have considered the matter, the genesis of this intense ambivalence has not often been linked, as there is evidence it should be, with the bereaved having suffered previous and perhaps repeated separations or rejections, especially in childhood. This is a main plank in my explanation of why it is that some individuals become prone to respond to loss in a pathological way.

I believe the hypothesis here advanced provides a satisfactory explanation of the presence of angry reproach in pathological mourning and thus of its presence too in depressive illness. Nevertheless, it casts light neither on the reasons for the hatred being so often diverted away from the object and toward the self nor on the processes by which that occurs. These I see as a separate set of problems. Since their solution requires an examination of theories of identification, I shall make no attempt in this series of papers to tackle them.

Care of Vicarious Figures

In the case reported by Root (39) and described earlier the girl, although failing to express grief for her mother, had, by contrast, frequently "felt sad for someone else." For example, she used to "shed tears for an orphaned beggar girl."

A similar case was reported a little more fully by Helene Deutsch (10) in the same paper from which the case of the man with the dog fantasy has already been quoted. This patient was "a middle-aged woman without symptoms but with a curious disturbance in her emotional life. She was capable of the most affectionate friendships and love-relationships . . . [and] had the potentiality for positive and negative feelings but only under conditions which subjected her and her love-objects to disappointment. . . . She found vicarious emotional expression through identification, especially with the sad experiences of others. The patient was capable of suffering a severe depression because something unpleasant happened to somebody else. She reacted with the most intense sorrow and sympathy, particularly in cases of illness and death affecting her circle of friends."

At the beginning of every analytic hour the patient wept bitterly and for no apparent reason. During the course of treatment, however, it became possible to discover "how the displaced emotional discharges were related to early unresolved experiences. The original grievous experience was not a death but a loss in the divorce of her parents. It gradually became clear," Helene Deutsch concluded, "that she had actually sought out the situations in which she had an opportunity to share the unhappiness of others, and that she felt a certain envy because the misfortune happened to another and not to herself."

In the lives of persons such as these, two characteristics stand out. One is the way in which they appear to be dogged by ill-fortune, and the other their compulsion to take pity on and to care for other unfortunates like themselves. Often they surround themselves with a succession of "lame ducks." Although much charitable work of value springs from these sources, when the motivation is uncontrolled it is apt to be as much a burden to the receivers as to the bestower.

This tendency of a bereaved person to limit the expression of his own grief and instead to concentrate on succoring some other individual who has also been bereaved is a response that calls on the mechanism of projective identification and is one about which Greene (25) has recently written. This other individual, Greene points out, serves as a vicarious figure [3] onto whom the bereaved person projects both awareness of loss and his own affects of grief and helplessness. In addition, I believe, he projects onto the vicarious figure both his yearning for the lost object and his anger at its desertion of him. As such it is a special elaboration of the patterns already discussed.

For an individual to fill the role of vicarious figure it is necessary either that he himself should have been bereaved or that he be perceived as in some other way both helpless and looking for help. Those who are younger or sick are often picked; occasionally it is an elderly person. In the case of children animals are often selected. By devoting himself to the care of vicarious figures a bereaved person may sometimes seem almost entirely to avoid experiencing sorrow and suffering himself.

Greene suggests tentatively that this proxy response may be a component even in normal mourning. I suspect this to be true: Eliot (12) has described it as frequent among the immediate responses to loss. There can be no doubt, however, that when it plays a dominant role in the reaction the mourning process becomes so distorted as to be pathological. In such cases sorrow, yearning, and despair remain unexpressed; disorganization and reorganization are avoided; salvation is sought through works; and behind a bright and busy exterior lurks depression. Whether in this form it is usefully described as a variant of mourning or whether it is better seen as an alternative to mourning is perhaps a matter of taste.

Although from the psychodynamic point of view the response of succoring a vicarious figure can be seen as part of a defense against the frustration of trying to recover a permanently lost object and the pain of sorrow and disorganization, it can sometimes be seen also from a sociodynamic point of view as filling a role vacuum. In every social group roles are distributed asymmetrically among individuals so that, when one is removed, disequilibrium results. In such circumstances there is pressure on one or other of those remaining to assume the role of the absentee. When a father dies, mother or elder son are likely to assume his role; when a mother dies or deserts it may be an elder daughter who takes her place. In addition, therefore, to internally determined motivation to assume the right of someone who is dead or absent, externally determined social pressures may encourage or even demand it. Thus when an elder daughter on her mother's death assumes the role of "little mother" to her younger siblings, and perhaps also "wife" to her father, and thereby experiences little overt sorrow herself, it is often the outcome of pressures from the family group as well as an expression of her own oedipal wishes.

It is evident that both succoring a vicarious figure and filling a role that is left vacant by the departure of another are important aspects of identification with the lost object. How large a part they play in it, however, remains to be determined.

Denial That Object Is Permanently Lost

In 1927 in a paper on "Fetishism" Freud (22) described two young male patients, each of whom "had refused to acknowledge the death of his father" who in each case had been lost in the patient's childhood. The two cases led Freud to develop his theory of defense in a critical way; he did not, however, relate his findings to the theory of mourning.

Since then a number of cases have been reported in which, secretly but nonetheless consciously, a patient has retained an active belief in the living existence of the figure who has been lost, albeit combined with a public acceptance of the reality of the loss. Since it is a state of mind that was demonstrated very vividly by a mother, Mrs. Q., to whom I gave once-a-week treatment over a long period, I shall draw on her case for illustration.[4]

After making good progress over a period of three years, during which her very intense ambivalence toward each of her parents (overtly positive to her mother and overtly negative to her father) was partially analyzed, Mrs. Q lost her father unexpectedly following an elective operation. Her first intimation of anything untoward was a message from the hospital that he had died suddenly in the night. During the ensuing months she was again intensely depressed, again had ideas of suicide, and described also symptoms of depersonalization. It was unfortunate that at the time of the loss treatment was suspended owing to my absence, and not until the anniversary of the loss was drawing near did she confess to me certain feelings and ideas she had been hiding but which throughout seem to have been conscious.

During the weeks following her father's death, she now told me, she had lived in the half-held conviction that the hospital had made a mistake in identity and that any day they would phone to say he was alive and ready to return home. Furthermore, she had felt specially angry with me because of a belief that, had I been available, I would have been able to exert an influence on the hospital and so enabled her to recover him. Now, twelve months later, these ideas and feelings persisted. She was still half-expecting a message from the hospital, and she was still angry with me for not approaching the authorities there. Secretly, moreover, she was still making arrangements to greet her father on his return. This explained why she had been so angry with her mother for redecorating the flat in which the old people had lived together and why too she had continued to postpone having her own flat redecorated: it was vital, she felt, that when at last her father did return he should find the places familiar. Nevertheless she was not deluded. Side by side with the dynamic system concerned to recover her absent father was a recognition that he was dead and never would return.

Among similar patients described in the literature, Krupp (30) reports the case of another mother, also in her early thirties. Here again there were difficulties with the children, and it was on this account that she had been referred to a social agency. At the age of fifteen years this woman had lost her father overseas. A few months later she had become promiscuous, but shortly afterward had married. From what she said it seemed that, from the first, she had refused to believe her father was dead and so had experienced no grief. For the next eighteen years, moreover, she had persisted in the illusion that her father might still be alive; accordingly she was forever searching for him, for example, in restaurants and other public places. For a time she had had an intensely emotional but platonic extramarital relationship with a man who reminded her of her father; and at the time of referral she was still excessively preoccupied in fantasy with him, to the neglect of her children. In the course of casework, she began to accept the idea that her father was really dead and for the first time began to cry and go through the work of mourning. Following this, fantasies of her extramarital relationship diminished and she developed a more satisfactory relationship with her children.

In the method adopted for meeting loss the mental state of this patient closely resembles Mrs. Q. By both of them the object is recognized to be missing but is judged nevertheless to be recoverable. Given energy and perseverance, the husband or father can be found again and reunion attained. There is loss admittedly, but it is only temporary. It is the permanence of the loss that is denied.

A variant of this is when the bereaved develops a fantasy that, despite everything, he is still in touch with the object. Pollock (35) refers to three such cases, all adults, and each of whom had suffered the death of a parent prior to the sixth birthday.[5] One woman's mother had died when she was four and a half years old. "This woman actually retained her mother in heaven as a live figure. Each night she spoke to her, and the patient knew that mother heard her." She had been unable to mourn, states Pollock, because that would have meant that her mother was dead. Pollock notes that "in all three instances the patients denied ever visiting the cemetery where the deceased parent is buried, and [that] there was a period of amnesia that extended from the moment when the patient was told of the death of the parent until many months later."

Nothing is more important for psychopathology than an understanding of the precise conditions internal to the patient and external to him that promote splits of this kind to occur in the ego. While Freud does not give particulars of the external circumstances surrounding the deaths of the parents in the childhoods of his patients, in the cases reported by Pollock and Krupp and in that of my own patient, Mrs. Q., they were known. In all five cases the loss had not only occurred in the absence of the bereaved but had been sudden. If, as I suspect, these conditions do in fact promote splits, it may be a step to understanding why such splits are so apt to occur in childhood; for young children are usually banished from the scene of death and, since they have little foresight, the event of death is almost bound to be experienced by them as sudden.

There is no problem, however, in understanding why these splits, once begun, persist and why they are kept so secret. To confess to another belief that the object is still alive is plainly to court the danger of disillusion. Only by refusing to match the belief with the beliefs of others can the illusion of the object's presence, immediate or potential, be retained. Every intimate relationship which may tempt the sharing of precious memories and hopes is therefore fraught with risk. No wonder patients of this kind find analysis and all other close relationships such a threat.

As with the other variants of pathological mourning that have been described, denial that the object is permanently lost is consistent with and contributory to a number of different clinical syndromes. Mrs. Q was predominantly depressive though she had also much manifest anxiety and occasional outbursts of hysterical behavior. The mother reported by Krupp seems to have been more psychopathic. One of Pollock's patients suffered principally from depression, another from anxiety, and a third alternated between periods of each. All five were married but, except for Mrs. Q., had severe marital problems.

Although in the literature there has been a tendency to link denial especially with manic conditions, this clearly needs qualification. Denial that the object is permanently lost can be combined with many other defense mechanisms and so lead to a variety of clinical conditions. Depression and also wandering, as in Krupp's case, are common. Indeed, as Stengel (41, 42, 43) has shown so clearly, it seems likely that a large proportion of cases in which pathological wandering is a feature belong here: these people are searching, sometimes consciously, sometimes unconsciously, for the lost figure they believe still exists somewhere. It is when differentiation between self and object is blurred or absent and is replaced by unconscious identification, I suspect, that a manic condition develops. In such cases there is often not only strong identification with the lost object, but also, by means of a demonstration of activity and joy, a brave effort to deny the possibility that the lost object is really gone. This view is consistent with that of many analysts, e.g., Helene Deutsch (9), Lindemann (33), and Lewin (32).

We are now in a position to compare the denial that the object is lost with the repression of yearning with which we began. In both types of case one part of the self believes the lost object to be alive and recoverable. When there is denial of loss, it is believed consciously; when there is repression of yearning, it is believed unconsciously. Here lies the difference between the two. It is a parameter that permits of many degrees of difference, from complete unconsciousness of yearning, as in the case of Helene Deutsch's male patient, to complete consciousness as in the case of Mrs. Q. As a result cases fall on a continuum between the two extremes and present a variety of clinical pictures. Irrespective of which end they tend to lie toward, however, they share one feature in common: grief is only partially experienced because loss is only partially admitted.

COMPARISON OF PATHOLOGICAL WITH
CHILDHOOD MOURNING

In a previous paper (4), a systematic comparison was made between responses to loss as they are commonly exhibited on the one hand by adults and on the other by infants and young children. The conclusion reached ran as follows: "Since the evidence makes it clear that at a descriptive level the responses are similar in the two groups, I believe it to be wiser methodologically to assume that the underlying processes are similar also, and to postulate differences only when there is clear evidence for them. That certain differences between age groups exist I have little doubt, since in infants and small children the outcome of experiences of loss seems more frequently to take forms which lead to an adverse psychological outcome. In my judgment, however, these differences are best understood as being due to special variants of the mourning process itself, and not to processes of a qualitatively different kind.''

Having now examined the nature of the processes at work in mourning and some of the common pathological variants of these processes we are in a position once again to make a comparison. This time it will be between the pathological variants described in the earlier part of this paper and the responses to loss that are commonly to be seen in infancy and early childhood. When this is done the conclusion is reached that many of the features that are characteristic of one or another pathological variant of mourning in adults are found to be almost the rule in the ordinary mourning responses of young children. Yearning for the lost object and also angry reproaches against it readily become unconscious; while vicarious objects are often cared for. Only in respect of denial of permanent loss is direct evidence lacking. Let us consider them one by one.

In the earlier paper I described some of the common patterns of response that were to be observed when healthy young children between the ages of about six months and three or more years are removed from their mother figures and placed with strangers. In particular I emphasized that yearning for the lost object is not only common but also that it is both more intense and more prolonged than is generally supposed. Its relative neglect is no accident, however. On the one hand, the adults in charge of a child find this yearning painful to perceive; on the other, it is subject to processes of distortion and repression which quickly obscure the scene. Thus Laura, aged two years four months, the subject of Robertson's film *A Two-Year-Old Goes to Hospital,* ''would interpolate without emotion and as if irrelevantly the words 'I want my Mummy, where has my Mummy gone?' into remarks about something quite different'' (37, 38). At other times the wish was displaced to another object, as when she chanted, ''I want to see the steam roller, I want to see the steam roller, I want to see my Mummy, I want to see the steam roller.''

Distortions of these kinds start early in the separation period and progress fairly rapidly to a state in which it is only the sensitive observer who will notice them. For example, it will be recalled how a small boy, Patrick, aged just over three years, after he had been in the Hampstead Nurseries for some weeks, ''would stand somewhere in a corner moving his hands and lips with an absolutely tragic expression on his face.'' By this time the movement of hands and lips had ceased to signify anything to anyone unfamiliar with the history of their development. Those who were familiar with it, however, knew that the lip movements were the remnants of a formula that earlier he had repeated over and over again—of how his mother would come for him, would put on his overcoat, and take him home with her; and that the hand movements were the fragments of a mime in which he had demonstrated how she would put on his overcoat, zip up the zipper, and put on his pixie hat.[6] The yearning for the lost object persisted but was in course of undergoing repression and so of becoming unrecognizable. A record of this kind is of special value for the light it throws on cases in which the process has already progressed far, for example, the male patient reported by Helene Deutsch who had ceased to yearn for his mother and had instead taken to leaving his bedroom door open in the hope that the large dog would come to him. In all such cases the yearning persists; but the object of it becomes obscured and changed, and the yearning itself may become repressed and unconscious.

When eventually this repressed yearning for the mother comes into the open again the full force of the affect and of the motivation of which it is a part becomes apparent. In the adult this will happen in the course of success-ful analysis. Angry reproaches for being deserted will alternate with sorrow-ful yearning for the object lost, a sequence that is likely first to be experi-enced within the transference. In the case of young children whose separation has been of limited duration the affect and motivation will become apparent soon after return home. If he has been away only a few weeks, the usual sequence is as follows: initially he seems strangely remote from his mother. In spite of the angry protests at her departure and tearful yearning for her return that he showed following separation, now that he has recovered her he seems unmoved. He may fail to recognize her or simply avoid her; alterna-tively he may respond to her as though he were an automaton. Sooner or later, however, his remoteness ceases and is replaced by clinging, often accompanied by a torrent of tears and reproaches. Thenceforward he insists on never letting his mother out of his sight. Below the facade of remoteness the yearning for the lost object has lived on as a dynamic, ready for active expression as soon as external conditions permit. It is a mental state identical with that seen in the adult patient in all features save its reversibility: whereas in the adult patient suffering from pathological mourning we know it to be very slow and difficult to reverse, in the young child, provided the separation has been limited to weeks only and has not been repeated, it usually reverses spontaneously after a few hours or days.

It is because the yearning for the lost object remains an active dynamic that I find myself unable to agree with the conception of the process recently proposed by Anna Freud (15). In her comments on my earlier paper, while agreeing that the responses to separation can usefully be divided into three phases, protest, despair, and detachment, she calls in question my use of a term[7] that implies a defensive process. In its place she proposes the term "withdrawal," because, she holds, it covers both the manifest behavior and "the internal process of libido withdrawal by which we believe this behavior to be caused." This picture of the processes at work, however, does not square with the observed data. Instead of the child's attitude to his mother developing again gradually and steadily as such a formulation would lead us to expect, it sometimes erupts with a suddenness and intensity which makes it plain that it has been potentially active all along. It is on this evidence that the hypothesis is advanced that, when a young child is in a phase of detachment, strong defensive processes are at work: in the terminology commonly in use, there is counter-cathexis, not withdrawal of cathexis. It is of interest that in an earlier publication (jointly with Dorothy Burlingham [16]) Anna Freud has herself advanced a view of this kind. Since, however, this issue is more closely connected with the theory of defense than with the present topic, a full discussion of it is postponed to a later publication.

Not only is there this evidence of a persistent but unconscious yearning for the lost object during the detached phase of separation,[8] but there is evidence also that after reunion a residue of reproach larger than is suspected may remain. This was shown dramatically by Laura six months after her return home, by which time she had seemed to be her normal self. Late one evening when her parents were viewing a rough version of the film, through a mischance Laura came in to see the final sequences. When the lights went up she was found to be agitated. Suddenly she flushed, turned angrily to her mother and exclaimed, "Where *was* you all the time, Mummy, where *was* you?" then she burst into loud crying and turned to her father for comfort. Not unnaturally her parents were astonished by the strength of the feelings she revealed and were disturbed also that she turned angrily away from her mother.

This episode illustrates not only the length of time after a separation that the feelings aroused by it may persist in latent form but also how much anger

is elicited. Here Laura's anger took the form of reproaches against he:
mother. At other times the anger is directed toward third persons. An example occurred just as Laura and her mother were departing from the hospital
Before leaving the ward, Laura had insisted on taking all her possession:
home with her; even a tattered old book she refused to leave behind. On the
way out she accidentally dropped this book and a nurse, trying to be helpful
picked it up. At this Laura screamed in temper and snatched the book away—
the fiercest feeling she had shown during her whole stay.[9] The function o
the outburst was clear: insistence that she was going home with her mothe
and refusal to be detained in the hospital by the nurse. It is an ange
comparable to that of bereaved persons who feel that would-be comforter:
are trying to rob them of the object they have lost. Mrs. Q.'s anger with me
for not approaching the hospital authorities to arrange for her father's retun
is not very different.

   In these examples the function of the anger is clear; in others it is more
obscure. As I have repeatedly emphasized, young children separated from
their parents in a hospital or residential nursery are notoriously destructive
Often it seems to the onlooker to be both wanton and pointless. If the
hypothesis I am advancing is right, however, it is neither. It is simply ar
expression, gravely intensified and distorted, of the child's anger with hi
mother for deserting him and anger with third parties for detaining him. A
such it is the equivalent in childhood of the intense, persistent, and misdi
rected anger of the melancholic patient and, though expressed in a ver
different way, of the affectionless psychopath also.

   So far, in drawing the comparison I have concentrated attention on th
two variants of pathological mourning first described, repressed yearning fo
the loved object and repressed reproaches against it. Each, it is seen, is o
regular occurrence in childhood. The third and fourth variants occur also bu
are perhaps more limited in incidence.

   Of the third variant, care for a vicarious figure, once again Laura provide
an illustration. Although she herself cried little, Laura was much concerne
when other children cried. On one such occasion a small boy was screamin
piteously. Laura's immediate response was to become solicitous and t
demand that the boy's mother be brought. A little self-righteously she ex
claimed, "I not crying, see!" and then emphatically, "Fetch that boy'
Mummy!" A couple of days later she exhibited a related response, directe
toward another figure. To a nurse who was talking to her she insisted
"My Mummy's crying for me—go fetch her!" Here Laura's grieving wa

projected onto the lost mother herself. This is a mental process identical, I suspect, to that underlying a belief that "lost souls" are searching for their loved ones (14), to which further reference is made in the next section.

Care for a vicarious figure appears to be specially common when siblings suffer loss together. One of them usually mothers the others. Though probably the elder most frequently fills this role, Robertson has recorded cases when it was the younger. For example, another little girl, Paula, who like Laura was under two and a half, when taken away by ambulance with her weeping brother, two years her senior, put her arm round him and said, "I'll look after you."

It seems not unlikely that girls and women respond in this way more often than do boys and men. Both the illustrative adult cases reported earlier were of women. That it is a response that can be evoked early in a little girl's life is brought home to us by both Laura and Paula, and also by observations made in the Hampstead Nurseries during the war (17, pp. 32–33). Plainly in these children, as in adults, the care of a vicarious figure is a response alternative to seeking care from the lost object for themselves.

This brings us to the fourth pathological variant of mourning, denial that the object is permanently lost. Because all the children whom Robertson has observed had lost their mothers only temporarily, he has had no opportunity to observe a development of this kind; the same is true of my other colleague, Christoph Heinicke. That denial can originate during the third year of life, however, is attested by Freud in his paper on "Fetishism" (22). One of the two young men, each of whom "had refused to acknowledge the death of his father," is reported to have lost his father when he was two years of age. (The other was ten.) Of the patients reported by Pollock, all three had lost the parent in question before the sixth birthday. There can be no doubt, therefore, that this variant too originates in childhood even though it may do so less regularly than the first two variants.

Thus we can conclude that responses similar to the first two pathological variants of adult mourning are the rule when young children lose a loved object; that the third, care for a vicarious figure, is common especially in girls; and that the fourth, denial that the object is permanently lost, undoubtedly occurs though with what frequency is not known. There are findings, I believe, that go far to explain why losses occurring in infancy and early childhood have a pathogenic potential. Should loss prove prolonged or permanent, it is now plain, there is great danger that one or more of the pathological variants of mourning will not only be set in train but, once present, will persist, and that as a consequence the child's object relatior will come to be permanently organized on this pattern. Even when loss only temporary danger remains. Once one or more of these pathologic; responses to loss has been active in a personality there is increased likelihoc of its being evoked afresh following further loss. This, I believe, accoun for the development of at least some personalities prone to respond to loss(in later life by pathological mourning.

Nevertheless not every child who experiences either permanent or tempt rary loss grows up to be a disturbed person. To understand why in som cases the experience is pathogenic and in others not so requires that tt conditions which favor reversal and those which promote an overt or late; persistence of the pathological patterns be identified. Among those that a; probably relevant in cases of temporary loss are the length and frequency (the separation, the conditions of care during it, and the attitude of the moth toward the child after his return, especially perhaps the extent to which st accepts and meets his demands for her presence or, on the contrary, forbit and punishes them. The phase of the child's development and the nature (his previous relationship with his mother, while obviously relevant, m; each be of less significance than is usually believed by analysts.

REVIEW OF LITERATURE

In an early section of the previous paper (5) I discussed seven themes the theory of mourning about which there had been controversy in tl psychoanalytic literature. In considering the sixth, ways in which patholog cal mourning is believed to differ from healthy, I gave reasons for n accepting the criteria for pathological mourning that have commonly be(advanced, prominent among which has been anger and reproach against tl lost loved object; and in later parts of that paper and earlier parts of this have explored other criteria. It is time now to consider what place h hitherto been given in the psychoanalytic literature to the first of the ne criteria proposed, the inability to accept and express yearning for and ang reproaches against the lost object.

A reading of the literature shows that an unconscious effort to recover t lost object has not previously been singled out as being, in most pathologic variants of mourning, the principal dynamic at work. Naturally it has n escaped attention altogether, and there are indeed many references to

Nevertheless, although a few are explicit, a majority are only implicit, and it is striking in how many formulations it is virtually absent.

Among many possible reasons for this neglect three stand out. One is the overwhelming emphasis given by Freud to identification with the lost object as the key concept in mourning, an emphasis that has obscured processes which I believe to be more fundamental. A second reason is the tendency of much analytic theorizing to be concerned, not with motivation and with objects and situations in the external world toward which motivation is directed, but with quantities of excitation and with affects as conditions that lead these quantities to become excessive. As a result there are plentiful references to affects, such as unconscious sadness and anger and unresolved grief, and correspondingly few to unconscious striving to recover a lost object and to unconscious reproach designed to discourage repetition of loss.

A third reason for this neglect is the weight given by Melanie Klein and her school to the bereaved's sense of guilt, arising, it is held, from his belief that he was the agent of the loss, and to her emphasis also on his desire in consequence to make reparation. Although the concept of reparation bears some relation to the concept of striving to recover the object, the two are different: reparation springs from a sense of guilt, the effort to recover from a sense of loss. Each is important, but they must be kept distinct.

Let us now consider how individual analysts have treated this theme. In his discussion of the dynamics of healthy mourning, it will be recalled, Freud attached much importance to persistent and insatiable yearning for the lost object. In *Inhibitions, Symptoms and Anxiety,* for example, he emphasizes the unappeasable nature of bereaved longing and attributes to it the pain-fulness of mourning and the onset of defensive processes (21, pp. 171–172). Yet in his discussion of the dynamics of pathological mourning as it mani-fests itself in melancholia there is little reference to this longing. Indeed, by suggesting that the object is abandoned, he seems to take an almost opposite view. In the case of melancholia, he maintains, "the object-cathexis proved to have little power of resistance and was brought to an end. But the free libido was not displaced on to another object; it was withdrawn into the ego. There [it] . . . served to establish an *identification* of the ego with the abandoned object" (19, p. 249). Ever since this time there has been preoccu-pation with identification as the key concept in mourning.

At about the same date Freud makes a brief reference to the inability of the Wolf Man to mourn his sister (20, p. 23). This sister was two years older than the patient and was for him "the most dearly loved member of his family.'' She had committed suicide in her early twenties. Nevertheless, "when the news of his sister's death arrived, so the patient told me, he felt hardly a trace of grief. He had to force himself to show signs of sorrow, and was able quite coolly to rejoice at having now become the sole heir to the property.'' Analysis, however, showed that soon afterward there had been a "substitute for the missing outburst of grief'': he had made a pilgrimage to the burial place of a great poet, to whom his sister had been compared, and had shed bitter tears on the grave. In this account, it will be noticed, though Freud recognizes the repressed and displaced grief, it is at no point linked to motivation. An unconscious desire to recover the object lost is not referred to.[10]

In his published papers the nearest Freud seems to have come to a recognition of the role of striving to recover the lost object is in the paper on "Fetishism'' in which he referred to the two young men each of whom had refused to acknowledge the death of his father. Nevertheless, these cases belong to the category of "denial that the object is permanently lost'' rather than to "unconscious urge to recover the object.'' In a letter of 1921 to Weiss, however, Freud does seem to refer to it (44). Weiss had reported on the case of a man of twenty-seven who had been sent for analysis by his mother because of intense apathy. The patient himself described how he felt himself "separated from the outside world by an impenetrable isolating layer.'' Weiss had diagnosed it as "a case of simple depression without melancholic trait.'' Freud concurred. "The affection is little studied,'' he continues, "I should say, as a surmise, that it is a matter of a simple fixation of high degree on the mother, whom he rejects from time to time, so that nothing then is left him.'' From the rather meager details given it appears that the dynamics of the case were the same as in Helene Deutsch's case, described earlier, of the man whose unconscious longing for his mother was manifest only in his fantasy of the big dog visiting him.

Edith Jacobson's position resembles Freud's. Like him she has, on the one hand, drawn attention to the role that yearning to retain the lost object plays in normal sadness and grief and, on the other, given it relatively little place in her account of pathological mourning. Yet, as with Freud, it is a concept which is readily compatible with her theoretical position. This is well illustrated in her paper "Denial and Repression'' (27), in which she reports a case that seems, like Weiss's, to have much in common with Helene Deutsch's case of the man with the dog fantasy. The man reported by Edith Jacobson is described as similarly detached in all his relationships; in addition he maintained that his only feeling toward his mother was one of "cold resentment." Progress in his analysis, Edith Jacobson reports, was signaled by "waves of affection toward his mother [which] were permitted to appear and to replace his symptoms." Though Edith Jacobson's terminology is one of affect, not motivation, the one is easily translated into the other. In terms of motivation, it is evident, these "waves of affection toward his mother" are equivalent to a longing for her; and it is this longing which had been unconscious until released during the analysis.

Edith Jacobson's case follows the pattern of Helene Deutsch's in another respect also. In both cases the disturbance was thought by the analyst to have had its origin in a separation experience of early childhood. In commenting on her case Edith Jacobson expresses the opinion that "the trauma that had broken up his relationship to his mother" had occurred when the patient was three and a half years old. At this time his mother had had a miscarriage. His father was absent and, although his mother remained at home, she "had been physically sick and depressed for many weeks after. . . . Left in the hands of a maid, he had felt lost and confused."

The theoretical position taken by Helene Deutsch in her paper "Absence of Grief" (10) is not dissimilar to that of Edith Jacobson: once again there is implicit recognition that unconscious longing for the lost mother is at the heart of the psychopathology. For example, when discussing the man with the dog fantasy, Helene Deutsch remarks: "apart from this one revealing fantasy there was no trace of longing or mourning for his mother" (who, it will be remembered, had died when he was five years old.) Despite this reference in the case report to longing as an unconscious motive, however, in the notes at the end of the paper theory is cast in the terminology of affect. "I believe that every unresolved grief is given expression in one form or another," she writes. I "am convinced that the unresolved process of mourning as described by Freud must be expressed in full." Referring to "suppressed affect following loss," she continues: "We must assume that the urge to realization succeeds under the impetus of an unconscious source of affect-energy exactly as in the case of the criminal who is at the mercy of his guilt feelings. I suspect that many life stories which seem to be due to a masochistic attitude are simply the result of such strivings for the realization of unresolved affects."

This mode of theorizing, as Helene Deutsch herself points out, is not unlike that employed by Freud in his reference to the Wolf Man's inability to mourn his sister. It is a mode of theorizing, moreover, that has been followed by both Landauer (31) and Lindemann (33), each of whom has taken mourning and its pathological variants as his focus of attention. In each case a use of the language of affects has had the result that in their formulations the unconscious longing that is part of the urge to recover the lost object, although implicit, has tended to be obscured.

More explicit references to the longing for the lost object are to be found in a contribution by Anna Freud (14) and also in a number of clinical writings that report on cases of compulsive wandering, depression, and suicide. In a paper "About Losing and Being Lost" Anna Freud discusses the connection between wishes to possess and tendencies to lose as they refer to parent figures and to material possessions respectively. In the third part she discusses dreams of the return of the dead during phases of mourning and likens them to "the well-known folklore of the 'lost souls,' i.e., dead people who are supposed to find no rest and [to] wander at night in search of their former loved ones. In both cases," she comments, a libidinal process in the mourner, i.e. longing, appears as projected into the image of the lost object." So long as the ghost is believed searching for his lost loved ones the bereaved continues mourning. In other words, mourning ends when conscious or unconscious searching stops.

The truth of this generalization is well illustrated in the papers by Stengel on compulsive wandering, a symptom, he found, that is commonly associated with pseudologia, episodic depression, and impulses to commit suicide. In his reports of thirty-six cases (42, 42) Stengel draws special attention to two closely connected features. The first is the high frequency of serious disturbance in the patients' relation to their parents in childhood, in particular losses due to death or separation. The second is the desire to seek the lost parent that is often present during the actual episodes of wandering. "Almost all these patients had suffered consciously from the failure of the normal child-parent relation," he writes. "Many felt even in childhood that they had missed something which could never be replaced. In a number this feeling became particularly acute during their periodic depressions, i.e. at the time when the wandering compulsion arose. A few became conscious of the desire to seek for the dead or absent parent. Some imagined immediately before or in this state that the dead parent was not really dead but alive, and perhaps to be met in their wanderings" (41).

Though Stengel gives a central place to the unrealistic urge to seek a lost parent, he does not recognize it as a sequel of childhood mourning having taken a pathological course. As a result, whereas elsewhere in the literature we find attention to mourning and its pathology but without reference to the unconscious urge to recover the object, in Stengel's work we find attention to the urge but without reference to mourning and its pathology.

Elsewhere in the clinical literature Gerö (24), in describing two patients suffering from "neurotic depression bordering on melancholia," emphasizes both the unconscious longing for mother and her care and also the unconscious rage against her for not having provided it that was present in both of them. Analytic progress, he found, turns on the patient becoming conscious "that he desires the breast—that is to say—the mother,"[11] and also on his recognition that his rage is directed against her for having neglected him. In both the cases he reports there was evidence that they had in fact been neglected. One patient is described as having been an unwanted child, "starved of love." The other had been sent to a residential nursery until he was three years old: "he seems never to have forgiven his mother for this separation."

Weiss (44) in his discussion of different forms of depressive illness also refers to the yearning for a former love object. In his view, however, it is not so much the lost mother who is longed for but "the parent or sibling of the opposite sex." Felix Deutsch (8) reasons on the same lines.

In Melanie Klein's writing and that of many of her followers the emphasis is so firmly on the sense of guilt and the need to make reparation that the sense of loss and the striving to recover the lost object tend to be obscured. Indeed, in his comprehensive discussion of the literature on the theory of depression, particularly as it supports Melanie Klein's views, Rosenfeld (40) omits all reference to it. Nevertheless it is not missing from Melanie Klein's own work. For example, she describes how a male patient, unable to experience sorrow, during his analysis "increasingly experienced the grief and longing for [his mother] which he had repressed and denied from his early days onwards." Earlier in the same paper she refers to the need for the ego "to develop methods of defence which are essentially directed against the 'pining' for the lost object" (28).

These same concepts underlie her interpretation of the personality of Fabian, the hero of a story by the French novelist Julian Green (29). Fabian is represented as an unhappy, dissatisfied man, full of resentment, incapable of sympathy, able to make only brief and frustrating liaisons with girls, full of insatiable desire for wealth and success and intense envy for those who possess more than himself. In the course of the story Fabian is enabled to assume the personalities of other people. In one such personality he murders the girl, Berthe, whom the man he has now become was trying, unsuccessfully, to win. In another he becomes fascinated by the eyes of a second girl, Elise, who has for long been hopelessly in love with the man he now is. Her eyes, he finds, have "in them all the tragedy of a longing that can never be satisfied"; and at that moment he realizes they are the eyes of Fabian. Finally, he becomes himself again and, with his mother sitting by his bedside, is overcome by longing to be loved by her and to be able to express his love for her, which he can never do.

In the light of her experience with patients like Fabian and drawing on the other dramatic details of the story Melanie Klein builds up an interpretation of Fabian's personality and the mode of development that lay behind it. A main component of it, she suggests, is that all his life he had been "unconsciously searching . . . for the ideal mother whom he had lost," and unconsciously expressing resentment at the deprivation he had felt "in the earliest feeding relation." While the resentment is expressed in the murder of Berthe, which Melanie Klein suggest was "an expression of the infantile impulses to murder the mother," the longing is to be found in the longing eyes of Elise, the girl whose eyes were Fabian's. Elise, she suggests, "represented the good part of his self which was capable of longing and loving." "The search for the lost ideal self," she continues, "inevitably includes the search for lost ideal objects; for the good self is that part of the personality which is felt to be in a loving relation to its good objects. The prototype of such a relation is the bond between the baby and his mother. In fact, when Fabian rejoins his lost self, he also recovers his love for his mother." In this interpretation it will be seen, although Melanie Klein places more emphasis on orality and the feeding relation and, by implication, the first year of life than I would, her picture of the dynamics underlying this type of personality resembles closely the picture I am advocating and also the ones that lie behind the thinking of Edith Jacobson, Helene Deutsch, and Gerö. By each author unconscious longing for the loved object is thought to coexist with unconscious resentment against it for its earlier neglect. One of the external factors to which Melanie Klein attributes Fabian's condition is the same also: "his mother's lack of affection."

There are at least two other analysts, both influenced by Melanie Klein, in whose thinking about pathological mourning the role of unconscious yearning for, and reproach against, the object can be discerned; in neither case, however, are they placed at the center of the stage.

Referring to pathological self-reproach, Anderson (2) writes: "These self-reproaches have their obverse for there is a plaint, an accusation against the dead person for having left and deserted the mourner."[12] It is a complaint, he points out, that enters also into certain peasant mourning rituals. Nevertheless, in his case histories this insight is little exploited.

Throughout his writing Winnicott shows a deep appreciation of the place of sadness and grief in psychiatric disturbance. In one of his papers (45) he describes his approach to "an intelligent girl of twelve who had become nervous at school and enuretic at night. No one seemed to have realized," he remarks, "that she was struggling with her grief at her favourite brother's death. This little brother had gone away supposedly for a week or two with an infectious fever, but he had not come home immediately as he developed a pain that turned out to be due to a tuberculous hip. The sister had been glad with the rest of the family that he was placed in a good tuberculosis hospital. In the course of time he suffered much more pain, and when at last he died of generalised tuberculosis, she had been glad again. It was a happy release, they had all said."

"Events," comments Winnicott, "had taken place in such a way that she never experienced acute grief, and yet grief was there, waiting for acknowledgment. I caught her with an unexpected 'You were very fond of him, weren't you?' which produced loss of control, and floods of tears. The result of this was a return to normal at school, and a cessation of the enuresis at night."

In another paper (46) Winnicott describes three sessions he had with a boy of nine who was given to compulsive stealing. Disturbances in Philip's home life had begun when he was two years old; and at six he had been sent to an uncle and aunt while a sister was born. During the first interview Winnicott asked him if he was ever sad. To this Philip replied that the worst sadness had happened "a long time ago," a phrase that referred to the time of his sister's birth. "My mother went away," he continued. "I and my brother had to live by ourselves. We went to stay with my aunt and uncle. The awful thing that happened then was that I could see my mother cooking in her blue dress and I would run up to her but when I got there she would suddenly change and it would be my aunt in a different coloured dress." Although Winnicott links the stealing to Philip's desire to find the mother he had lost, in his commentary he seems to place more weight on the birth of the baby, Philip's jealousy of it and envy of his mother's capacity to have it, than on the real loss that Philip had suffered. Philip's hallucination of his mother cooking, it can be inferred, was the result of a split in the ego of the kind described above in the section ''Denial That Object Is Permanently Lost.''

Although striving to recover the lost object has never been at the center of attention in theoretical formulations regarding pathological mourning, it is not without interest to note the place that yearning of other kinds has been given in psychopathology generally. Many analysts from Abraham (1) and Rado (36) to Melanie Klein have emphasized a fixation on the mother's breast and a longing to recover it. Others, including Freud (22, 23), Helene Deutsch (9), and Anny Angel (3) have emphasized the longing in female patients for a penis. Another line of theorizing, favored among others by Rado (36) and Weiss (44), has explored the notion that the missing object is wanted not so much for itself but for its value in restocking the ego with ''narcissistic supplies.'' A review of these hypotheses in the light of further knowledge of object relations and of processes of mourning, healthy and pathological, may lead to their being reappraised.

The resemblance that the mourning processes of childhood bear to pathological variants of mourning in the adult is discussed in the literature of only one main school of psychoanalytic theorizing, that of Melanie Klein. Inevitably it is missing from the literature of those schools which either overlook the possibility or reject the idea that mourning occurs in infancy and childhood. In the work of Melanie Klein and her colleagues, on the other hand, the reality of childhood mourning and of its relatedness to adult mourning is not only recognized but made a central pillar of theory construction. The way in which Melanie Klein treats the connection is at many points very different from the one presented here, however. In the first place, her ideas rest not on the empirical studies of the actual behavior of young children but on reconstructions. In the second, the picture she has of the dynamics of mourning, whether healthy or pathological, in the adult or the child, derives from a theoretical schema that is based on the death instinct, the primacy of persecutory and depressive anxiety, and the overwhelming importance of orality. Since in earlier papers I have given reasons for not accepting this framework, no purpose would be served in describing Melanie Klein's conception further. Nevertheless, trained in this school of thought as I have been, I remain deeply indebted to it for an emphasis on the reality of childhood mourning and its implications for understanding psychiatric illness.

CONCLUSION

In this paper I have had two aims. The first has been to delineate the dynamics of four of the commoner pathological variants of mourning; the second to demonstrate that patterns of response that are typical of these pathological variants in adult life resemble closely the patterns that are typical of mourning processes when they are evoked in infancy and early childhood. The implications of this finding for the theory of childhood pathogenesis will be clear.

Once again the ground traversed has proved controversial. As a result much of the paper has been concerned with clarifying the dynamics of pathological mourning, especially the roles in it of unconscious yearning and unconscious reproach. In presenting clinical material, therefore, I have deliberately selected that which throws into relief the parts played by these two powerful motives; often, it has seemed to me, the original case report has not given them sufficient weight. This I believe to be due partly to their role in healthy mourning not having been fully appreciated and partly to the preoccupation with affect, guilt, and processes of identification, which has marked so much of the psychoanalytic theorizing about pathological mourning. There is no evidence, we have seen, that Freud recognized the part played by the urge to recover the lost object in pathological mourning, despite the fact that he recognized its role in healthy mourning and also detected that self-reproach is often a turning toward the self of reproach originally aimed at the object.

The function of reproach directed against the object seems to have been little discussed. The hypothesis advanced here is that it is to discourage the object from deserting again. It is within this functional context also, I believe, that both the extraordinary bitterness and the persistence of the anger that follows prolonged or permanent loss are to be understood. When separation is only temporary opportunity soon comes for the anger and reproach felt toward the deserting object to be expressed and for love to be revived. When separation is prolonged or permanent, anger and complaint fester while love lies dormant. Though therapeutic technique is outside the scope of these papers, the therapeutic implications of these hypotheses are not negligible. What they imply is that a principal goal in the treatment of many sorts of patient, including some who are anxious and depressed and others who suffer from various forms of character disorder, is to assist them to experience each one of the impulses that are directed toward recovering and retaining the lost object and of the ambivalent feelings associated with them—on the one side the urge to recover, with its accompanying yearning, weeping and sadness; and on the other the complaints and reproaches with their accompanying anger and bitterness.

If this account of the dynamics of pathological mourning is valid, their resemblance to patterns of response commonly seen following loss in early childhood is unmistakable. Although Melanie Klein had also laid much emphasis on the relatedness of childhood mourning to adult mourning, the theoretical context within which she has drawn the comparison is one that in earlier papers I have given reasons for rejecting. In none of the details of her exposition, therefore, do I follow her.

In the case histories recounted in the course of the paper, all but one derived from the writings of others, pathogenesis has again and again been attributed by the analyst reporting them to a loss, temporary or permanent, that occurred in the patient's early years. What appears in each case to have happened is that processes of mourning, having been evoked in early childhood, took a pathological turn in a way typical of them in that period of life; and that, over the years, the pathological processes have either persisted substantially unchanged or, having temporarily modified, have been evoked afresh by a further loss. The extensive evidence that shows that a loss of a parent in the early years is especially frequent in persons who later suffer from psychiatric illness is reviewed elsewhere (6).

Repeatedly during the discussion of pathological mourning it has been necessary to refer to defense. I have described repression of yearning for the lost object, displacement of reproaches against it, denial of the reality of loss, splits in the ego, the role of projective identification, and the use as defenses both of aggression and of the care of a vicarious figure. Loss, it is clear, can readily evoke defense. Furthermore, observation of young children who either temporarily or permanently lose their mothers furnishes us with information on how some of these defenses originate. Do these observations, we may ask, throw fresh light on the nature of defensive processes? It is my belief they do, and it is to exploring this possibility that further publications will be directed.

NOTES

1. Throughout this series of papers I am using the concept of function in a way that is nonteleological. Thus the function of aggressive thought and action following loss is conceived on the same model as the physiologist conceives the function of inflammation following infection. In one case the function is to achieve reunion, in the other to repel bacteria: in both the concept of purpose is absent. "In order to emphasize that the recognition and description of end-directedness does not carry a commitment to Aristotelian teleology as an efficient causal principle," the term *teleonomic* has been proposed by Pittendrigh (34): it denotes any end-directed system.

2. Although a response of this kind may result from the projection onto another of the bereaved person's own unconscious hostile wishes toward the lost object, and so be truly eligible for the adjective "paranoid," I do not believe this is always so. At times I suspect such behavior to be no more than the fury of frustration at loss being more or less irrationally expressed. For this reason I term it "quasi-paranoid." Lindemann (33) appears to make the same distinction.

3. Greene's term is "vicarious object." Since, however, the person in question is acting as a substitute for the self and not the loved object, the term "vicarious figure" is preferable.

4. Mrs. Q had been referred for help with her little boy of eighteen months because he had been refusing to eat and was seriously underweight, and her own emotional disturbance had seemed to be contributing to his condition. This had been confirmed by psychiatric investigation which had found her to be in a sub-acute agitated depression with ideas of suicide and of killing the baby, a condition that appeared to have developed during the puerperium. For many years previously, however, she had had isolated episodes when she went berserk and threw saucepans and crockery about her flat. Otherwise she was a conscientious housewife, notably house-proud, excessively shy, and attached to her own mother with pathological intensity. She was thirty-five at the time of referral.

5. One was two and a half years old when his father died and was later in an orphanage for a time. A second was five years old when her father died. The third, referred to above, was four and a half years old when her mother died. (Personal communication from Dr. George Pollock.)

6. The material on both Laura and Patrick is reported in (4, pp. 22–23).

7. Although in her comments Anna Freud is referring to my earlier formulation in which I employed the term "denial" instead of "detachment," the change of term does not materially alter the burden of her criticism.

8. The evidence is clearest in children who have not yet progressed far into the detached phase and whose feelings for their mother, therefore, emerge fairly readily after reunion.

9. Accounts taken from Robertson (38).

10. In view of Freud's current interest in mourning and its vicissitudes, including his remark in the *Introductory Lectures* that "there are neuroses which may be described as morbid forms of grief," it is curious that the patient's pathological grief response, which is described early in the case history, is not once referred to again, and that it is accounted for by Freud without reference either to any previous experience of loss the patient may have had or to the patient's relation to his mother and mother substitutes, about which some fragmentary and suggestive information is given (20, pp. 13–15).

11. Gerö's conception of the pace of orality resembles my own: "The importance of the oral experience in infancy," he writes, "lies in my opinion in the mother-child relationship.

... The specifically oral pleasure is only one factor in the experience satisfying the infant's need for warmth, touch, love and care."

12. In "Mourning and Melancholia" Freud remarks of melancholic patients that "their complaints are really 'plaints' in the old sense of the word" (19, p. 248). He does not discuss their origin or function, however.

BIBLIOGRAPHY

1. Abraham, K. A short study of the development of the libido, viewed in the light of mental disorders (1924). In: *Selected Papers on Psycho-Analysis*. London: Hogarth Press, 1927, pp. 418–501.

2. Anderson, C. Aspects of pathological grief and mourning. *Int. J. Psychoanal.*, 30:48–55, 1949.

3. Angel, A. Einige Bemerkungen über Optimismus. *Int. Z. Psychoanal.*, 20:191–199, 1934.

4. Bowlby, J. Grief and mourning in infancy and early childhood. *The Psychoanalytic Study of the Child*, 15:9–52. New York: International Universities Press, 1960.

5. Bowlby, J. Processes of mourning. *Int. J. Psychoanal.*, 42:317–340, 1961.

6. Bowlby, J. Childhood mourning and its implications for psychiatry. *Amer. J. Psychiat.*, 118:481–498, 1961.

7. Breuer, J. & Freud, S. Studies on hysteria (1895). *Standard Edition*, 2. London: Hogarth Press, 1955.

8. Deutsch, F. *Applied Psychoanalysis*. New York: Grune & Stratton, 1949.

9. Deutsch, H. Zur Psychologie der manisch-depressiven Zustände, insbesondere der chronischen Hypomanie. *Int. Z. Psychoanal.*, 19:358–371, 1933.

10. Deutsch, H. Absence of grief. *Psychoanal. Quart.*, 6:12–22, 1937.

11. Engel, G. Is grief a disease? *Psychosom. Med.*, 23:18–22, 1961.

12. Eliot, T. D. Bereavement: inevitable but not insurmountable. In: *Family, Marriage, and Parenthood*, ed. H. Becker & R. Hill. Boston: Heath, 1955.

13. Fleming, J., Altschul, S., Zielinski, V. & Forman, M. The influence of parent loss in childhood on personality development and ego structure. Read at the American Psychoanalytic Association, May, 1958.

14. Freud, A. About losing and being lost. Abstract in *Int. J. Psychoanal.*, 35:283, 1954.

15. Freud, A. Discussion of Dr. John Bowlby's paper [Grief and Mourning in Infancy and Early Childhood]. *The Psychoanalytic Study of the Child*, 15:53–62. New York: International Universities Press, 1960.

16. Freud, A. & Burlingham, D. *War and Children*. New York: International Universities Press, 1943.

17. Freud, A. & Burlingham, D. *Infants without Families*. New York: International Universities Press, 1944.

18. Freud, S. *Introductory Lectures on Psycho-Analysis* (1916–1917). London: Allen & Unwin, 1922.

19. Freud, S. Mourning and melancholia (1917). *Standard Edition*, 14:243–260. London: Hogarth Press, 1957.

20. Freud, S. From the history of an infantile neurosis (1918). *Standard Edition*, 17:3–122. London: Hogarth Press, 1955.

21. Freud, S. Inhibitions, symptoms and anxiety (1926). *Standard Edition*, 20:75–174. London: Hogarth Press, 1959.

22. Freud, S. Fetishism (1927). *Collected Papers*, 5:198–204. London: Hogarth Press, 1950.

23. Freud, S. Splitting of the ego in the defensive process (1938). *Collected Papers,* 5:372–375. London: Hogarth Press, 1950.
24. Gerö, G. The construction of depression. *Int. J. Psychoanal.,* 17:423–461, 1936.
25. Greene, W. A. Role of a vicarious object in the adaptation to loss: I. Use of a vicarious object as a means of adjustment to separation from a significant person. *Psychosom. Med.,* 20:344–350, 1958.
26. Jacobson, E. Normal and pathological moods: their nature and functions. *The Psychoanalytic Study of the Child,* 12:73–113. New York: International Universities Press, 1957.
27. Jacobson, E. Denial and repression. JAPA, 5:61–92, 1957.
28. Klein, M. Mourning and its relation to manic-depressive states (1940). In: *Contributions to Psycho-Analysis.* London: Hogarth Press, 1948, pp. 311–338.
29. Klein, M. On identification. In: *New Directions in Psycho-Analysis,* ed. M. Klein, P. Heimann & R. E. Money-Kyrle. London: Tavistock, 1955, pp. 309–345.
30. Krupp, G. R. The bereavement reaction. *The Psychoanalytic Study of Society,* 2:42–74. New York: International Universities Press, 1962.
31. Landauer, K. Äquivalente der Trauer. *Int. Z. Psychoanal.,* 11:194–205, 1925.
32. Lewin, B. D. *The Psychoanalysis of Elation.* New York: Norton, 1950.
33. Lindemann, E. Symptomatology and management of acute grief. *Amer. J. Psychiat.,* 101:141–148, 1944.
34. Pittendrigh, C. S. Adaptation, natural selection and behavior. In: *Behavior and Evolution,* ed. A. Roe & G. G. Simpson. New Haven: Yale University Press, 1958, pp. 390–416.
35. Pollock, G. H. Mourning and adaptation. *Int. J. Psychoanal.,* 42:341–361, 1961.
36. Rado, S. The problem of melancholia. *Int. J. Psychoanal.,* 9:420–438, 1928.
37. Robertson, J. *A Two-Year-Old Goes to Hospital* (film). London: Tavistock Child Development Research Unit. New York: University Film Library, 1953.
38. Robertson, J. Guide to the film *A Two-Year-Old Goes to Hospital.* London: Tavistock Child Development Research Unit, 1953.
39. Root, N. A neurosis in adolescence. *The Psychoanalytic Study of the Child,* 12:320–334. New York: International Universities Press, 1957.
40. Rosenfeld, H. An investigation into the psycho-analytic theory of depression. *Int. J. Psychoanal.,* 40:105–129, 1959.
41. Stengel, E. Studies on the psychopathology of compulsive wandering. *Brit. J. Med. Psychol.,* 18:250–254, 1939.
42. Stengel, E. On the aetiology of the fugue states. *J. Ment. Sci.,* 87:572–599, 1941.
43. Stengel, E. Further studies on pathological wandering. *J. Ment. Sci.,* 89:224–241, 1943.
44. Weiss, E. Clinical aspects of depression. *Psychoanal. Quart.,* 13:445–461, 1944.
45. Winnicott, D. W. Shyness and nervous disorders in children (1938). In: *The Child and the Outside World,* ed. J. Hardenberg. New York: Basic Books, 1957, pp. 35–39.
46. Winnicott, D. W. Symptom tolerance in pediatrics: a case history (1953). In: *Collected Papers,* New York: Basic Books, 1957, pp. 101–117.

Introductory Notes to Chapter 13

Rita V. Frankiel

In this early paper, Helene Deutsch begins the exploration of varieties of pathological mourning—an activity that engaged the interest of psychoanalysts for the next three or four decades. She states here that every unresolved grief is given full expression in the subsequent behavior and character development of the person who cannot grieve. This expression can be manifested in as extreme a form as criminal behavior (stemming from a sense of guilt); it can be obviously pathological, disguised, or displaced—transformed into hysterical, obsessional, narcissistic, schizoid, or depressive symptoms. However, the necessity to mourn persists psychically, and unless a process can be initiated that will enable the person to contact the absent grief directly and thereby "complete" the process of mourning, it will continue without abatement and indefinitely. I have put the word "complete" in quotes because we know today that in some ways, it may never be completed. What we can hope for is a restoration of function, an undoing of the frozenness and somatic displacements that today seem ubiquitous in many cases.

13. Absence of Grief

Helene Deutsch

In publishing this paper I am fulfilling the wish of my beloved friend, Dorian Feigenbaum. It is a tragic coincidence that my last interchange of ideas with him was largely concerned with the problem of death and with mourning. In his last letters to me he pressed me repeatedly to send this paper, incomplete as it is, for the Quarterly. At that time we had no suspicion that this man, so full of the joy of life, so deeply and actively interested in everything intellectual, would himself become so soon an object of mourning to all those who knew and loved him.

Mourning as a process is a concept introduced by Freud [1] who considers it a normal function of bereaved individuals, by which the libido invested in the lost love-object is gradually withdrawn and redirected toward living people and problems.

It is well recognized that the work of mourning does not always follow a normal course. It may be excessively intense, even violent, or the process may be unduly prolonged to the point of chronicity when the clinical picture suggests melancholia.

If the work of mourning is excessive or delayed, one might expect to find that the binding force of the positive ties to the lost object had been very great. My experience corroborated Freud's finding that the degree of persisting ambivalence is a more important factor than the intensity of the positive ties. In other words, the more rigorous the earlier attempts to overcome inimical impulses toward the now lost object, the greater will be the difficulties encountered in the retreat from that ultimately achieved position.

Psychoanalytic findings indicate that guilt feelings toward the lost object, as well as ambivalence, may disturb the normal course of mourning. In such cases, the reaction to death is greatly intensified, assuming a brooding,

Reprinted by permission of the author's estate and *The Psychoanalytic Quarterly* 6 (1937): 12–22.

neurotically compulsive, even melancholic character. Indeed the reaction may be so extreme as to culminate in suicide.

Psychoanalytic observation of neurotic patients frequently reveals a state of severe anxiety replacing the normal process of mourning. This is interpreted as a regressive process and constitutes another variation of the normal course of mourning.

It is not my purpose to dwell at length upon any of the above mentioned reactions. Instead, I wish to present observations from cases in which the reaction to the loss of a beloved object is the antithesis of these—a complete absence of the manifestations of mourning. My convictions are: first, that the death of a beloved person must produce reactive expression of feeling in the normal course of events; second, that omission of such reactive responses is to be considered just as much a variation from the normal as excess in time or intensity; and third, that unmanifested grief will be found expressed to the full in some way or other.

Before proceeding to my cases I wish to recall to your minds the phenomenon of indifference which children so frequently display following the death of a loved person. Two explanations have been given for this so-called heartless behavior: intellectual inability to grasp the reality of death, and inadequate formation of object relationship. I believe that neither of these explanations has exclusive validity. Should an intellectual concept of death be lacking, the fact of separation must still provoke some type of reaction. It is also true that although the capacity for an ultimate type of object relationship does not exist, some stage of object relationship has been achieved. My hypothesis is that the ego of the child is not sufficiently developed to bear the strain of the work of mourning and that it therefore utilizes some mechanism of narcissistic self-protection to circumvent the process.

This mechanism, whose nature we are unable to define more clearly, may be a derivative of the early infantile anxiety which we know as the small child's reaction to separation from the protecting and loving person. The children of whom we are to speak, however, were already of a sufficiently advanced age when the loss occurred that suffering and grief were to be expected in place of anxiety. If grief should threaten the integrity of the ego, or, in other words, if the ego should be too weak to undertake the elaborate function of mourning, two courses are possible: first, that of infantile regression expressed as anxiety, and second, the mobilization of defense forces intended to protect the ego from anxiety and other psychic dangers. The most extreme expression of this defense mechanism is the omission of affect. It is of great interest that observers of children note that the ego is rent asunder in those children who do not employ the usual defenses, and who mourn as an adult does. Under certain circumstances an analogous reaction occurs in adults, and the ego takes recourse to similar defense mechanisms. The observations serve to show that under certain conditions forces of defense must be set in operation to protect a vitally threatened ego, when the painful load exceeds a threshold limit. Whether these defense mechanisms are called into operation depends upon the opposition of two forces: the relative strengths of the onrushing affects, and of the ego in meeting the storm. If the intensity of the affects is too great, or if the ego is relatively weak, the aid of defensive and rejecting mechanisms is invoked. In the first instance quantitative considerations are of greater importance; in the second, special circumstances render the ego incapable of working through the mourning process. This might be the case, for example, should the ego at the time of the loss be subjected to intense cathexis on some other account. For instance, the ego might be in a state of exhaustion by virtue of some painful occurrence just preceding the loss or conversely, be engrossed in some narcissistically satisfying situation. In brief, if the free energies of the ego have been reduced by previous withdrawals for other interests, the residual energy is unable to cope with the exigent demands of mourning.

We speak then of a relative weakness of the adult ego induced through experiences, as compared with the child's ego which is weak by virtue of the stage of its development. We assume, therefore, that a particular constellation within the ego is responsible for the absence of a grief reaction; on the one hand the relative inadequacy of the free and unoccupied portion of the ego, and on the other hand a protective mechanism proceeding from the narcissistic cathexis of the ego.

But all considerations of the nature of the forces which prevent affect are hypothetical and lead into the dark realms of speculation. The questions— whether the psychic apparatus can really remain permanently free from expressions of suffering, and what is the further fate of the omitted grief— may be better answered by direct clinical methods.

Among my patients there have been several who had previously experienced a great loss and who exhibited this default of affect. I should like to present their stories briefly.

Case 1: The first case is that of a young man of nineteen. Until the death of his mother, when he was five years old, this patient had been a very much petted youngster with an affectionate and undisturbed attachment to his mother, and with no special neurotic difficulties. When she died, he showed no grief whatsoever. Within the family this apparently "heartless" behavior was never forgotten. After his mother's death he went to live with his grandmother where he continued to be a thriving, healthy child.

His analysis revealed no special conflicts in his early childhood which could explain his affective behavior. He could remember from his early years having been angry with his mother for leaving him, but this anger did not exceed the normal ambivalent reaction common to children under similar circumstances. The young man brought no other material which could throw light on the unemotional behavior of his childhood. His later life, however, revealed certain features which indicated the fate of the rejected affect. Two characteristics of his behavior were particularly striking: he complained of depression which had first appeared without apparent cause during puberty and which had recurred with no comprehensible motivation, and he was struck by the fact that he could break off friendships, and love-relationships, with amazing ease, without feeling any regret or pain. He was, moreover, aware of no emotional disturbance so long as the relationships lasted.

These facts rendered comprehensible the fate of the repressed affect in childhood which interested us. Lack of emotion repeatedly recurred in analogous situations, and the rejected affect was held in reserve for subsequent appearance as "unmotivated depressions." The service performed by the postulated defence mechanism was purely in the interest of the helpless, little ego and contented itself with a displacement in time, and a dynamic distribution of the mourning.

Case 2: A thirty-year-old man came into analysis for the treatment of severe neurotic organic symptoms[2] of purely hysterical character and, in addition, a compulsive weeping which occurred from time to time without adequate provocation. He was already grown up when his very dearly loved mother died. When the news of her death reached him, in a distant university city, he departed at once for the funeral but found himself incapable of any emotion whatsoever, either on the journey or at the funeral. He was possessed by a tormenting indifference despite all his efforts to bring forth some feeling. He forced himself to recall the most treasured memories of his mother, of her goodness and devotion, but was quite unable to provoke the suffering which he wanted to feel. Subsequently he could not free himself from the tormenting self-reproach of not having mourned, and often he reviewed the memory of his beloved mother in the hope that he might weep.

The mother's death came at a time in the patient's life when he was suffering from severe neurotic difficulties: inadequate potency, difficulties in studying, and insufficient activity in all situations. The analysis revealed that he was having severe inner conflicts in relation to his mother. His strong infantile attachment to her had led to an identification with her which had provided the motive for his passive attitude in life. The remarkable reaction to his mother's death was conditioned by several factors. In his childhood there had been a period of intense hate for the mother which was revived in puberty. His conscious excessive affection for his mother, his dependence upon her and his identification with her in a feminine attitude, were the neurotic outcome of this relationship.

In this case, it was particularly clear that the real death had mobilized the most infantile reaction, "she has left me," with all its accompanying anger. The hate impulses which had arisen in a similar situation of disappointment in his childhood were revived and, instead of an inner awareness of grief, there resulted a feeling of coldness and indifference due to the interference of the aggressive impulse.

But the fate of the omitted grief is the question of chief interest for us in the analytic history of this patient. His feeling of guilt towards his mother, which betrayed itself even in conscious self-reproaches, found abundant gratification in severe organic symptoms through which the patient in his identification with his mother repeated her illness year after year.[3] The compulsive weeping was the subsequent expression of the affect which had been isolated from the concept—"the death of mother." Freud in "From the History of an Infantile Neurosis,"[4] describes a similar fate for an inhibited expression of grief. In this history the patient relates that he felt no suffering on hearing the news of his sister's death. The omitted suffering, however, found its substitute in another emotional expression which was quite incomprehensible, even to the patient himself. Several months after his sister's death he made a trip to the region where she had died. There he sought out the grave of a well-known poet whom he greatly admired, and shed bitter tears upon it. This was a reaction quite foreign to him. He understood, when he remembered that his father used to compare his sister's poems to those of this poet.

The situation in which the affect of Freud's patient broke through to expression had direct bonds of association with the factors which had originally been repressed. In my patient the compulsive affect had been completely isolated from the original situation.

The identification with the mother which was such a preponderant factor in the libidinal economy of our patient was perhaps the most important motive for the refusal of the ego to grieve, because the process of mourning was in great danger of passing over into a state of melancholia which might effect a completion of the identity with the dead mother through suicide. When the analysis succeeded in bringing the patient into the situation of omitted affect, the danger of suicide became very actual. So we see, that in this neurotic individual there developed in addition to the existing pathological emotional conflict, a process of defense serving as protection to the severely threatened ego.

Case 3: A man in his early thirties without apparent neurotic difficulties came into analysis for non-therapeutic reasons. He showed complete blocking of affect without the slightest insight. In his limitless narcissism he viewed his lack of emotion as "extraordinary control." He had no love-relationships, no friendships, no real interests of any sort. To all kinds of experiences he showed the same dull and apathetic reaction. There was no endeavor and no disappointment. For the fact that he had so little success in life he always found well-functioning mechanisms of comfort from which, paradoxically enough, he always derived narcissistic satisfaction. There were no reactions of grief at the loss of individuals near to him, no unfriendly feelings, and no aggressive impulses.

This patient's mother had died when he was five years old. He reacted to her death without any feeling. In his later life, he had repressed not only the memory of his mother but also of everything else preceding her death.

From the meager childhood material brought out in the slow, difficult analytic work, one could discover only negative and aggressive attitudes towards his mother, especially during the forgotten period, which were obviously related to the birth of a younger brother. The only reaction of longing for his dead mother betrayed itself in a fantasy, which persisted through several years of his childhood. In the fantasy he left his bedroom door open in the hope that a large dog would come to him, be very kind to him, and fulfill all his wishes. Associated with this fantasy was a vivid childhood memory of a bitch which had left her puppies alone and helpless, because she had died shortly after their birth.

Apart from this one revealing fantasy there was no trace of longing or mourning for his mother. The ego's efforts of rejection had succeeded too well and had involved the entire emotional life. The economic advantage of the defense had had a disadvantageous effect. With the tendency to block out unendurable emotions, the baby was, so to speak, thrown out with the bath water, for positive happy experiences as well, were sacrificed in the complete paralysis. The condition for the permanent suppression of *one* group of affects was the death of the *entire* emotional life.

Case 4: This was a middle-aged woman without symptoms but with a curious disturbance in her emotional life. She was capable of the most affectionate friendships and love-relationships, but only in situations where they could not be realized. She had the potentiality for positive and negative feelings but only under conditions which subjected her and her love-objects to disappointment. In order not to complicate the presentation I shall confine myself to describing the phenomena pertinent to our problem. For no apparent reason the patient wept bitterly at the beginning of every analytic hour. The weeping, not obsessional in character, was quite without content. In actual situations which should produce sadness she showed strikingly "controlled," emotionless behavior. Under analytic observation the mechanism of her emotional reactions gradually became clear. A direct emotional reaction was impossible. Everything was experienced in a complicated way by means of displacements, identifications, and projections in the manner of the "primary processes," described by Freud in "The Interpretation of Dreams." For example: the patient was highly educated and had a definite psychological gift. She was very much interested in the psychic life of others, made a study of it, and used to bring detailed reports of her observations. On investigation one discovered that what she had observed in the experience of another individual did not really pertain to him but represented a projection of her own unconscious fantasies and reactions. The true connection was not recognized for want of a conscious emotional reaction.

She found vicarious emotional expression through identification, especially with the sad experiences of others. The patient was capable of suffering a severe depression because something unpleasant happened to somebody else. She reacted with the most intensive sorrow and sympathy, particularly in cases of illness and death affecting her circle of friends. In this form of experience we could trace the displacement of her own rejected affects.

I am inclined to regard this type of emotional disturbance as schizoid and have the impression that it is a not infrequent type of reaction, which in its milder form usually passes unnoticed.

In the analysis of our patient one could discover how the displaced emotional discharges were related to early unresolved experiences. The original grievous experience was not a death but a loss in the divorce of her parents.

It gradually became clear that she had actually sought out the situations in which she had an opportunity to share the unhappiness of others, and that she even felt a certain envy because the misfortune had happened to another and not to herself. In such instances one is inclined to think only of masochistic tendencies as responsible. Certainly the gratification of masochism must play a role.

Observation of this patient, however, directed my attention in another direction. I believe that every unresolved grief is given expression in some form or other. For the present I limit the application of this *striving for realization* to mourning and am convinced that the unresolved process of mourning as described by Freud[5] must in some way be expressed in full. This striving to live out the emotion may be so strong as to have an effect analogous to the mechanism which we see in criminal behavior from feelings of guilt,[6] where a crime is committed to satisfy unconscious guilt feelings, which preceded the crime instead of following it. Analogous is the situation in which suppressed affect following a loss seeks realization subsequently. We must assume that the urge to realization succeeds under the impetus of an unconscious source of affect-energy exactly as in the case of the criminal who is at the mercy of his guilt feelings. I suspect that many life stories which seem to be due to a masochistic attitude are simply the result of such strivings for the realization of unresolved affects. Our last-mentioned patient was a particularly clear example of this assumption.

The process of mourning as reaction to the real loss of a loved person *must be carried to completion.* As long as the early libidinal or aggressive attachments persist, the painful affect continues to flourish, and *vice versa,* the attachments are unresolved as long as the affective process of mourning has not been accomplished.

Whatever the motive for the exclusion of the affect—its unendurability because of the ego's weakness, as in children, its submission to other claims on the ego, especially through narcissistic cathexis, as in my first case, or its absence because of a previously existing conflict with the lost object; whatever the form of its expression—in clearly pathological or in disguised form, displaced, transformed, hysteriform, obsessional, or schizoid—in each instance, the quantity of the painful reaction intended for the neglected direct mourning must be mastered.

I have already postulated a regulator, the nature of which is not clear to me. I have thought that an inner awareness of inability to master emotion, that is, the awareness by the ego of its inadequacy, was the motive power for the rejection of the emotion or, as the case may be, for its displacement.

In any case the expediency of the flight from the suffering of grief is but a temporary gain, because, as we have seen, the necessity to mourn persists in the psychic apparatus. The law of the conservation of energy seems to have its parallel in psychic events. Every individual has at his disposal a certain quantity of emotional energy. The way in which emotional impulses are assimilated and discharged differs in each individual and plays its part in the formation of the personality.

Probably the inner rejection of painful experience is always active, especially in childhood. One might assume that the very general tendency to "unmotivated" depressions is the subsequent expression of emotional reactions which were once withheld and have since remained in latent readiness for discharge.

TRANSLATED BY EDITH JACKSON

NOTES

1. Freud: *Trauer und Melancholie*. Gesammelte Schriften, Bd. V. (Trans. by Joan Riviere in Coll. Papers, Vol. IV.)
2. This case has been previously described as an example of conversion hysteria. See, Deutsch, Helene: *Psycho-analysis of the Neuroses*, Part I. London: The Hogarth Press, 1932.
3. Fenichel speaks of a "repression" in intense grief "wherein perhaps the mechanism of identification with the lost (dead) object plays a role." Fenichel, Otto: *Hysterie und Zwangsneurose*. Vienna: Int. Ztschr. f. Psa., 1931.
4. Freud: Coll. Papers, Vol. III.
5. Freud: *Trauer und Melancholie*. Gesammelte Schriften, Bd. V. (Trans. by Joan Riviere in Coll. Papers IV, 152.)
6. Freud: *Das Ich und das Es*. Gesammelte Schriften, Bd. VI (Trans. by Joan Riviere, *The Ego and the Id*. London: The Hogarth Press, 1927.)

Introductory Notes to Chapter 14

Rita V. Frankiel

Jacobson, in this paper, examines the ubiquitous "family romance" fantasies developed by patients who have lost a parent in early childhood. She observes that patients who have suffered such losses often refuse to accept the actuality of their origins or the nature of the circumstances surrounding the death of the lost parent. In the three cases included here, distortion and denial were carried to the point of expecting that one day the dead parent would actually appear. The lost parent was idealized, whereas the surviving parent was the object of deprecation and devaluation. Jacobson generalizes that "children experience the loss of a parent in early childhood not only in terms of loss of love or of a love object, but also as a severe narcissistic injury, a castration." Her observations in this paper have been supported in numerous subsequent reports and surveys (see Lerner, Chapter 25).

Jacobson's interest in the development of the self in relation to its objects led her repeatedly to think about mourning and loss in relation to the transitions involved in the emergence from the oedipal crisis (see particularly her paper on disappointment in a loved parent and its devastating effects on ego and superego development [1946]). She also invoked these ideas in trying to understand the moody transitions and black moods of adolescence (1957, 1961, 1964).

14. The Return of the Lost Parent

Edith Jacobson

In the course of my psychoanalytic practice I have treated a number of patients who in early childhood had lost either one or both of their parents.

From observational and clinical studies of motherless or parentless children we have learned much about the tragic effect of early object loss. As could be expected, all of my orphaned or semiorphaned patients showed the emotional scars left by their infantile psychic injury. In most of them the old wounds had never healed. Their object relations were seriously affected. They suffered from depressive states and other symptoms in which these traumatic infantile experiences played a decisive role.

From the multifaceted problems presented by such patients, I have selected for discussion one specific response to the early object loss which I observed in three of the patients who had lost one parent in early childhood. It bears special reference to the well-known "family romance."

Almost all of my orphaned or semiorphaned patients had built up a florid family romance in their childhood. It involved daydreams about admirable families or persons—wealthy, gifted, and of noble origin—who would turn out to be their real parents, from whom they had once been forcibly separated, and with whom they would one day be reunited.

A few of these patients gave up such daydreams in the course of adolescence. Others merely modified their fantasies and, bringing them closer to reality, tried to search for families or individuals to whom they could attach these fantasies. They looked for superior, "worthy"—and frequently wealthy—people who might be willing to "adopt" them. Naturally, such attempts were bound to fail. The persons they selected could not live up either to the part they were supposed to play or to the patients' glorified imagery. The patients would usually react to their disappointment with great

Reprinted by permission of International Universities Press, Inc., from *Drives, Affects, Behavior*, Vol. 2, edited by M. Schur, 1965.

anger, followed by a period of grief and depression, after which their search would often start anew.

Three of those patients who had lost only one parent had reacted to the loss with fantasies of this kind, which for certain reasons led to particular complications in their adult life.

The predominant feature in their reaction to the loss was their stubborn refusal to accept the reality of the actual events. They remained doubtful about them, distorted them, or even denied them altogether. In "A Type of Neurotic Hypomanic Reaction" (1937) Lewin described such patients in terms of their glorification of the lost parent, their unconscious belief that he did not die, and their particularly intense ambivalence conflicts with the surviving parent. These traits were characteristic of my patients, too. However, my patients carried their denial to the point of preconsciously, and at times consciously, expecting that one day the lost parent would actually reappear. Their fantasies and expectations of a return of the lost parent were mostly coupled or alternated with daydreams of the familiar "family romance" type.

In the first case that I wish to report, the patient's hope to find her lost father had a more realistic basis than in the others, since her father had not died: he had deserted her mother before the patient was born, and for all practical purposes had disappeared forever. In this patient as well as in the two others, the attitudes and behavior of the surviving family were apt to support the denial of the significant real events. These other two patients suspected, indeed, that their parents had not died but abandoned their families and lived in some faraway places. In the minds of all these patients this—actual or supposed—desertion had not been the fault of the lost parent who, they were sure, had been a wonderful person. It had been caused by the surviving parent's intolerable character traits or moral worthlessness.

CASE 1

From the clinical point of view, the most impressive of the three cases was that of Mary. She entered treatment with me because of a monosymptomatic hysteria and a depressive state of about two years' duration. Her history showed immediately that she also suffered from a "fate neurosis" that threatened to ruin her life.

Mary was a thirty-year-old, rather attractive, unmarried secretary. She lived with an older spinster sister, who had a similar job. This sister exercised a considerable influence on Mary's opinions and decisions, and never separated from her even for a single day.

However close the sisters were to each other, there was an area in Mary's life about which she had been secretive to her sister, to friends, and also to the various physicians whom she had consulted before she came to me. The reason for her previous consultations and treatments had been her main symptom, which had been caused by an accident. The patient had fallen down the subway stairs without suffering any serious physical injury. But, at home, when she tried to use her hands, she discovered that her right index finger became stiff, erect, and could not be bent. Treatment by several orthopedists and physiotherapists did not help. She was finally sent to a psychiatrist who, after a brief period of psychotherapy, referred her to me for psychoanalytic treatment.

Mary wept when she told me her story and complained bitterly how much this symptom interfered with her secretarial job. But when I questioned her more specifically, I discovered that for many years she had actually worked as an executive secretary, with a sufficient number of typists at her disposal. At this point Mary became very embarrassed and responded as if I had caught her in a lie. At last she began to tell me the "true story," which she had carefully managed to conceal.

In her early twenties, Mary, who had a remarkable musical talent, had decided to obtain in her free time serious training as a pianist, and to become a professional musician. In her daydreams she would see herself as an admired successful concert pianist, in close contact with other prominent musicians. To some extent Mary had carried through her plans. She had vigorously practiced every night, and regularly attended concerts and rehearsals, where she was introduced to a number of musicians. On such an occasion she had met Karl, the concertmaster of a well-known symphony orchestra. Karl was about twenty-seven years her senior. He was married and had two daughters who were close to her age. A strange friendship sprang up between Mary and Karl, whom she had told about her vocational plans. It was understood that every week after the last big orchestra rehearsal they would secretly spend a few hours in a little restaurant with each other and talk— mostly about music. This was all. Karl had never tried to make passes at her or to change their relationship in any way. But in spite of the very limited gratification which such a friendship could offer, Mary devoted herself completely to it. She loved Karl very intensely. When at concerts she saw his family in a box, she would feel terribly jealous—not of his wife, but of his two daughters. She did not look at any other man and rejected the idea of marriage, now or in the future. She wanted nothing but this friendship and her piano.

One night, about six years after their friendship had started, Karl at last expressed the desire to play sonatas with her in her home. Mary became anxious, evasive, finally angry, but her friend insisted and they made a date for one of the following days. On that day, on her way home from work, Mary suddenly began to feel very dizzy. Walking down to the subway platform, she fainted, lost her balance, and fell down the staircase. When she came to, she immediately thought, with a feeling of relief: "I broke my arm, so now I cannot play with Karl." Actually, she had not suffered any physical harm, except for a few bruises. Hurrying home in a state of shock, she sat down at her piano. Trying to bring her fingers down on the keys, she found that her right index finger could not be used. She was unable to play. Mary immediately called up her friend, reported what had happened, and canceled the date. He responded with an expressive silence, and from then on never again attempted to visit her in her home. Since her symptom did not subside, it naturally prevented her from continuing her piano studies. But her day-dreams did not break down completely. She went on hoping for a cure, keeping her interest in music alive, and seeing Karl every week, who accepted the situation on this basis as he had done before.

To the analyst, this story of a girl's hopeless love for a married man old enough to be her father and of her symptom formation under the threat of a sexual temptation sounds rather transparent. But no analyst could have guessed at the unusual infantile history and exceptional experiences of this patient, which were actually responsible for the development of the neurosis.

Mary's life as a musician had not been her only "secret." What she had also tried to conceal all her life was the fact that she had been adopted, and was the illegitimate daughter of a peasant girl who, a few weeks after the delivery, had put the child into a foster home. The foster parents, very nice, lower-middle-class people with one little girl of their own and a second one to be born a year later, nevertheless fell in love with this pretty baby and decided to adopt her. The real mother seemed glad to get rid of her. She became a seamstress, settled down nearby in the same city, and never got married. From time to time she visited Mary, brought her a little gift, but never showed any signs of genuine interest or made attempts to gain her love. Mary regarded her as a "stranger." During latency, when Mary learned from other children that she was an adopted child and that this woman was her mother, she began to despise her more and to detach herself completely from her. In these years, under the influence of her parents' attitude and of their silence about her background, her denial mechanisms began to flourish. She developed what one might call a special version of the family romance. She could not believe that she was the child of her true mother and had been adopted by her parents, who had spoiled and adored her more than their own children. Being so clearly the "favorite" child, especially of her father, made her feel that they must be her true parents, while her real mother might once have been her nurse.

In her adolescence, Mary's fantasies took a new turn. She and her older sister had always been serious, strict, and moralistic as her adoptive mother. But the youngest girl, for whom they never had had much respect, showed increasing signs of waywardness. Thus Mary developed a fantasy, which returned to awareness in her analysis, that perhaps *this* girl was actually the adopted one, and was really the seamstress's illegitimate child. Evidently Mary repressed this fantasy after her adoptive mother, quite unexpectedly, had given her serious warnings regarding her relations to boys. These warnings implied that her adoptive mother was afraid Mary might repeat the misdeeds of her real mother.

The girl reacted with feelings of shock and confusion, of hurt and resentment, to her mother's revelations and implied lack of trust in her. But she soon managed to re-establish her self-esteem and her good relationship with her mother by displacing her anger and contempt to her true mother and her younger sister; they were the ones who needed moral guidance. When at the age of eighteen this younger sister became engaged to a rather attractive though not very solid young man, the whole family felt relieved. But in Mary's opinion, this worthless girl did not deserve a husband, since, like her real mother, she was no better than a prostitute. These hostile, derogatory thoughts made Mary feel guilty. She began to suspect that she might possibly be jealous of this sister and might want as much sexual freedom as this girl and her own mother had permitted themselves. What happened next was that one day, when nobody was home, her sister's fiancé dropped in, made passes at her, and tried to seduce her. At this moment her defenses broke down and so did her identification with her adoptive mother's and her older sister's virtues. If this man behaved toward her as to a prostitute, she must be one. She must be the true daughter of her real mother. Whereupon Mary yielded to the seduction. When the incident was over, Mary felt guilt-ridden, sinful, and disgusted at this boy and at herself. Neither she nor the boy ever confessed to anybody what had happened. But she made a solemn vow to herself that she would never let herself be seduced by a man again. She kept her promise and renounced sex and young men in general. A few years later Mary lost first her adoptive mother, then her father. The younger sister had married, and she was left with her older sister as a moral guardian.

In her analysis Mary described how, after a period of sincere grief, she began to plan to take up music as a profession and to develop daydreams about her future career. At this point she suddenly mentioned a strange screen memory, which turned out to be of singular significance. She remembered that at the age of about five or six she had been visited by a wonderful stranger, who had brought her candies. He held an odd big gadget in his arm that he put in a corner. She had never forgotten it, but never raised any questions about him. After having told me this story, Mary decided to ask her sister whether she could recall this visit and knew who this man had been. The sister was flabbergasted. She was sure Mary knew that this had been her true father and the mysterious gadget had been a musical instrument, a trumpet. Her father had been a trumpet player in a military band stationed in her mother's home town. Mary reacted to this revelation with the feeling that she had known this all along. It turned out that after the loss of her adoptive parents she had built up a colossal daydream, which was unconsciously centered on a glorified image of her lost musician father. She remembered having had fleeting fantasies during this period about actually meeting her real father one day. Her repression of her father's vocation permitted her to keep these thoughts apart from her plans and daydreams about her musical career, and from her relationship with Karl, the married musician, old enough to be her father. With great anxiety Mary now began to realize that her musical interests had been in the service of her secret search for the lost father. It finally occurred to her that Karl's affectionate attachment and secret relationship to her might have a special reason: he might actually be her father who, in his turn, had searched for her and found her. In fact, as with her adoptive father, she felt he preferred her to both of his legitimate children, who had not inherited his musical talents. In regard to this identification with her real father, the analysis finally disclosed the idea that her real father might have married her real mother, if the latter had been decent; or else, if Mary had been a boy. Her adoptive father, too, had been sorry that none of his children was a boy. Only by being musically gifted and more intelligent than the others, which meant closest to being a boy, had she become his favorite child.

Only now can we understand the causes for Mary's symptom formation. In her mind, a sexual relationship with Karl might have been a real incestuous act. Thus Karl was not, or only partly, a "transference" object. She suspected him of actually being her lost real father who had abandoned her and her mother, married another "decent" woman, but had secretly looked for her and finally found her. She could regain him and keep him forever if she could prove to him and to herself that she was worthy of him: indeed, his worthiest child, the opposite of her prostitute mother, and even better than his legitimate children. Since "playing" sonatas with Karl in her home meant to Mary a sexual play, her friend's suggestion threatened to destroy her idealized father image as well as that of her own virtuous self. For this reason she reacted to his proposal not only with great anxiety but with intense anger at him, which subsided only when he calmly accepted the results of her accident.

Going back to Mary's various fictitious stories and the denial and projections on which they rested, we can at least define their main defense functions. They were not merely supposed to keep alive and even gratify Mary's desire to regain the lost love object. They were also attempts at mastery of the castration and guilt conflicts whose normal vicissitudes and solution her special situation had precluded. Undoing the narcissistic injury of her illegitimate birth and adoption, Mary's stories served the warding off of her unacceptable unconscious identifications with the sinful (castrated) "prostitute" mother who was responsible for the harm done to her. At the same time her fantasies aimed at the solution of the guilt conflicts arising in part from these very identifications and in part from the severe hostility toward her real mother. Needless to say, Mary's illusory fantasy productions and the primitive defenses which they employed did not have the desired effect. They brought about an untenable situation and led to neurotic symptom formation.

I shall conclude Mary's story by adding that the analysis gradually helped her to liberate herself from her masochistic enslavement to her musician friend and from her puritanic attitudes in general. She began to look for a suitable partner, started a sexual relationship, and became more independent of her moral guardian, the sister, who promptly followed her example. After her symptom subsided, Mary took up her piano studies again, but gave up her ideas of a musical career.

In the other two cases that I shall briefly report, the denial was of quite a different order. If Mary had refused to accept the fact that she was an illegitimate adopted child and the daughter of her seamstress mother, these two patients, who were semiorphans, could not admit that their parent had really died.

CASE 2

Robert, a married man in his thirties, had lost his mother in childbirth toward the end of his oedipal period. The newborn child, a boy, also died on the same day.[1]

In the first years of his life Robert had been very closely tied to his mother and, besides, had been thoroughly spoiled by his nursemaid. When his mother tried, during her pregnancy, to send him to kindergarten, he developed such separation anxiety that she finally had to take him back home.

When the tragic event occurred, the child was completely ignored. He knew that his mother had left for the hospital to have a baby, but nobody informed him about what had happened. The next day he was taken to relatives, where he stayed for some time. Suddenly deprived of his mother and his nursemaid, of his home and, for some time, also of his father, placed in a new environment with grieving adults, the little boy went through a period of anxiety and helpless confusion, and then of deep loneliness and depression, with feelings of self-estrangement.

Neither his father nor his relatives ever gave Robert an explanation of his mother's disappearance. Later on whenever he asked his father what had happened to his mother, the only answer would be: "Your mother was an angel." Unsatisfactory though it was, this answer helped the child to create an utterly glorified, rather mystical picture of his lost "angelic" mother. Thus his hostility could be readily diverted to the surviving members of the family.

Robert's former nurse became a special target for his negative derogatory feelings. When she came to visit him, he found her "disgusting," turned away from her, and completely detached himself from her. Robert's father did not remarry. He moved with his son into his mother's home. But even though in general he took loving care of his son, neither he nor the grandmother, a gloomy, overly strict woman, was able to gratify the child's passionate emotional needs. Robert reacted to the lack of understanding with considerable ambivalence and feelings of loneliness. His conflicts increased when his father took a city apartment, where he would spend his evenings with various mistresses. The situation became even worse when he introduced his son to some of them. There was again an unpleasant aura of secrecy and mystery about these women, their role, their appearances and disappearances. As soon as Robert began to guess the nature of his father's relationships to them, he became very critical of his father's immoral and materialistic attitudes, and began to build up a reactive, overly strict superego and high ego ideal, modeled after the image of his "saintly" mother.

During this period, the lonely child began to develop a family romance. It revolved around fantasies of being the son of an aristocratic British family. In his family romance, a mother figure did not play a particular role. It is of interest that these fantasies had a considerable influence on his appearance, bearing, and behavior, which suggested a British upper-class background.

When Robert lost his father in his early twenties, he immediately married a well-bred, very intelligent girl, who came from a family socially higher than his own. His rather large inheritance actually permitted him to live the life of a gentleman. He detached himself from his less educated, simple, and simple-minded relatives, and accepted his wife's family as his own. Subsequently, Robert, a very gifted man with broad intellectual and aesthetic interests, made a successful career in a vocational field related to that of his father-in-law.

Up to the time of his marriage, Robert had never had any sexual affairs. Like Mary, he was and he remained a Puritan in his convictions, his attitudes and, with certain exceptions, also in his actions.

Robert had come for treatment because of his recurring states of depression and depersonalization. The analysis revealed an intensely cathected sadomasochistic fantasy life, which had its origin in violent primal-scene fantasies, aroused by his mother's pregnancy and death. Robert had managed to find secret gratification of these unconscious fantasies in certain aesthetic pursuits, and also in repetitive stormy scenes with his very charming and intelligent but temperamental wife and his impulsive children. Having totally idealized both his marriage and his particular aesthetic interest, Robert was very disturbed by the discovery that under the guise of his ideals his striving had found expression in his fantasies and behavior.

As in Mary's case, this made him feel that he was actually no better than his "immoral" father. The analytic material showed that Robert's sadomasochistic fantasies were linked up with unconscious suspicions that his father might have killed mother and child in the sexual act. These fantasies were so unacceptable that they had to be warded off by a denial of his mother's death. The secrecy that surrounded his mother's sudden disappearance could be explained just as well by the assumption that mother had left his father because of his immorality and worthlessness. This interpretation would still hold father responsible for the loss of the mother, but it did not make him a sexual murderer, and the mother a victim of her sexual passion for the father. How firmly Robert believed this story became clear when he told me that every morning he would run down to the mailbox, expecting to get a "special" letter. Each time he would return very much disappointed that again "the letter" had not arrived. The mysterious letter, for the arrival of which he had stubbornly waited as long as he could remember, was a letter from his mother and brother who, as he suspected, lived somewhere in a faraway place, and would one day write and return to him.

It is noteworthy that Robert's family romance about being the son of a British nobleman was completely disconnected from the set of fantasies which denied his mother's death and sustained his hope for her return and their final reunion.

The first was a conscious daydream, expressive mainly of his wish for a worthy ideal father with whom he could identify. The patient had always been fully aware of the fantastic quality of this part of his family romance, in spite of its influence on his ego and superego development and on his object relations. The ideas about his mother's and brother's survival were of a different nature. They were not daydreams but vague suspicions, hopes, and expectations, which would only occasionally come close to awareness. They reflected Robert's ambivalence toward his father and grandmother, and had been provoked by their secrecy about his mother's death. Later on, these ideas found support in the mysterious sudden appearances and disappearances of his father's mistresses, and in the father's partly exhibitionistic, partly secretive "bad" sexual behavior.

Of course, Robert's unconscious denial of his mother's death, and his expectation of her return in some distant future helped him to keep up the illusory belief that he might get back his first love object, to whom he had been so closely attached. But in particular they served as a defense against his murderous primal scene fantasies, his identifications with his sinful parents, and the guilt feelings aroused by these sadomasochistic identifications. His belief certainly enabled him, during those unhappy, lonely years in his grandmother's home, to maintain a certain optimistic, hopeful outlook on life and himself. His optimism probably had its origin in the ineradicable happy memories of his early childhood years. But being quite illusory, his optimistic expectations failed in preventing the development of recurring depressions, which repeated his original response to his mother's sudden death, and remobilized the guilt conflicts caused by his hostile reactions to her pregnancy and his death wishes toward his future rival.

CASE 3

Paul was a married man in his late twenties. His father had died a short time before he was born. But even though the patient did not go through the traumatic experience of early object loss, he could not escape the fate of a fatherless child. His father's illness and death had exhausted the financial resources of his mother and compelled her, after Paul's birth, to take over the support of the family. She first worked at home and, as Paul grew a little older, held regular jobs. The mother's oldest sister, likewise a widow, moved in and took care of the home and the two children—little Paul and a sister several years older. Thus Paul was brought up with three rather aggressive females around him. The old aunt, who was quite a character, was the most loving one of the three. But both she and her sister did not seem to care much for the other sex. Neither of them ever talked about their past lives or seemed to want a second marriage. Both showed little respect for Paul's uncle, their brother, who frequently visited the family on week ends.

Thus, the little boy's situation at home was a very unhappy one. In his preschool years he was very lonesome. None of the three females seemed to be aware of his needs and would ever play with him. Paul's mother, a very dutiful mother but a rather narcissistic, compulsive person, would make constant complaints about her hard life. She impressed on him very early that she expected him to compensate her for all her losses and sacrifices and to assume the responsibilities of a "man" in the home. At the same time she did her best to tie him to herself and to prevent him from ever becoming independent. In response to these contradictory maternal attitudes, Paul developed the conviction that as a fatherless boy he had no chance of ever becoming a real man. Thus, on entering school, he felt different and rather estranged from other boys who had "normal" families. His uncle tried to play the role of a father, which Paul eagerly accepted for some years. Once the uncle invited Paul for a vacation with his own boys in his home in the suburbs. Paul immediately began to hope that his uncle might keep him forever in his family. He was very disappointed when his uncle neither "adopted" him nor ever invited him again. Later on, this uncle became very critical of him, evidently being jealous because Paul was much brighter than his own sons. His uncle's behavior did much to lower Paul's self-esteem still further. Some years later Paul began to develop a series of friendships with boys who seemed to have admirable, loving parents. Trying to establish himself as a member of their families, Paul spent as much time as he could in their homes. During this period he began for the first time actively to compete with other boys. But in the end his renewed efforts to find a family that would adopt him proved to be as futile as the attempt with his uncle.

In his own home, the situation had become intolerable. The three women constantly fought with him and with each other, playing off one against the other. The atmosphere became even more hostile when Paul began to rebel, to assert his masculinity and independence, and to show the three women his physical and mental superiority.

Paul was, in fact, by far the most gifted member of the family. He was a brilliant, ambitious boy, but forever doubtful about the extent of his physical and intellectual abilities. This did not change when he became financially independent. After working his way through college and law school, he attained a very good position in a law firm and married. At this point, in his early twenties, Paul at last felt able to detach himself from his family in the same way as Robert had done.

Paul soon achieved a financially and professionally successful career. He had a charming, devoted wife and a lovely, bright child. In reality, he had accomplished everything he could have wished to attain at this age, yet he was constantly dissatisfied and depressed. Although his wife and his law firm gave him all the freedom he wanted, he felt as much trapped in his professional and marital situations as he had once felt at home with his mother.

He expressed continuous complaints about his wife, his firm, his jobs, and his own work. At the same time he would have daydreams about drastic changes in his life in the future. In fact, he was forever in search of the right people and work to help him find his real self at last.

This leads us to Paul's fantasy relationship to the father he had lost before he was born. In Paul's case, the family behavior had not supported any glorification of the late father. Paul knew the bare outlines of his father's background, of his vocation, and of his fatal illness and death. Even this account had been incomplete, confusing, and contradictory. His mother had never talked with him about his father as a person. She had never arranged for him to meet any of the surviving members of his father's family. As far as she was concerned, Paul's father seemed never to have existed. His mother's eloquent silence about her former husband profoundly affected Paul and caused him to create a myth about his father. He had built up a highly glorified but rather lifeless, abstract paternal image. Since he had no personal memories of his father or even stories about him, Paul himself thought that his image of a brilliant, great man might have nothing to do with his real father. He thought it might be a product of his own imagination and even felt quite triumphant about the fact that he had not needed a realistic model but had created his goals and ideals, which this image reflected, independently and out of himself.

This spiteful feeling, which denied his urgent need for a father, was expressive of his rejection of the mother's attitudes and behavior and, especially, of her hypermorality and her scales of value in general. His reactive ego ideal and his ambitious ego goals were, in fact, the product of a permanent struggle against his unconscious identifications with her and with his sister and aunt (Greenson 1954).

Unfortunately, this struggle had resulted in marked identity conflicts and prevented Paul from ever developing a feeling of continuity and firm direction. But his constant search for an identity did not simply reflect his need for a realistic parental figure whom he could accept as a model for himself. Apparently no person—man or woman—had ever been acceptable in this role, since part of him believed that his father might be alive and would return and take over the part of the model that Paul so urgently needed.

If Paul had greater doubts than Robert about the correctness of this assumption, he was far more specific in his elaboration of the story about his father. He wondered whether his father had not left his intolerable, hostile wife and founded a new family on the West Coast where his relatives lived. Moreover, he thought that probably for this reason mother had never let him meet his father's relatives. He suspected that she always kept him so close to herself because she did not want him to discover the truth and to find and join the father and his new family. There was also a vague implication that he might not really be his mother's son. While Paul never made the slightest move to write to these relatives or to see them, it turned out that he had developed the same habit as Robert. He, too, expected every morning to get an exciting "special" letter, which never came: the letter from his father. And he also continued to hope that one day in the future father would write to him and they would be reunited.

The intensity of Paul's hopes for his father's return was illuminated when he acted them out during his analysis. Paul developed a sudden, very strong emotional involvement with an impressive, much older lawyer, until he found out that this man closely resembled the only picture of his own father that he owned. For a brief period Paul had evidently hoped that this man might actually be his real father.

Paul's suspicions about his father's desertion of his family and his life in California had always been on a preconscious or, at time, even conscious level. What he had not known, however, was that his feelings of being trapped, his compulsive urge to run away from his mother, his wife, from his jobs and his superiors, and to look for the right persons and the right work were an expression of his search for his father and of his wish to join him and his new family.

His father's supposed new wife did not play any part in his conscious fantasies. Her role in his unconscious became clear from his fantasies about certain older married women who might be able to give him something very "special." The "special" gift he expected to get and never could get from them was obviously a real father, and hence his real own manly self.

All these fantasies, hopes, and expectations, which we may call a family romance, centering on the figure of his real father, began to develop in his latency period. They arose concomitantly and were interwoven with his desires and his disappointing attempts to be "adopted." Paul's denial of his father's death, his ideas about the latter's desertion and life with a new family, and his hopes for a final reunion were likewise in the service of his defenses, predominantly of his attempts at a solution of his narcissistic conflicts. Since the loss of his father was experienced as a narcissistic injury, in fact as a castration, the survival and future return of his father meant to him a potential recovery of his own lost masculine identity. As in Robert's case, however, the additional function of his myth was to ward off deeply unconscious fantasies about his father's violent death. Sadomasochistic primal scene material involving Paul's mother disclosed fantasies—similar to those of Robert—that mother might have vengefully killed his father when the latter tried to rape her. Paul remembered that as early as the age of six he had developed fantasies in which his mother was assaulted and disrobed by a man on the street. Being a helpless little boy, he could only watch the scene but do nothing to help his mother. As he grew up, the fantasy changed, inasmuch as he would now try to save her by attacking the aggressor. The analysis of his fantasies showed that Paul was clearly identified with both partners' roles and crimes. He suffered, indeed, from guilt feelings borrowed from both parents. Since Paul felt that his mother had wanted and tempted him to usurp his father's place, he felt in particular that he shared with her the responsibility for his father's death.

DISCUSSION

A comparison of the three cases shows rather striking resemblances and also interesting differences, not only in the patients' direct response to the object loss but also in the broader psychopathology which they gradually developed on the basis of this loss.

It was not accidental that all three patients entered treatment in a state of depression. But it is significant that Mary became depressed only after she had developed her hysterical symptom, and that her depression showed conspicuous features of true grief. Its obvious cause was the sad recognition that she could no longer anticipate any satisfaction or happiness in the future, either as a woman or as a musician. As to the conflicts leading to her depression, the analysis showed that they were of a hysterical rather than of a profound narcissistic type: they revolved essentially around her incestuous problems. Of course, the fact that Mary was an adopted, illegitimate child was a profound narcissistic injury. It readily directed all her hostility to the "prostitute" mother, who had abandoned her. But we must not forget that since early infancy Mary had been brought up by very loving adoptive parents. Probably her readiness to act out her incestuous impulses was caused by the very fact that her adoptive father had been less inhibited in giving her physical affection than with his own children. The love she received could not prevent the development of a fate neurosis that cut her off from a normal heterosexual love life, but Mary's general capacity for object relations had not been seriously affected. The disgraceful fact of her illegitimate birth and adoption was so intolerable for her that she built up fictitious stories which not only denied this fact but projected it onto the younger sister, thus reversing the situation. However, despite the extent to which her denial and projection mechanisms went, they remained limited to this specific problem. Her secrecy about her vocational plans and her friendship with Karl were also linked up with that.

While Mary did not deny the loss of her father but denied only the fact of her illegitimacy and adoption, the two semiorphaned patients had to resort to a denial of their parent's death. Both of them had a rather lonesome, unhappy childhood. Robert at least had memories of his happy early childhood years, even though his happy life ended with the traumatic experiences which I have described. This accounted for the fact that, except for recurring states of depression and his prolonged adolescence with detachment from his relatives, Robert had developed stable emotional relations and interests, and was able to enjoy life. He was basically a hysterical personality, though with obsessional-compulsive features. His narcissistic vulnerability was caused by the abrupt traumatic change from the life of a protected, overindulged child to that of a motherless, emotionally deprived one.

There were striking resemblances in the cases of Robert and Paul: their surmise that the parent had not died but deserted the unworthy partner and lived in another city, and their expectation of a confirming letter and a future reunion. In both cases, the denial of the lost object's death had been provoked by the surviving parent's refusal to talk about the late partner. And in both patients their stories served the same function: to ward off not only the intolerable fantasy that the lost objects had been killed by their partners in the sexual act, but in particular the guilt feelings caused by the patient's unconscious fantasy identification with the surviving parent's supposed criminal act.

In Robert's case, the murderous primal scene fantasies had been provoked by his knowledge that during childbirth something terrible had happened to mother and infant. Paul's corresponding fantasies had been stimulated by the close temporal link between his own birth and his father's illness and death.

In view of Paul's early emotional deprivations, it is not surprising that, in contrast to Mary and Robert, he had become an obsessional-compulsive, chronically depressive person, with marked identity conflicts.

I have intentionally pointed to the differences in the personalities of these three patients and in the structure of their conflicts, provoked by the early object loss. The question arises why two of these patients developed such similar stories about the survival of their parents and the reasons for their loss, and why all of them lived on their hopes for a return of the lost object.

With regard to the similarity of Robert's and Paul's stories and the hope of these patients for the return of the lost parent, it appears to be of utmost importance that in all three cases the stories were, above all, supposed to aid the patients in the mastery of the narcissistic injuries caused by the loss of the glorified object, and to help them in the solution of their castration and guilt conflicts. Their expectation of getting back the lost object in the distant future is certainly reminiscent of little girls' hopes of getting back the lost penis. One feels tempted to speak in these patients of an "illusory parent," in analogy to women's "illusory penis."

Evidently, children experience the loss of a parent in early childhood not only in terms of loss of love or of a love object, but also as a severe narcissistic injury, a castration. Since children, in their first years of life, depend on their parents for narcissistic supplies and participate in their supposed grandeur, to be fatherless, motherless, an orphan or an adopted child is felt to be utterly degrading. The fact that in such children the hostile and derogatory feelings caused by their losses are so commonly diverted to the surviving parent or the parent substitutes, while the lost object becomes glorified, tends to raise that object's narcissistic value and meaning to the point of turning it into the most precious part of their own self which has been lost and must be recovered. This is the reason why such children refuse to accept, and struggle against identifying with, their surviving (castrated) parent or the parental substitutes, and are apt to develop a florid family romance serving their own aggrandizement.

In Mary, the disgraceful fact of her illegitimacy and adoption, and of her father's desertion of her mother, had indeed been unconsciously considered as a castration, a punishment for her mother's—and her own—sexual sins. Her struggle against her unconscious identification with her true mother and her hope for the return of the lost father—and the lost penis—rested on her unconscious expectation of getting them back as a reward for her outstanding sexual virtuousness.

Although Robert had lost his mother, he also regarded this loss, which compelled him to live with his grandmother and his "immoral" sinful father, as a degradation and, unconsciously, as a castration. The glorified angelic mother was in his unconscious the most precious part of himself, the penis which he and his father had lost as a punishment for their sinfulness. As in women's denial of castration, his denial of the mother's death and his hope for her return were intended to assert that this most valuable part of himself had not really been lost, that he would get it back as a reward for his saintliness.

In Paul's mind, the loss of his father was even consciously equated with his supposed lack of manliness. His doubts and his fantasies about his father's greatness, about his death or survival, were interchangable with his doubts about his sexual identity. His supposed castration was considered to be a punishment for his unconscious sadomasochistic identifications with his parents against which he had so desperately struggled. His search for his glorious father—and the latter's worthy second wife—was expressive of his unconscious wishes for a mother, who, being able to be both father and mother to him, could have turned him into a powerful, great man.

NOTES

1. I discussed this case from a different perspective in a former paper (1959).

BIBLIOGRAPHY

Bonaparte, M. (1928), L'Identification d'une Fille à sa Mère Morte. *Rev. Franç. Psychanal.*, 2:541–565.

Greene, W. A., Jr. (1958), Role of an Object in the Adaptation to Object Loss. *Psychosom. Med.*, 20:344–350.

Greenson, R. R. (1954), The Struggle against Identification. *J. Amer. Psychoanal. Assn.*, 2:200–217.

Jacobson, E. (1959), Depersonalization. *J. Amer. Psychoanal. Assn.*, 7:581–610.

Lehrman, P. R. (1927), The Fantasy of Not Belonging to One's Family. *Arch. Neurol. & Psychiat.*, 18:1015–1023.

Lewin, B. D. (1937), A Type of Neurotic Hypomanic Reaction. *Arch. Neurol. & Psychiat.*, 37:868–873.

Meiss, M. L. (1952), The Oedipal Problem of a Fatherless Child. *The Psychoanalytic Study of the Child*, 7:216–229.

Neubauer, P. (1960), The One-Parent Child. *The Psychoanalytic Study of the Child*, 15:286–309.

Tarachow, S. & Fink, M. (1958), Absence of a Parent as a Specific Factor Determining Choice of Neurosis: Preliminary Study. *J. Hillside Hosp.*, 2:67–71.

Introductory Notes to Chapter 15

Rita V. Frankiel

Tyson suggests that three components of narcissism be assessed in order to understand the nature and extent of narcissistic damage that often follows object loss in early childhood: lingering infantile omnipotence, disorders of self-constancy, and defective self-esteem regulation. The developmental basis of each is described and a clinical example is offered for each component. This paper uses Margaret Mahler's separation-individuation theory, tracing the lingering effects of early object loss in the etiology of pathological narcissism and showing how narcissistic damage can be perpetuated unless ameliorative steps are taken by focusing the treatment on the narcissistic issues. Tyson leans heavily on Mahler's observations in explicating the diminution of omnipotence in the practicing subphase of normal development.

What is suggested is a developmental assessment of the three proposed components of narcissism in order to differentiate the immediate effect of the loss, the influence of earlier factors, and the effects of loss on later development. These three constituents are proposed as a clinically useful framework for assessing narcissistic damage.

15. Some Narcissistic Consequences of Object Loss: A Developmental View

Robert L. Tyson

A sizable psychoanalytic literature is concerned with the libidinal aspects of object loss and the stages in adaptation to it, but there are only a few studies which specifically consider relevant narcissistic factors, particularly those of developmental significance (Jacobson 1965; Rochlin 1953a, 1959; Wolfenstein 1969; and especially Perman 1979). Most often general mention is made regarding ego impoverishment, narcissistic injury, mortification, supplies, or depletion, but there is little or no reference to the specifically narcissistic sources of psychic pain attendant on object loss. In what follows I will suggest a way to identify these sources and to make a developmental assessment of the patient's narcissistic status at the time of object loss or subsequently. Such an assessment can be an aid in the formulation of accurate, appropriate, and tactful interpretive interventions as part of the psychoanalytic process. For the purposes of this exposition, aspects of drive development, conflict, and defenses essential to a complete assessment will not be considered, but should, of course, not be neglected in practice.

INTRODUCTION

Most writers on the subject of object loss deal with the inner or psychic consequences of the total loss of an external object. Loss through death of the object is held to be essentially different from the experience of other kinds of losses (E. Furman 1974; Pollock 1961). Whether or not children can mourn, as distinct from having other reactions to loss, has been debated chiefly on the grounds of whether or not they possess adequate psychic structure with which to accomplish the work of mourning. In an extensive review, E. Furman (1974) described the circumstances in which mourning in

Reprinted by permission of the author and *The Psychoanalytic Quarterly* 52 (1983): 205–24.

childhood can be carried on, and how the child analyst can facilitate the process, utilizing the available psychic structures. Because of the realistic dependence of children on their primary objects, the trauma of primary object loss in childhood with its obvious effects on libidinal development and psychic structure formation has commanded the attention of both child and adult analysts (Fleming and Altschul 1963; E. Furman 1974; Meiss 1952; Neubauer 1960; Pollock 1961, 1978). Reactions to losses and impairment of the mourning process in adolescence and later tend to be understood either in terms of the repetition of reactions to early losses or as the investment of the current reality with unconscious meaning derived from persisting wishes, fantasies, conflicts, and defenses.

To separate out the narcissistic constituents in reaction to object loss and to develop the context for the discussion to come, I will give special emphasis to the *loss of a significant relationship* and to the consequences of this loss for the individual, depending on the stage of development at the time. Considering *relationship loss* will also facilitate the study of links between the external object and the self and object representations conceived of as structures which encompass role relationships, conflicts, and affective tendencies as well (Eisnitz 1981; J. Sandler 1976; Sandler and Sandler 1978). Thus, whenever the loss of a significant relationship occurs at any age, whether by death, disaster, or divorce, there are *internal* and *external* implications of the experience which need to be assessed. The assessment of the internal factor is concerned with evaluating the current level of functioning and with estimating the highest developmental level achieved by the person along various developmental lines (A. Freud 1963, 1965). Such an assessment allows for distinctions between the person's current functioning and immediate reactions to the loss itself, and the impact of earlier influences on development (Rangell 1967); it also helps us to evaluate the effects such a loss might have on personality structure, function, and further development. For example, Charlie, age five and a half, was placed in the custody of his mother following a divorce. Within six months, there was an eruption of psychotic behavior in Charlie which was thought to be a direct and simple consequence of the divorce until one of Charlie's older sisters fearfully described how the father would fondle Charlie's penis when the children visited him on weekends. One of the reasons the mother had sought the divorce was the father's sexual approaches to his daughters. Neither they nor Charlie had previously provided information about the homosexual incest. Clearly, the divorce affected Charlie, but the two years of precocious sexual excitement preceding that event could be seen in retrospect to have played a crucial role in his early enuresis, sleep disturbances, and behavioral problems at nursery school, as well as the later catastrophic regression.

Children react to loss differently in different developmental stages (A. Freud 1960). For example, a very young child's loss of a parent may result in a developmental interference (Nagera 1970), because the loving attachments made between the child and the parent are the basis for harmonious personality growth, and the disruption of these attachments inhibits and distorts subsequent further development. It is true that sometimes adequate substitutes can be found, but if the lost relationship was a good one, it takes time to re-establish the kind of interchange between child and substitute which allows for the resumption of optimal personality development. Also, as Freud (1926, 169) pointed out, the infant is unable to distinguish the mother's temporary absence from a permanent one and needs to develop the capacity to anticipate her return. Slightly older children may experience the loss of a parent as a confirmation of their hostile omnipotence, based on the ambivalence inherent early in the process of separation-individuation (Mahler, et al. 1975). This early ambivalence is increasingly accompanied by death fantasies about the targets of the child's rage. Clinical experience teaches us that with development the overt expression of anger may come to be better controlled, but that death wishes persist in one form or another (Freud 1928). Other children may feel the loss of a parent as a narcissistic wound of some sort, for example, by feeling that the parent has left—died or divorced—because the child himself was not lovable enough for the parent to stay.

Another advantage in assessing developmental level is that we are less likely to be misled by chronological age. For example, children need a concrete explanation of death and the attendant circumstances; they often miscontrue abstract, philosophical, or religious explanations (R. A. Furman 1970). However, it is insufficiently appreciated that the stress of anxiety, conflict, or psychic pain often results in a regression even in older children and adults, and the capacity for abstract thinking may be compromised (e.g., Barnes 1964).[1]

External factors encompass the particular circumstances of loss and the external resources available to help in coping with the inner consequences. These factors will not be examined here in detail, a task which would require an examination of the effects of *impaired* relationships in addition to the effects of total object loss (e.g., Mahler 1961; Rochlin 1953b). However, in taking a close look at the narcissistic constituents of the personality and examining how they are variously affected by object loss, I will attempt to maintain a link between intrapsychic factors and the external circumstances and resources, between inner reality and outer reality.

NARCISSISM

For convenience here it will be assumed that theories are attempts to explain the clinical events and feelings with which we must deal every day, and perhaps to predict a little. It is a technical truism in analysis that it matters both what is said and how it is said. Indeed, much of what is now encompassed in contemporary theories of narcissism seems to have been understood long ago. For example, Kierkegaard declared in 1849 (in *The Sickness unto Death*):

Despair is never ultimately over the external object but always over ourselves. A girl loses her sweetheart and she despairs. It is not over the lost sweetheart, but over herself without the sweetheart. And so it is with all cases of loss. . . . The unbearable loss is not really in itself unbearable. What we cannot bear is in being stripped of the external object. We stand denuded and see the intolerable abyss of ourselves (*cf.* Gaylin 1968, 15).

Freud's (1914) well-known remark added a developmental dimension to the topic: "The development of the ego consists in a departure from primary narcissism and gives rise to a vigorous attempt to recover that state" (100). The term "primary narcissism" is usually understood as referring to a hypothetical state of early undifferentiated mother-infant unity in which all the infant's needs are said to be met and which is lost as a consequence of development; at least the degree of gratification associated with that state is thought to be lost and sought for in subsequent phases.

Kierkegaard emphasizes the egocentric aspect of the pain consequent on the object loss; Freud's comment, in contrast, points to the narcissistic losses inherent in growth and development and to the strenuous efforts expended in compensating for them. Freud's remark also suggests the persistence of narcissistic elements in the developmental line of object relationships which begins, in Freud's terms, in the state of "primary narcissism" during the first few weeks of life. Mahler (Mahler, et al. 1975) names this beginning period the "normal autistic phase" (it has also been called the "quasi-autistic phase" [Harley and Weil 1979, xiiin.] and the "undifferentiated phase"

[Hartmann, et al. 1946]), referring to a time before the infant makes any enduring differentiation representationally between the infant's self and another person, that is, before self-object differentiation. Of course, such a differentiation is quite a separate developmental achievement from the exercise of the newborn's built-in capacity to make distinctions between different sources of external stimuli. From the infant's point of view one cannot speak of object loss at this early stage of life because there is no object nor any "self" in terms of durable mental representations. Gradually, building on the child's biological dependence, a complex reciprocity between mother and infant provides a basis for a progressively more psychological relationship, leading into the stages of separation-individuation.

Optimally, the child will eventually attain a notably increased ability to tolerate separation from the mother without great distress or impact for longer and longer periods of time. The progressive consolidation of object constancy enables the child to look to the mother's return with a confident expectation which the good-enough mother will meet as she has met the child's expectations often enough in the past. The durability or constancy of the mental and emotional structure underlying such object constancy is only relative (McDevitt 1975), and the death of, or excessively prolonged separation from the mother or substitute will break it down or seriously alter it and profoundly affect object relations thenceforward (A. Freud 1952; McDevitt 1967, 1971; Robertson and Robertson 1971).

Clearly, the development of object relations is closely interwoven with narcissistic factors both in interpersonal relationships and in the relevant mental representations. Prior to self-object differentiation, during the time the biological relationship continues to be primary from the point of view of the infant, the departure of the mother or primary caretaker means death unless a substitute is provided. This provision can be made easily over a relatively brief period after birth, but many constraints are soon imposed by ongoing development, limiting the changes the infant can sustain without disturbance (A. Freud 1952; Mahler 1961). These constraints indicate the increasing number and strength of links between the infant and the specific primary object, links which also come to facilitate progressive self-object differentiation and the dawning awareness of feeling-states both pleasurable and unpleasurable. Elaborating an idea of Spruiell's (1975), I suggest that the clinical understanding of narcissistic phenomena is helped by separating out three metaphorical strands or components of narcissism: feelings of *omnipotence,* feelings of *self-constancy,* and feelings of *self-esteem.*

OMNIPOTENCE

Mahler refers to the gradual decrease in age-appropriate feelings of grandeur and magical omnipotence which ordinarily takes place from about the fifteenth month onward (Mahler et al. 1975, 213): "In boys and girls alike, the repeated experience of relative helplessness punctures the toddler's inflated sense of omnipotence." Benefits from the optimal experience of this process include first the recognition and tolerance of the primary loved person as increasingly separate. This achievement offers the child a reassurance that the expression of hostile or nonhostile aggression does not result in loss of objects, thus facilitating the elaboration of further relationships with them (Winnicott 1969). A second benefit is the important step thus taken toward the ultimate, but much later recognition that the primary loved person is *also* not omnipotent (Jacobson 1946). A third advantage from the gradual loss of omnipotent feelings is a resulting protection from a "basic depressive mood" (Mahler 1966), a mood which might otherwise result in intensive yearnings to restore the feelings of narcissistic well-being experienced in the earlier stages of individuation (Sandler and Joffe 1965). Fantasies of omnipotence play an important role in the course of development as well as in pathological states (Ritvo, in Panel 1974). Thus, if identification with the presumed omnipotence of the object has not taken place, then to the extent that feelings of omnipotence and power remain important in the person's narcissistic equilibrium and depend on the loved one for their persistence and potency, there exists a vulnerability to narcissistic injury in that area, by disappointment in or loss of the object.

Object Loss and Omnipotence

The impact of object loss on the metaphorical narcissistic constituent of omnipotence is given early focus in development because of crucial vulnerabilities first peaking, according to Mahler, about the fifteenth to sixteenth month as the practicing period comes to an end (Mahler 1966, 63). There are children who fail to experience the age-appropriate, properly dosed series of disillusionments and deflations of their grandeur and omnipotence. They are consequently more vulnerable to loss of the loved object later on in life, since they have not had the phase-appropriate inoculations of loss beforehand. There are those children, too, whose experience of object loss coincides in time or in other ways with destructive fantasies and who consequently feel themselves to be responsible for the loss and are terrified by what appears to be their dangerous omnipotence. The cognitive egocentricity appropriate to younger age groups combines with the intense, phase-appropriate conflicts over aggression to make such younger children especially vulnerable to being frightened by the apparent potency of their hostility. As an example of the effort to ward off the feared destruction while feeling responsible, a six-year-old boy with a three-year-old brother said, "Mommy, I wish I never said I wanted a baby, then we never would have gotten Eddie!" Another example of how small children assume themselves to be all-powerful is provided by a four-year-old boy; this child, in sad response to the sudden disappearance of his beloved nursery school teacher who had quit, tearfully asked, "Mommy, what did I do bad?"

These examples illustrate how early one may react more to the threat of apparent destructiveness than to the loss of the object alone. In addition to expressing feelings of responsibility or guilt at the time of the loss, a child may seek to escape these uncomfortable feelings by regressing to what feels safer, to a more infantile and helpless way of relating. In addition to the frightening evidence of their presumed power, both the regression and guilt will secondarily have the effect of lowering the child's self-esteem. Regression has this effect because the child wants to be big and grown up, but a regression is in the opposite direction. Therefore, in order to understand the nature of a person's reaction to object loss in terms of his feelings of omnipotence, it is important to assess what his developmental status was in regard to his ideals for himself, and the degree to which he attained a realistic view of his powers prior to the loss.

SELF-CONSTANCY

Self-constancy, the second metaphorical strand of narcissism, is a more complicated idea which concerns the continuity of the sense of identity over time. Self-constancy may be defined as the enduring quality gradually acquired by the common elements in the many memories of oneself in many different experiences and situations. These mental representations have "both structural and experiential aspects, just as the object has, in the mind of the child" (A.-M. Sandler 1977, 199). The emerging sense of self is reflected in the gradual attainment of self-constancy, which is an open-ended process just as is the attainment of object constancy (Mahler, et al. 1975, 112). Furthermore, the establishing of the emerging sense of self requires the ability to maintain an image of one's self which integrates different affectively toned "good" and "bad" self-representations; it also requires an ability to sustain this integration in the face of the relative lack of pleasurable, or of an excess of unpleasurable, reflections about one's self from a variety of sources.

To the extent that this integration has been achieved and to the extent that it retains its durability, this constant mental image of the self serves as an inner support, nourishing the child's sense of safety, autonomy, and mastery just as does the constant representation of the mother and others. Given reasonable object and self-constancy, the capacity for constant relationships (Burgner and Edgcumbe 1972) becomes possible; a constant relationship is one in which the person maintains predominantly the same feeling about another individual regardless of the vicissitudes to which their relationship may be subjected. The real loss of a person with whom one has an important constant relationship affects the ability to sustain unchanged the mental representation of that person. The reason for this is that even in adulthood, apparently, some "refueling" (Mahler and Furer 1963) from the real object is needed from time to time in order to maintain the corresponding mental representation. "Out of sight, out of mind" is a phrase which might describe the fate of this mental structure without sufficient "refueling." There is also evidence to indicate that the real object serves to "refuel" the constant self as well, as Kierkegaard has so sensitively described. The integrated self-image is no longer the source of comfort that once it was after some period of absence of the real person, the refueling object. This bereft self-image may now become rather more a source of pain, especially in proportion to the degree to which the lost person served to bring about an agreeable integration in the face of otherwise deficient positive feelings about the self.

Object Loss and Self-Constancy

Let us turn now to the effects of object loss on the emerging sense of self. One frequently hears a comment made some months after a divorce or other loss, to the effect that it was "really a growth experience."[2] While it may reflect defense activity, such a comment could just as well signal both a sense of alteration in the self-representation and a challenge to one's self-constancy. Clearly, this experience is distinct from an injury to feelings of omnipotence and from alterations in self-esteem. To some extent, changes in the sense of self may take place as a consequence of identifications with the lost person (Freud 1917), identifications which are usually not made very selectively. Since most, if not all, relationships are ambivalent to some degree, a loss of self-esteem will occur to the extent that identifications are made with hated aspects of the lost object.

Identifications with the lost object are made by children (Birtchnell 1969; Jacobson 1965) as well as by adults, and these childhood identifications may either facilitate or impede subsequent development (E. Furman 1974, 59–66; Jacobson 1971). The usual motivations for making identifications with the lost object are to defend against the pain of the loss and to compensate for it by keeping the person through identifying with her or him, thereby denying the loss. In childhood these motivations also include efforts to avoid and to repair the painful state of self-without-the-object which threatens the constancy of the self and the not yet stabilized sense of self. The widely recognized value of staying in the familiar environment and of keeping things the same serves to lessen these fears and to restore a sense of safety to the child. The wish to maintain the *status quo* appears to be much more explicitly stated and striven for by children suffering from object loss than by adults, or by the remaining parent of bereaved children; it is the adult who seems more prone to seek change. In addition to the pain of self-without-the-object, the threat to children lies in a painful menace to their self-constancy, since identifications with a lost object tend to be regressive, their self-object boundaries are not so secure as in adults, and the process of establishing self- and object constancy has not gone on so long or withstood as many trials. In contrast, adults in seeking change are not fearful of a loss of self-constancy, but they seek a person to assuage the pain of a change in their self-representation of the self-without-the-object. This is commonly referred to as "being on the rebound," and many authors describe the phases of adaptation to painful loss (e.g., Pollock 1961).

An example to illustrate both aspects of this point is provided by the treatment of Doug, a fifteen-year-old boy who was precipitated into a painful state of despair, and thus into treatment, when his well-educated mother suddenly moved them to another house shortly after divorcing his father, an illiterate janitor who had left to live alone elsewhere. In what could be understood as signs of threatened self-constancy, Doug felt "changed inside," "neither fish nor fowl"; he lost all ambitions and goals, and he began to do poorly academically. He developed fears of being approached homosexually and complained bitterly of the apparently never-ending nature of his painful state. Doug also lamented the fact that his mother had not consulted him about this move. He was fearful of even hinting at his discontent with her, but gradually over the next year he began to lay plans to move out into an apartment. Doug always shared all his plans with his mother, and so he mentioned that a place had now become available that he was considering taking. He was devastated anew to find on return from school the very next day that all his belongings were efficiently packed up in boxes and waiting for him by the front door. Doug barely survived this further challenge; he was bedeviled by fantasies of suicide which gradually dissolved with the expression of his rage at his mother and with their appearance and interpretation in the transference. However, he dropped out of school, eventually took a menial job, and began a long series of affairs and liaisons with a number of girls. In the course of these relationships he attempted with some success to work through conflicts over hostility and over sexual identity and genital activity. While in the first phase of treatment Doug's sense of self-constancy was painfully threatened by the almost simultaneous loss of father and of familiar surroundings, in the later phase he came to grips with the task of finding an object to replace those he had lost. These efforts were discernible in, among other things, his choice of girlfriends, the earlier choices being uneducated, irresponsible, and impulsive girls who occasionally did unskilled jobs; his later choices gradually came to represent an amalgam of idealized representations of himself (having artistic and literary interests and talents similar to his own), and more realistic representations of his mother (in being educated, efficient, and with a steady, managerial job). In the transference I served these functions one after the other, as if I were being used as the leading edge of his development. When Doug found a girl who seemed to him to reciprocate his feelings adequately, he felt no longer in need of me or of treatment, and he brought it to an end.

SELF-ESTEEM

To the areas of narcissistic vulnerability in feelings of omnipotence and in feelings of self-constancy, a third and last strand, that of self-esteem, may now be added. The appearance of feelings of greater or lesser self-worth developmentally follows close on the establishment of self-constancy. Mahler feels that early roots of self-esteem lie in the mother's ''quasi-altruistic surrender of the infant's body to himself'' during the practicing phase (1974, 98).[3] Clearly this ''surrender'' is not an abandonment, and the mother's continued and interested real presence is crucial to the development and maintenance of adequate feelings of self-esteem. These feelings of self-regard are closely intertwined with, but not identical to, the evolution and taming of omnipotent feelings; both the child's self-esteem and his feelings of omnipotence are linked to the mother's feelings about herself and her child, and to his emerging self-constancy.

An increased understanding of the development and functions of the superego (e.g., Beres 1958) has clarified the part played by ideals in the inner regulation of self-esteem (Jacobson 1954; Reich 1960; J. Sandler 1960; Sandler, et al. 1963; Tyson and Tyson 1982). We have also been made aware of the importance of the "loving and beloved superego" in the attainment of an inner, durable sense of self-worth and comfort which is relatively independent of the presence of the object (Schafer 1960).

The "ideal state of the self" may be thought of as one in which feelings of well-being and heightened self-esteem are a function of the discrepancy between the ideal state of the self and the perceived, actual state of the self; the greater the discrepancy, the greater the amount of mental pain suffered (Joffe and Sandler 1965). The ideal state of the self can be shown to contain significant aspects of early, pleasurable experiences with the mother or primary caretaker; thus we would expect that the presence of the loved object or substitute in the external world would be an essential condition for approximating the actual self-representation to this inner ideal. At any age, the person's loss of such an important object must then inevitably result to some degree in mental pain and in a loss of self-esteem, offering thereby an explanation of Kierkegaard's observation. To the degree that the stable internalization of these ideals and these functions has been attained, and an external "policeman" is no longer needed to prompt the conscience, one may speak of superego autonomy. We usually see signs of this beginning by age five to seven years. To the degree that these ideals and functions are dependent on the presence of an external object, need to be refueled, or are subject to excessive enlargement, there exists an extra measure of narcissistic vulnerability in the area of self-esteem.

To reiterate this last point, prior to the establishment of superego autonomy, the child's self-esteem is closely linked with the mother's loving and concerned accessible presence, with her own self-regard, and with the esteem and pride with which she invests her child. With the progressive attainment of superego autonomy and thus of an inner means of regulating self-esteem, the child acquires some degree of insulation from the most crude assaults to self-esteem which result from object loss at this early age. The formation of ideals offers the child an opportunity to nourish the sense of self-worth by approximating to an inner ideal which is not so directly affected by object loss. However, these ideal self-representations are vulnerable to disruption if the loss occurs in the course of their formation. In addition, they may be subject to a magnification or overidealization, resulting in even wider discrepancies between the actual self-representation and the ideal, or they may be subject to erosion to the extent that they need to be "refueled" by the presence of the external object.

Object Loss and Self-Esteem

Once the issues of self-esteem have been distinguished from those of self-constancy and omnipotence, the clinician must assess to what degree the individual's self-esteem regulation is relatively independent of other people and based on the adequate functioning of the superego and its ideals, and to what extent the level of self-esteem is dependent on the presence of external objects who are relied upon to perform the observing, judging, and praising and rewarding, or criticizing and punishing functions. On close inspection, most references to "external narcissistic supplies" are actually references to circumstances in which the individual's self-regard is dependent in this way on external objects. However, the previous discussion has pointed to two other uses to which "supplies" from an external source may be put, namely, in adding to feelings of omnipotence, and in maintaining an adequate sense of self-constancy. Therefore, some caution is needed not to confuse these issues, since the effectiveness of interventions will be in proportion to the accuracy with which the particular "needs" are assessed and responded to.

Mention has already been made of Freud's (1917) classical formulation regarding identifications with the ambivalently regarded lost person and the consequent loss of self-esteem. The discovery of additional components of the reaction to object loss has in no way decreased the frequency with which the identifications described by Freud occur. As a final illustration, Donald was eight yeas old when his manic-depressive father, a "practical joker," a "clown" at parties, and an embezzler, committed suicide. Prior problems with Donald were known to have existed. For example, he did not learn to urinate standing up until age four, and then only when his father made a point to teach him, urged on by his wife. Later evidence from his treatment, begun at age eleven years, suggested both a struggle against an identification with his father and identifications with his mother and an older sister made at that early age. Always an intensely passive boy, after his father's death Donald was found wandering down some train tracks, and he described a wish to commit suicide by throwing himself under a bus. Later, he indulged in various delinquencies, chiefly as a member of a gang which stole cars. From these activities he obtained a boost to his self-esteem from external sources—his co-delinquents—and confirmation from others of his own persistently highly critical view of himself. In early adolescence he became a "clown" in school where he was mimicked and teased, and he expected the same denigration from the therapist and from his mother and sister who had ridiculed the father. The low state of Donald's self-esteem can be seen to be derived from several sources. Not only did the family place a low value on being male, but Donald's early identifications with his father were amplified subsequently by the loss of his father and by the identifications he made with the disturbed aspects of his father following his death.

SUMMARY

The pain of narcissistic injury is most often referred to in general terms which give only descriptive information. The experience of object loss offers an opportunity to investigate more closely the dynamics and constituents of narcissistic pain, especially in relation to the development of self-object differentiation and the progressive establishment of mental representations, and of self- and object constancy. Prior to some degree of self-object differentiation, loss of the primary caretaker does not result in object loss in the sense that such an experience will come to have later—that a meaningful relationship has been lost. A disruption in the equilibrium of the progressively more complex mother-infant reciprocity becomes progressively more difficult to repair, and complete substitution progressively less satisfactory. A developmental assessment is required in order to distinguish between the immediate impact of object loss, the influence of earlier factors on development, and the effects of object loss on subsequent development. Focusing on specifically narcissistic elements, three narcissistic constituents or strands are described as providing a clinically useful framework for such an assessment. These constituents are referred to as feelings of omnipotence, of self-constancy, and of self-esteem. Important landmarks along the developmental path of each element are described, linked to the relevant consequences of object loss, and illustrated by clinical examples.

NOTES

1. Children as young as three years of age can be taught about death through the child's normal contacts with animals and insects, at home and at nursery school (E. Furman 1974). There seems to be a great discrepancy between the eagerness with which some adults instruct children in the sexual area, and their reluctance to give children factual explanations about death and dying commensurate with the children's capacity to understand and in appropriate response to their questions. One too often hears, "Oh he is too young to know about those things."
2. This kind of remark seems to be made much more often by adults than by children or adolescents.
3. Fenichel (1945, 40) states that the first supply of satisfying nourishment from the external world restores "self-esteem and revives the narcissistic state" by removing a disturbing displeasure.

REFERENCES

Barnes, M. J. (1964). Reactions to the death of a mother. *Psychoanal. Study Child*, 19:334–357.

Beres, D. (1958). Vicissitudes of superego functions and superego precursors in childhood. *Psychoanal. Study Child*, 13:324–351.

Birtchnell, J. (1969). The possible consequences of early parent death. *Brit. J. Med. Psychol.*, 42:1–12.

Burgner, M. & Edgcumbe, R. (1972). Some problems in the conceptualization of early object relationships: Part II, The concept of object constancy. *Psychoanal. Study Child*, 27:315–333.

Eisnitz, A. J. (1981). The perspective of the self-representation: some clinical implications. *J. Amer. Psychoanal. Assn.*, 29:309–336.

Fenichel, O. (1945). *The Psychoanalytic Theory of Neurosis*. New York: Norton.

Fleming, J. & Altschul, S. (1963). Activation of mourning and growth by psychoanalysis. *Int. J. Psychoanal.* 44:419–431.

Freud, A. (1952). The mutual influences in the development of the ego and id: introduction to the discussion. In *The Writings of Anna Freud, Vol. 4, Indications for Child Analysis and Other Papers, 1945–1956*. New York: Int. Univ. Press, 1968, pp. 230–244.

——— (1960). Discussion of Dr. John Bowlby's paper. *Psychoanal. Study Child*, 15:53–62.

——— (1963). The concept of developmental lines. *Psychoanal. Study Child*, 18: 245–265.

——— (1965). *Normality and Pathology in Childhood. Assessments of Development*. New York: Int. Univ. Press.

Freud, S. (1914). On narcissism: an introduction, *S.E.*, 14.

——— (1917). Mourning and melancholia. *S.E.*, 14.

——— (1926). Inhibitions, symptoms, and anxiety. *S.E.*, 20.

——— (1928). Dostoevsky and parricide. *S.E.*, 21.

Furman, E. (1974). *A Child's Parent Dies. Studies in Childhood Bereavement*. New Haven and London: Yale Univ. Press.

Furman, R. A. (1970). The child's reaction to death in the family. In *Loss and Grief: Psychological Management in Medical Practice*, ed. A. C. Carr, et al. New York: Columbia Univ. Press, pp. 70–86.

Gaylin, W., Editor (1968). *The Meaning of Despair*. New York: Science House.

Harley, M. & Weil, A. P. (1979). Introduction. In *The Selected Papers of Margaret S. Mahler, M.D., Vol. I. Infantile Psychosis and Early Contributions*. New York: Aronson, pp. ix–xx.

Hartmann, H., Kris, E., & Loewenstein, R. M. (1946). Comments on the formation of psychic structure. *Psychoanal. Study Child*, 2:11–38.

Jacobson, E. (1946). The effect of disappointment on ego and superego formation in normal and depressive development. *Psychoanal. Rev.*, 33:129–147.

———— (1954). The self and the object world: vicissitudes of their infantile cathexes and their influence on ideational and affective development. *Psychoanal. Study Child*, 9:75–127.

———— (1965). The return of the lost parent. In *Drives, Affects, Behavior, Vol. 2, Essays in Memory of Marie Bonaparte*, ed. M. Schur. New York: Int. Univ. Press, pp. 193–211.

———— (1971). Normal and pathological moods: their nature and function. In *Depression: Comparative Studies of Normal, Neurotic, and Psychotic Conditions*. New York: Int. Univ. Press, pp. 66–106.

Joffe, W. G. & Sandler, J. (1965). Notes on pain, depression, and individuation. *Psychoanal. Study Child*, 20:394–424.

Mahler, M. S. (1961). On sadness and grief in infancy and childhood: loss and restoration of the symbiotic love object. *Psychoanal. Study Child*, 16:332–351.

———— (1966). Notes on the development of basic moods: the depressive affect. In *The Selected Papers of Margaret S. Mahler, M.D., Vol. 2, Separation-Individuation*. New York: Aronson, 1979, pp. 59–75.

———— (1974). Symbiosis and individuation: the psychological birth of the human infant. *Psychoanal. Study Child*, 29:89–106.

———— & Furer, M. (1963). Certain aspects of the separation-individuation phase. *Psychoanal. Q.*, 32:1–14.

————, Pine, F. & Bergman, A. (1975). *The Psychological Birth of the Human Infant. Symbiosis and Individuation*. New York: Basic Books.

McDevitt, J. B. (1967). A separation problem in a three-year-old girl. In *The Child Analyst at Work*, ed. E. R. Geleerd. New York: Int. Univ. Press, pp. 24–58.

———— (1971). Preoedipal determinants of an infantile neurosis. In *Separation-Individuation: Essays in Honor of Margaret S. Mahler*, ed. J. B. McDevitt and C. F. Settlage. New York: Int. Univ. Press, pp. 201–226.

———— (1975). Separation-individuation and object constancy. *J. Amer. Psychoanal. Assn.*, 23:713–742.

Meiss, M. L. (1952). The oedipal problem of a fatherless child. *Psychoanal. Study Child*, 7:216–229.

Nagera, H. (1970). Children's reactions to the death of important objects: a developmental approach. *Psychoanal. Study Child*, 25:360–400.

Neubauer, P. B. (1960). The one-parent child and his oedipal development. *Psychoanal. Study Child*, 15:286–309.

Panel (1974). Vicissitudes of infantile omnipotence. S. Kramer, Reporter. *J. Amer. Psychoanal. Assn.*, 22:588–602.

Perman, J. M. (1979). The search for the mother: narcissistic regression as a pathway of mourning in childhood. *Psychoanal. Q.*, 48:448–464.

Pollock, G. H. (1961). Mourning and adaptation. *Int. J. Psychoanal.*, 42:341–361.

———— (1978). Process and affect: mourning and grief. *Int. J. Psychoanal.*, 59:255–279.

Rangell, L. (1967). The metapsychology of psychic trauma. In *Psychic Trauma*, ed. S. S. Furst. New York: Basic Books, pp. 51–84.

Reich, A. (1960). Pathologic forms of self-esteem regulation. *Psychoanal. Study Child*, 15:215–232.

Robertson, J. & Robertson, J. (1971). Young children in brief separation: a fresh look. *Psychoanal. Study Child*, 26:264–315.

Rochlin, G. (1953a). The disorder of depression and elation. A clinical study of the changes from one state to the other. *J. Amer. Psychoanal. Assn.*, 1:438–457.

——— (1953b). Loss and restitution. *Psychoanal. Study Child*, 8:288–309.

——— (1959). The loss complex. A contribution to the etiology of depression. *J. Amer. Psychoanal. Assn.*, 7:299–316.

Sandler, A.-M. (1977). Beyond eight-month anxiety. *Int. J. Psychoanal.*, 58:195–207.

Sandler, J. (1960). On the concept of the superego. *Psychoanal. Study Child*, 15:128–162.

——— (1976). Countertransference and role-responsiveness. *Int. Rev. Psychoanal.*, 3:43–48.

———, Holder, A. & Meers, D. (1963). The ego ideal and the ideal self. *Psychoanal. Study Child*, 18: 139–158.

——— & Joffe, W. G. (1965). Notes on childhood depression. *Int. J. Psychoanal.*, 46:88–96.

——— & Sandler, A.-M. (1978). On the development of object relationships and affects. *Int. J. Psychoanal.*, 59:285–296.

Schafer, R. (1960). The loving and beloved superego in Freud's structural theory. *Psychoanal. Study Child*, 15: 163–188.

Spruiell, V. (1975). Three strands of narcissism. *Psychoanal. Q.*, 44:577–595.

Tyson, R. L. & Tyson, P. (1982). A case of "pseudo-narcissistic" psychopathology: a reexamination of the developmental role of the superego. *Int. J. Psychoanal.*, 63:283–293.

Winnicott, D. W. (1969). The use of an object. *Int. J. Psychoanal.*, 50:711–716.

Wolfenstein, M. (1969). Loss, rage, and repetition. *Psychoanal. Study Child*, 24:432–460.

TECHNICAL ISSUES IN THE TREATMENT OF COMPLICATED MOURNING IN ADULTS

Introductory Notes to Chapter 16

Rita V. Frankiel

This much-cited paper summarizes findings from a research project originally centered at the Chicago Institute for Psychoanalysis that gathered data on the personal characteristics and transference resistances of a population of patients in analysis who had suffered serious early object loss.

The case report included in this paper provides a vehicle for discussion of clinical phenomena commonly encountered in these cases. It is the report of the treatment of a woman who was separated from her parents in the Holocaust when she was an adolescent. The parents, she later learned, were killed; she was safe in another country. Fourteen years later, at age twenty-nine, she entered treatment for help with difficulties that centered around her unresolved mourning and an adolescent development so incomplete as to seriously limit her capacities for work and love. This patient remained in the grip of her rebellious attitudes and unresolved conflicts over her sexuality. From the perspective of treatment technique as thought of today, some analysts might question the analyst undertaking to discourage the patient's affair with an older man, which was interpreted as acting out that was interfering with the treatment. Whereupon the patient gave up her lover. The effect of this interdiction on the subsequent unfolding of the transference was not discussed in this article. Others might have continued to analyze without interdicting.

The reports of this research group have emphasized that these patients' reactions were characterized by absence of grief and denial of the reality of the death. Further, they were thought to show special forms of resistance and deficit that required a therapeutic atmosphere fine tuned to helping them recover from their immature ego organizations (Fleming 1972). In a subsequent publication, Fleming (1974) provided evidence that these patients almost uniformly showed serious arrests of personality development originating in the stage of development the patient was in at the time of the loss, presenting with markedly uneven development. At one point, Fleming recommended that an adaptation of Anna Freud's developmental profile be used to highlight the specific areas of deficit and immaturity in these patients (1978). This immaturity persisted until the uncompleted mourning could in fact be resumed and completed. Stolorow and Lachmann (1975) reported on the treatment of a patient who also suffered early parent loss in the Holocaust; in their judgment she manifested quite different patterns of behavior in the transference and greater personal strengths than those described by Fleming and her colleagues. E. Furman (1974) and Bowlby (1980) commented on their particular views of the case.

16. Activation of Mourning and Growth by Psycho-Analysis

Joan Fleming and Sol Altschul

In this paper we intend to present clinical evidence (1) for phenomena associated with pathological mourning as an adaptation to object-loss; and (2) showing how psychoanalytic treatment activated the mourning process and facilitated resumption of arrested development.

This paper is presented as part of the work of a group of analysts[1] studying the effect of object-loss in childhood on adult personality structure. This group research, called the Parent-loss Project, has been described in another paper (Fleming 1963) which defines the special population of patients and the method of study. All the patients are chronological adults who have lost a parent by death in childhood. They are being treated by psychoanalysis, which offers an excellent method for observing the effect of various childhood experiences on the development of adult personality structure.

In the psycho-analytic situation childhood events are relived in the transference, and the vicissitudes of the ego's adaptation to the stresses of normal growth as well as to pathogenic experiences can be subjected to close scrutiny. Regressive and integrative processes become observable, and various developmental influences on the structuralizing of the ego can be studied through the testing of reconstructive inferences.

Our study has focused on the adaptation to loss of a significant object prior to maturity when the structure of the personality is more vulnerable to deprivation of an object needed to supply experiences essential for normal growth and development. In recent years there has been increasing emphasis on the importance of the object in the development of personality. This has been documented in both clinical and theoretical studies. Many authors have written on the function of the object in normal development, and others on

Reprinted by permission of the authors' estates and *The International Journal of Psycho-Analysis* 44 (1963): 419–31. Copyright © Institute of Psycho-Analysis.

the effect of object deprivation as an interference with the developmental process. Most of these studies have been made on the mother-child relationship in early infancy, on longitudinal studies of child development, or on institutional or foster-home placement as it affects the growth of children. Very few reports have been made of observations on adults who have suffered the loss of an important libidinal object during the formative stages of the child's development. One of these studies, conducted by Hilgard and Newman (1959), was an important stimulus to our own work. They investigated anniversary reactions in adult patients who had lost a parent in childhood and who, after becoming parents themselves, developed a psychosis.

In a preliminary report (Fleming, et al. 1958), evidence was presented from the analyses of the first three cases in our series, which demonstrated a disturbed adaptation to the death of the parent. The immediate reaction was characterized by absence of grief at the time of loss, and denial of the reality was manifested in various forms. Efforts to adapt to the trauma resulted in uncompleted mourning work and what appeared to be a persisting immaturity. Patterns of immature behaviour seemed to be correlated with the level of development achieved by each patient at the time of loss. In our preliminary report, very rough correlations were made with generally accepted descriptions of phase-specific behaviour.

Since then, in a larger series of patients, correlations of adult behaviour patterns with developmental phases point towards an arrest of the normal process, especially in the area of ego-object relations. A striking picture of immaturity in self-image and in the development of ego-ideal and superego structures is apparent. Reality-testing, impulse control, object-need, and self-object awareness are not adequate for adult functioning in the patients studied. These manifestations of ego deficiencies seem to belong to levels of functioning more appropriate to different stages of childhood development. We encountered many difficulties in attempting to make an accurate diagnosis of phase-specific behaviour, as well as in formulating metapsychological concepts of age-adequate progress along significant lines of development. The recent work being done at the Hampstead Clinic by Anna Freud and her colleagues on profiles of development promises to be of great assistance in our investigation of adults (Freud, A. 1962; Sandler 1960; Sandler, et al. 1962; Sandler and Rosenblatt 1962).

It was with the first case in our series, a 29-year-old woman who had lost both parents in middle adolescence, that recognition of these phenomena and their dynamics began to occur. The first clue was apparent in the failure of the transference to develop after the usual pattern. For some time this situation prevented our clear understanding of the patient's dynamics and the dynamics of the therapeutic relationship.

In the analytic situation, the defensive denial of the reality of loss was manifested in two ways; first, by negating the significance of the analyst in present reality, and second, by insistence on repeating with the analyst the fictional relationship with the lost parent. This state of affairs produced a transference resistance which interfered with the establishment of a therapeutic alliance as a basis for interpretation and working through. The patient's defensive balance demanded that no relationship with a new object could exist, especially on a new basis, because it would disturb the protective illusion and require the patient to face the painful fact of parental death and to resume the mourning work successfully avoided up to this time.

When we realized that giving the analyst any significance in her present life meant to her the establishment of a new relationship that would force her to give up her fantasy that her parents were still alive, we began to see the fixation and its defensive function, and knew the therapeutic task was to break through the defensive denial of loss and to complete the work of mourning. The mourning process had to be set in motion before analysable regressive transference neurosis could develop. In a number of cases we have observed, once the resistance against mourning has been overcome, the analyst becomes important not only as a transference figure but as a new object useful in new integrations.

In this paper we offer clinical evidence from the analysis of one patient to show: (1) how the defence structure she had built up in response to the trauma of separation and loss of her parents delayed the development of an analysable transference in the first 270 hours of therapy; (2) how this serious resistance was broken through; (3) how the patient's investment of energy in a therapeutic relationship activated the mourning process with the recall of previously repressed memories and the experiencing of grief; (4) how, when the mourning for the dead parents had been partially accomplished with much of the guilt for the ambivalence resolved, the patient began to work through her adolescent sexual conflict, which had continued to exist for fourteen years on an early adolescent level; (5) how growth and change began to occur with the achievement of insight into the denial mechanisms. Termination of the analysis reproduced the traumatic separation in the transference, but with a more integrated ego which could grieve and mourn for old losses and new separations without trying "to make time stop." Lastly, we would like to discuss the theoretical aspects of mourning derived from this case and how it correlates with the work of previous investigators.

CLINICAL MATERIAL

The patient, a 29-year-old woman, was an only child born in Germany, who separated from her parents at age fifteen. Her parents remained behind and were killed in the European massacre sometime around her eighteenth year. She entered analysis because of anxiety and depression, precipitated by failure to pass an examination in graduate school, and disappointment in a love affair.

In the early hours of the analysis, the picture unfolded of the adolescent quality of her 29-year-old character structure. These adolescent patterns and the typical early adolescent conflicts dominated the analysis. The pre-oedipal and oedipal material which comes into sharp focus in the usual analysis played a very subordinate role in this one.

However, since she was twenty-nine years old, it did not occur to either of us to think of her as an adolescent in her character structure until the analysis had gone on for some time, and the difficulties in establishing an analysable transference became apparent. Even then we did not diagnose these difficulties as being born of the adolescent personality structure. The uncompleted mourning struck us first. The denial of the parents' death, the absence of grief for them, were observations which preceded the recognition of the extent and fixity of the persisting adolescent personality structure.

In the beginning of treatment, in what we later recognized as a characteristically adolescent attitude, the patient protested that she did not really need help—she was sure she could work out her problems by herself, although it might take longer. She felt that external circumstances were primarily responsible for her difficulties and insisted that everything would be all right if only she could have a satisfactory love affair.

In relating her history, she described her inability, up to the age of twenty-nine, to establish warm relationships with either men or women. She had a few girl friends her own age. With her aunt she was defiant and rebellious, feeling that the aunt was trying to dominate her as she felt her mother had tried to do. With men she carried on a buddy-buddy relationship even when she had intercourse with them. She tended to avoid any close contact except in her fantasies, but became easily hurt and felt rejected when men turned away from her.

Prior to the age of ten her memories were vague and meagre. The patient was fixed on the few years just before and after the separation from her parents, which she described as the longest span of her life. During the whole analysis very few memories were recovered that belonged to the earlier period, although it is more than likely that this period of time predisposed the patient to this type of defensive character structure.

Her emotional tone at the time of the separation from her parents appeared to be typical of some adolescents with a conflict over sexuality. Her romantic fantasies, which were about imaginary men, were always kept secret. Later she rejected any idea of having a man for herself and depreciated women whose only task is to have children and be housewives. She prided herself on her lack of breasts, her boyish figure, her masculine stride, and was considered arrogant, aggressive, and bossy by her friends. Keeping a diary was another pattern characteristic of her adolescence. She filled this diary with arguments between herself and her parents, and compared the need to write in the diary with "the need to have a friend to whom you can tell everything because after all there are some things that you can't discuss with your parents."

It was in this atmosphere that the separation took place. Little information was reported about the decision to separate or the events and affects surrounding the separation itself until much later when the process of mourning for her parents was far advanced. Letters full of arguments continued the old type of relationship with her parents which had existed in Germany. She did not hear of their fate until after the war, although after 1942 her letters brought no reply. When people sympathized on hearing about her parents' death, she felt guilty because of her lack of obvious mourning. In fact, she occasionally had the fantasy that if they did come to England she might have to support them, and this she did not want to do. In the last few years prior to therapy, any conversation which brought thoughts about her parents evoked tears.

One of the difficult problems was the resistance of the patient to letting herself be aware of her involvement in the analysis. She talked about being afraid that she would be overwhelmed if she became fond of someone, and said that her feelings about the analyst were amorphous. Continuing along this line, she expressed the idea that the treatment had become a nuisance: "It's silly to investigate some of these things; these are ideas I picked up in the course of my life and I just ought to shrug my shoulders about it."

Around the hundredth hour came the shift in the patient's recognition of the analyst as someone of importance to her. After being informed of the analyst's vacation, she had a dream of dying, being shunned and abandoned, and subsequently got depressed. When the relationship to the vacation was pointed out, she said she "almost had a desire to be taken care of." She thought of the analyst and then dismissed the thought. Shortly after this, she felt helpless and abandoned, and for the first time with any affect, began to talk about her parents. She began to realize that she was much more affected by their loss than she had thought.

Concurrent with her denial of the analyst's significance to her, she dreamed of her parents' being alive. In these dreams she was embroiled in arguments, trying to provoke them and feeling deprived. This seemed to support the defence of denial and to maintain the illusion of their existence. This illusion was continued in another form through the development of an affair with a married man. She acted out with him a fantasy of a relationship with an older man, and used it as a resistance against an awareness of feelings and fantasies about the analyst. As long as the patient was able to continue to confuse the analyst with her friend B., she was able to confuse both the analyst and B. with the image of her father, and so deny father's death. As she began to feel frustrated in the relationship with B. and to recognize a need to repeat frustrating experiences, she became better able to differentiate between the analyst and B.

At about the 270th hour, using this greater differentiation on her part as a wedge, a suggestion was made that she stop the acting out. It was felt that she could tolerate this prohibition because she had become a little more involved in the analytic relationship. The patient became depressed, but in response to a transference interpretation got some recognition of the struggle with her parents at age thirteen.

At this point, the 280th hour, she brought in a fragment of a dream, "I left the icebox door open and everything was defrosted. Things were beginning to spoil. I could not imagine why I had left it open." This dream seemed to indicate that the defence of repetition in fantasies was no longer as effective as before.

In the next series of hours, as the analyst became increasingly recognizable as an important figure in the transference, the grief associated with the loss of the parents came to the surface, but was pushed aside. The patient reacted to the second annual vacation with the idea that she would miss the analyst but that it was futile to talk about it.

After this vacation she expressed directly the feeling that she was beginning to feel towards the analyst as a child feels towards her father. Also in hanging up her coat in the office, she felt like an intruder and remembered arguments with her mother. She dreamt of her parents in Germany. They had gone out without her and she was in a rage. In association to this dream, memories of what the parents had been like returned. She wondered if father preferred mother. As this material unfolded it was associated with more grief. She remarked, "There are times when I wish my parents were alive and could see me now; it is agonizing to think that I will never see them again." She said at this point, "I've hit a new low," and reported a confused dream. "I didn't know where I was. I couldn't understand time." She compared this dream to one she had just before entering analysis in which she awoke one morning and couldn't get up because she "had forgotten her coordinates." In looking back this dream seemed to represent her fear of change, and an unconscious understanding of her problems, concurring as it did with her first step toward getting help for herself.

In relationship to feeling excluded and rejected in an affair, she wondered if this did not resemble some old feeling she had about her parents. When the analyst agreed, her response was, "I won't see them again, I'll never see them again." She began to cry and said, "I must have loved them. I never wanted to look at that." Then she wondered why she should have chosen that way to deal with her feelings about her parents—denial: "It's back to the death of my parents." This time the interpretation was made that as long as she could perpetuate the feelings of conflict with her parents, she could continue to reenact her pre-loss relationship with them and so continue to believe they were alive. In the 450th hour, on coming across a story of the War, the patient began to cry during the hour, with great affect, and asked, "Am I belatedly mourning my parents?"

At this point, longer in duration than in many analyses, the relationship in the transference had opened up and activated a grief reaction that had previously been repressed. The task, at this point, was the resolution of the mourning for her parents in addition to the resolution of the normal conflicts of adolescence. Both involved separation for the sake of growth.

In response to the third vacation, a shift in conflict appeared. The patient focused more on the wish to separate two people in contrast to her former fear of being abandoned.

Material in the hours dealt with envy of her mother's hair, and a desire to be more feminine. In a dream, she was in the middle between a man and a woman and felt squeezed out. She suggested it would be better "to walk with a woman on each side of the man," which was done. But she felt guilty because the man was holding her intimately. In association, she wondered if she ever felt this way about her parents, and then remembered the time when she got her own room. She felt both pleased and pushed out, "A feeling of suddenly finding out that you have grown."

This was very much the tone of her current life where she felt like a child on the fringe, and at the same time was able to act in a more feminine way with one of her male friends. Although she felt about to make a big jump, she still pictured herself in her fantasies with her parents hugging them and crying. She also had a fantasy of what it would be like to meet the analyst in ten or twenty years. Two events occurred concerning two friends she had known in London, where it was obvious to her that changes had taken place in them. She vigorously insisted that she herself was not going to grow. It was interpreted that she was having more and more difficulty in acting as if the world were the same as it had been when she was fifteen years old.

During the last eighteen months of treatment, there was an increasing elaboration and expression of the mourning process with recall of significant events related to the separation from her parents. Development of insight into her mechanism of denial was achieved, and with this achievement there was a more direct approach to her adolescent conflict. The patient no longer had to depreciate sexuality and competitive impulses. She began to talk about a man, C., with whom she had recently become intimate. She wanted the analyst to meet him, stating, "I, too, can have a man."

As she worked through this conflict of wanting a man of her own and choosing between C. and the analyst, she talked about her parents in a different way. "At times I think it's a shame that I never knew them when I was grown and they didn't know me." Here is evidence of acceptance of their death and movement towards the conflicts of later adolescence, with a beginning of detachment of libido from the parental images and making it available for new objects. Some of this energy was attached to the analyst as she used the latter for a transference object to work out her adolescent struggle for emancipation and growth. Here, on the stage of a basic positive relationship, she acted out her adolescent rebelliousness with simultaneous fears of steps towards adulthood. She was feeling rebellious towards the analyst as she planned to move into a new apartment. She reported a dream of some teen-age kids all behaving in a noisy, violent fashion, but she was different. She began talking about ending the analysis, but in no concrete way.

Much of the conflict at this stage of the analysis could be described as the patient's efforts to grow. Steps were made forward, followed by retreat, refusing temporarily to accept the real changes that were taking place in her job, personal life, physical characteristics, and general sense of well-being. In association to her rebellious feelings towards the analyst the patient talked about her rebellious feelings towards her parents with a new insight that in a later stage of development one can see one's parents as people. She had never felt this, but had always taken them for granted.

The conflict about growth continued. It was associated with the expression of grief and increasing perception of the present-day situation. She felt deprived of her parents, but "I refuse to have their place taken." In association to a dream of a power struggle with her mother, she said tearfully, "I don't let my parents die." She began to think about the separation for the sake of her own growth as excluding the parents. Around the time of the fourth vacation, she reported a dream of phoning her father in London, but with the perception that he should be dead. On a vacation of her own, she felt desolate although rebellious. This feeling was associated with the fear that the analyst would not be there on her return. This was interpreted as her fear of the repetition of the real experience. Once she left her parents and had never seen them again. Her reply was, "I thought it would only be for two or three months. How could I get so fouled up? This business of being stuck somewhere without wanting to grow. I feel ashamed of it. It makes me feel inadequate, that I'm not able to cope with my problems better than by refusing to grow up." The reality of the danger in the European situation in 1939 came up. It was interpreted to the patient that she needed to separate from her parents to survive, and that they sent her away so that she could survive. Her associations were, "They must have been more aware of the danger than I." "I have to live in the present, and I've never done this."

After the summer vacation, the patient informed the analyst that she had put in motion an application for restitution from the German government. This was possible because she was accepting the fact of their death. She had a feeling of being on the fence and did not want to jump. She began to bring up the idea of approaching the end of treatment, but "I have some things to work out. It's not a problem of growing up, but it's accepting myself as I am. I'm still not satisfied. If I'm still not satisfied it's too bad. I could always look to the future as before. I kept myself happy by this. Maybe I'm just postponing the moment when I may not like some of these things." She began to have a growing awareness of the passage of time, and made the remark, "I've lost a lot of time—eighteen years."

There was, concurrently with this, a growing awareness of the analyst as a person. "You must have got a lot of pleasure out of fixing this room up. You like it and spend a lot of time here. I'm very pleased, we have something in common. I fix my room, you fix yours." This whole period of struggle about growth culminated in a dream. The patient made a point of saying she dreamt her parents were alive. She was away somewhere on a camping trip. Then she got a phone call that was from her grandmother. Grandmother was beating about the bush regarding some bad news. Patient knew it was about her parents. Grandmother did not want to tell her. She asked the patient on the phone to come back and the patient said, "For Christ's sake tell me." She was in a panic—something had happened to her parents. Even in the dream she was amazed at her own feeling and was horrified when she learned that they had been killed in an automobile accident. She was grief-stricken even though she knew it was a dream, and she was amazed at the intensity of what she felt. When she awoke she said, "Good heavens, can you imagine such intensity of feeling so many years later?"

As the patient worked on the resolution of her mourning and her adolescent conflicts, the significance of the sense of danger previously experienced in the analysis became more apparent: namely, the importance of her guilt over her wish to separate from her parents, and the part it played in her need to deny their death which followed on leaving them. She talked about feeling guilty because of doing so well in her personal life and in her job. When the analyst remarked that she associated things going well with her to the loss of her parents, she replied, "I thought you meant that things were going well *because* I lost my parents." This she associated to a feeling of liberation. "It's a good idea at sixteen to separate from your parents," she said, but she was doubtful what she would say about it now because her separation was a "complete loss." But if her parents were alive this would limit her ambitions, and about this she felt guilty. At this time, the patient was concerned with the question, what is wrong with having loving or affectionate feelings towards the analyst or her father? At the same time she felt rage when she got no response from C., or the analyst, and remembered similar feelings towards her father when she was a small child. All this was related to thoughts of terminating the analytic relationship, which the patient compared to leaving her parents. She was afraid of being on her own, felt guilty about leaving the analyst behind, and had an increasing insight into the way in which she handled her fear and her guilt. "At some point when I left my parents there was something that was so unbearable, it stopped the clock. I couldn't keep the outward circumstances constant so I kept the inward ones constant." When the analyst remarked that it looked as if the clock was starting, the patient reported changes in her personal habits. She felt on her own now. She had the feeling that she had something to settle with the analyst, and remarked that as an adolescent she did not feel afraid. The analyst asked what she was afraid of repeating with him, and she replied, "That rings a bell, but what? Why was I stuck about feelings about father? It's O.K. for teens but why didn't I grow? Is the clock stopped? What was too painful? To avoid realizing that they were dead—did I have to stop everything?"

Under the pressure of guilt about termination, the patient retreated and again denied caring about people she might be leaving behind. "In due course I'll be leaving this city without caring the least about leaving anybody." But soon after this she began to talk about whether she was important to the analyst, would the analyst remember her? She felt she had grown beyond C. The analyst made a transference interpretation that she was repeating conflicts which existed before she separated from her parents, which had to do with the desire to surpass her mother. She was guilty about this and yet she wanted to be special. In a way she had been special because she was saved and they were not. Therefore she has to continue living over and over the conflict with her parents in order to master the guilt of her own survival and their death. The reaction to this interpretation was a wish to cry. "You hit it right. The guilt before separation—it's true, I wanted to be independent and I was not upset when I left them. When mother cried I was ashamed that I had no response." The analyst said, "But one of your wishes was to go away." Her remark was, "The final separation—there was a lot wrong with it, especially the way it occurred—it could have been such fun to go away and come home."

When the patient wanted to take a vacation from the analysis, the analyst questioned her motivations and wondered if it was advisable. Again she became rebellious, as if the analyst were holding her down and not giving her her freedom. This led to the recall of "After I left my parents, I was forever in rebellion. This is typical of teen-agers but not of the thirties, or should not be, but I enjoyed it. I was proud of it. I resent talking to you. I was glad when I left home, I felt free. But I was guilty later when my parents were killed. Every time something comes up about being glad to leave, it adds to the feeling that it had not been nice of me. It's a shame that my parents couldn't understand me as a teen-ager, but I guess they were just human too." It was interpreted that she did not want to change but wanted to keep herself in this position because to grow and be free meant something destructive to her parents and also to herself.

After this she began to have a more realistic approach to what father had mother had been like. Specifically, she began to talk about father, wondering why he did not get out of Germany. Everyone knew that the end was coming, even when he left he did not really get out. Then she remembered a picture of mother at her prayers, "Several times I caught her crying. I used to be pretty upset, but it's likely I pretended not to know." The patient began to cry and said, "It's strange, I never realized that I loved my mother until this minute." She had a picture of mother crying and praying and wished that she could do something for her, as though it were now.

Following this, she experienced an important transference reaction. She wondered about the separation from her parents. "For it to have had such an effect there must have been some weak spots in the relationship with them. Is that right?" she asked. When the analyst said, "It sure is," she had a feeling the analyst was laughing at her for trying to make interpretations and feeling able to do what the analyst does. "Will I ever be able to stand on my own two feet again? It's funny that I added 'again.' " She had the idea she was beginning to finish and realized she was afraid. She began to talk about giving up her own work and going into psychology instead. She was somewhat ashamed and embarrassed to talk about this. The analyst said she was talking about the same thing that he does, and that this was a problem never worked out with her mother, namely, being able to do the same thing as well or better. She continued to ruminate about feeling guilty about growing. "But I don't want to be an analyst," she protested. She then had a splurge of activity in which she functioned well but presented herself as afraid of finishing. She began to talk about the positive values of finishing—more time and money for herself. The analyst interpreted that she was afraid to face these feelings because of some idea that it was associated with destruction.

At this time she felt that the analyst had cancelled some hours deliberately as a way of cutting down without it seeming to be so. The analyst pointed out her need to see this as being done surreptitiously. This would solve the conflict about her wish to leave the analyst behind and make it seem as if there had been no parting.

The problem discussed here becomes clearer in another dream about doodling. She had a piece of paper and a pencil—she was talking and doodling, "It meant something to you because you took the paper and looked at it. It was very valuable because at that session things became clarified without my having to do much about it. The doodle was more important than what I had said." The analyst remarked that he thought she had already made her decision and that she could not communicate it directly but only by the doodle. The patient said, "I wonder what it could be. The only thing is how much longer am I going to come here?" She felt blocked and frightened at this point, but when asked, "What date did you have in mind?" she said, "It's very close, maybe by the time summer is over. The time that actually occurred to me was when you go on your vacation. I never put a date on it before. I thought about it being at the end of the summer before but this time it's different."

When she continued to talk about separation from her parents, the analyst asked her about that date. She gave the date and compared it to leaving the Zionist farm to go to London a year later. Going to London really was permanent, but she wanted it to look like a vacation. The analyst remarked, "It sounds like the problem you have about leaving analysis. You feel guilty about the idea that you might never see me again." She said, "I've done this for years," felt sad, depressed, and began to talk again about finishing. When the analyst interpreted that if someone is out of sight they do not exist any more, she remarked, "Something occurs to me: it seems I got stuck when my parents and I separated and I didn't see them any more. After a certain number of years they ceased to exist actually. This was a shock. It seems as though I got fixed on this reaction and I react to everyone in this way; why should I unless I was guilty or felt responsible for what happened? I had a thought—it just hit now—they did it for me. They sent me to England by myself and I was better off materially than if they came with me." The analyst remarked that she felt guilty about the mere fact that she had survived. She said, "That goes for the money and survival."

The subsequent material had to do with the patient's denial and delay in facing the termination, and her associations and interpretations about the meaning of this. Of equal importance is the patient's participation in setting the procedure for termination. On 3 June the patient was informed that the analyst's vacation was to begin on 15 July. Her reaction to this was, "It seems so soon. I just won't terminate then." She began to talk about "How do you finish? Do you come less frequently?" She did not want to decide because she would never be certain whether the analyst had approved. She wondered if she would be just as upset if she quit before the time to terminate. Her indecision about making a decision came up in association with the original idea of going to England. She realized that she had had quite a bit to do with it—her parents brought it up but she liked it since she was not the least bit eager to go to Poland with them. She wondered, "Will I actually finish on the fifteenth?"

She came in on the anniversary of her separation from her parents all tired out and depressed. She was about to repeat the dawdling of the day before, "What do you do at the end? Do you throw a party? C. said, 'Take a bottle of wine to the hour.' " The analyst felt the patient did not recognize the date and its significance. When he asked if she knew what day it was, she gave the date and remarked, "Good heavens, I didn't remember. Now I'm crying. That must be why I resented C. going home today."

This awareness enabled her to talk about the last day with her parents. She remembered them on the platform crying. She had no regret and felt terrible about this. It was necessary to change trains in Frankfurt and the officials were very disagreeable. When the refugees crossed the border, they were welcomed by a group of Dutch people, tea, food and great rejoicing. When she got to England she was confused and could not take care of her luggage. On this anniversary in 1957 she said, "I must have been remembering all of this yesterday without realizing it, and that's why I got up at six o'clock. I was thinking of father and mother, how old they would have been now. Father would be fifty-seven now. The last seventeen years have gone so fast—faster in memory than the first seventeen years. I don't remember, but this is sort of an anniversary—exactly eighteen years, or is it seventeen? I can't do the arithmetic! It's really eighteen."

She began to look more grown-up and feminine at this point, and continued to talk about terminating. "I can't visualize that this is the end. Yet it's going to be very soon. I'm not able to decide." She confused C. with the analyst frequently at this point, and it was interpreted that she was trying to avoid the intensity of her feelings about leaving the analyst. "I can't feel it's right—I should say, I can't feel it's wrong." She then talked about leaving England again, began to ruminate about a coat of her mother's and wondered whether it would fit her now. She talked about finishing in a month; "Maybe I will and then I'll just see you a couple of times." The analyst agreed with the wisdom of this procedure, which would in this way avoid a separation too identical with the separation from her parents.

Then came a long dream, indicating some integration of herself in time and in present reality. She was back in Munich with her parents. They left and called to her, "Aren't you coming?" She said, "I'm going to stay another day." Then she looked through the apartment, talked about the living-room with windows a little high, "I was surprised to be my present age in the dream but when I say this about the windows that might be how it would look to a child." Then she investigated the apartment and found a telephone which in reality they did not have. She wanted to call someone, but she did not quite know whom to call. Then she did not remember the number; "After all, it's been seventeen years." Then the dream changed and there was the idea that her parents were dead. She thought of looking up people who were still there. This was both pleasant and painful. She thought of some teachers, but they were old and might also be dead. Then she reported another dream, back in Munich, but it looked like London. She did not mind walking by herself after dark, but she was hungry. She talked to someone; German was spoken, but without any fluency on her part. There were lots of stands for snacks, but none seemed to have what she wanted. One had the remains of a sign in English. "It must have been from the war—an American hot dog stand, and I was annoyed that it was not there anymore."

She felt this dream meant, "I was finally making my peace; a final step." She continued to talk about her guilt for leaving her parents. The analyst pointed out the termination was difficult for her because it looked as if she took all of her mother's talent by growing. She said, "I can't remember, but what I think seems to confirm this. I'm pleased to look like a woman. I want everyone to notice my weight, my legs, my waist." Then she talked about being surprised that the analyst took her seriously about the termination date. "The status quo is over, I can't postpone any longer. Treatment is beyond the point of usefulness, it's prolonging the dependence relationship that's no longer necessary. I've grown fond of you and the idea of not seeing you is going to be painful. Now I want to cry." She then talked about setting a definite time to see the analyst after she terminated, and the analyst agreed that they would make an appointment sometime in September when she returned from her vacation.

In characteristic fashion her next remarks demonstrated the persistent drive to keep a separation from the analyst as identical as possible with the separation from the parents. She said, "Do I kiss you goodbye? I presume I kissed my parents goodbye." People suggested to her that she ought to celebrate about finishing treatment. She said there was nothing to celebrate. The analyst remarked that there was some sadness. She said she ought to be able to answer yes, but she feels none, as if she must again repress her emotions. "It's foolish to cry or be upset because one is finishing. Everyone else reacts that it's nice and they're happy, and so it is in a way, but on another level I have nothing to celebrate. It's odd to feel this way about someone that you know in such a limited contact."

It should be emphasized that five or six weeks prior to the termination of the analysis was the anniversary of the first weeks in England and the period immediately following the separation from her parents.

She began to talk about what she would do in the last hour. Would she sit up? It would be difficult. The analyst pointed out how she wanted to make the last hour like all the others. She said, "Sitting opposite you I'd be tongue-tied. When someone you're fond of leaves you get upset. I'm sorry that it's coming to an end; I can't face it. It's only half real—it isn't true. It's absurd to be upset on leaving one's psycho-analyst. I've tried to make a joke out of it. Maybe there is a parallel between leaving my parents. There's something inevitable about this separation just as there is with parents and children—only mostly they're not quite so drastic. But this is inevitable, natural and right, so I have no right to be unhappy." The analyst agreed with her that there was a parallel between her feelings for the analyst and her parents, but the same thing was actually not happening. She was close to tears, and said, "What difference does it make?" The analyst pointed out that unhappiness was not all she felt. When she had said it was inevitable, natural, and right, there was some gratification in leaving. She said, "It's true, I don't feel it when I'm here, but it's uppermost in my mind when I'm away. Do I feel guilty?" She would like to know the analyst socially. Separation and breaking up in any kind of contact one has valued had always been difficult for her. She thought it would be difficult to imagine not liking the analyst.

Patient then returned to the question about making an appointment after she had finished. She wondered what she was afraid of. The analyst remarked, "You're not really sure you'll ever see me again." The patient's response was, "It looks like it," and was close to tears.

The last hour the patient came in and emphasized the convenience of not having to come any more. "It's your turn to talk now." She said she had learned a lot "but that is not the primary purpose of treatment; the rest, I feel, is intangible. It would be funny to mention to C. that this is the most prolonged relationship I've had. The word I wanted was the first mature relationship. How do you say goodbye? Do you shake hands? I should have brought flowers. As I was coming I thought this was the last time and I was glad. When I'm here it's all so different—it's mostly sad at the parting and some fear. It's easier to talk to you. It stops me from deceiving myself." Then she talked about teenagers growing up whether they want to or not.

At the end of the hour an appointment was made for the last week of September, following the vacation. The analyst remarked that he had enjoyed working with her. They shook hands, the analyst wished her luck, and they said goodbye with some feeling of sadness on both sides.

When the patient returned in September she reported that she had "had a lousy summer." For two weeks she felt acutely bad and then the rest of the summer was generally miserable. She told about difficulties with C. till the last week when he was leaving town. This was interpreted as reliving the separation from her parents and wondering if the analyst would be able to survive the change in the relationship. "Even if I try to put you into a fantasy, there is no place for you." She had been thinking about her parents in the last three weeks, with sadness about never having known them as an adult.

Patient readily agreed to come a few times to talk the situation over. The analyst interpreted that what she called her relapse was due to a problem about leaving the analyst that she could not allow herself to feel because she had fears of a total dissolution of the relationship with the analyst rather than a change. She said, "But separations were always permanent, like with my parents, and leaving London."

The patient felt better immediately after the return visit and had a dream about two men in which she had to make a choice. She chose the man associated with C. and not the one associated with the analyst. She talked about wanting to know the analyst in the future, but had no regrets in the dream about her choice. She felt much better about herself at this point.

The patient was impressed with the change in her feelings following these return visits. She realized that the interruption and return had been necessary in order for her to accept the change in herself. She said not to return would have left something undone. In the treatment her idea that learning and growing meant the destruction of her parents "became untwisted." "The way I handled it then was maybe the only way but not very good. This is a better way."

DISCUSSION

We have described the course of an analysis of a 29-year-old woman whose maturation was complicated by the death of her parents during her adolescence. This traumatic event had intensified the adolescent development task of emotional and social emancipation from childhood parental relationships. The mechanisms by which she adapted to this experience included denial of the reality of her loss and of the passage of time. This adaptive effort resulted in a prolonging of adolescent behaviour patterns and a failure to complete either the mourning for her parents or the normal resolution of her developmental conflicts.

This arrested development and uncompleted mourning presented an unusually difficult resistance and distortion of the development of the transference neurosis. Our material confirmed what Anna Freud described in her article on adolescence (A. Freud 1958). Here she pointed out how attempts to analyse an adolescent often met this kind of resistance, an inability to cathect the analyst and so to establish a basic transference from which the analytic work can proceed. According to Anna Freud, growth in this period normally requires a withdrawal of cathexis from the parent similar to what is required in mourning work, but so much energy is needed for this adolescent developmental task that not enough is available to cathect objects involving new levels of relationship.

In our patient, the demands inherent in the tasks of emancipation and mourning occurred simultaneously and required an integrative capacity which the patient did not possess. She managed to function well for fourteen years as long as the pressures for further sexual and social growth remained fairly constant. However, when life forces urged adult sexuality and career roles on her, adaptations to stresses of adolescence and to the trauma of parental loss broke down. At this point she was able to seek and eventually use outside help. Only after the repressed grief and ambivalence for the parents was mobilized through the repetition of separation experiences in the analytic transference could a new resolution to her adolescent conflicts be achieved. Analysis of the initial transference resistance activated the uncompleted mourning process and permitted the patient to proceed with her interrupted development. The most significant working through was accomplished in the experience of termination and consequently separation with emancipation from the analyst. The termination of this relationship differentiated him and the analytic experience from what had occurred with her parents, and freed her from the defensive fixation which had arrested the process of maturation in this patient. She was able to accept the death of her parents without ambivalence and guilt and to gain a new self identity with an orientation in present time.

Repression of grief has been described by[2] Helene Deutsch (1937). She explains the absence of expressions of grief or awareness of the feeling as the ego's defensive attempt to preserve itself in the face of overwhelming anxiety. Death of a libidinal object is experienced as separation from a needed source of supply, the loss of which threatens the self. The intensity of the danger depends upon the degree of helplessness experienced in the separation. The more immature the ego, the more needed is the object and consequently, more intense anxiety will be experienced as a result of the loss. Deutsch emphasizes the importance of ambivalence and unneutralized aggression present in the pre-loss relationship as a factor in determining the quantity of stress to which the ego must adapt.

In *Mourning and Melancholia* (1917), Freud develops the concept of mourning as a process whose aim is adaptation to the loss of a loved object. It is a process which continues over a period of time, has stages in its operation, and a goal resulting in a modification of ego organization. He called this process mourning work, whose task is to shift libidinal cathexes from their attachment to the lost object and make this energy available for use in new relationships.

Partial and temporary separations from libidinal objects are experiences which from birth possess significance as activators of the adaptive mechanisms of the ego. To a large extent these separation experiences influence the rate and direction of growth, and play a part in organizing the developing ego structure. Thus the process of growth and maturation can be compared to mourning work in that every step towards maturation involves some adaptation to separation, and therefore some mourning work. In true mourning, however, the separation is total, whereas in normal growth the maturing separation more often involves detachment from an old pattern of relationship while the real object continues to exist and the step forward is in terms of change and giving up rather than losing something. Freud, in *The Ego and the Id* (1923), described this development process most succinctly when he said, "the character of the ego is a precipitate of abandoned object-cathexes and . . . contains the history of those object-choices."

Spitz (1957) and others have demonstrated that the presence of adequate objects is essential for the earliest organization of the ego. Many authors, A. Freud (1944), Benedek (1938, 1956), and others have described at length the importance of the mother as a part object, then as a differentiated object essential for the experiences which structure the child's sense of self and the ego's patterns of adaptation to reality. Meiss (1952), in reporting on a five-year-old boy whose father died when he was three, emphasizes the need for objects of both sexes when the integrative tasks of the oedipal period are at their height. She describes how her patient attempted to provide himself first with his own father through imagination and then with an actual substitute father in a transference triangle with her.

The disturbing effect of object loss on ego development has also been described by many other authors. Rochlin (1953) stresses the length to which the child's ego will go to make up for the deficiency caused by the absence of a needed object. In his case, the loss occurred very early in the little boy's relationship with his mother when his need for narcissistic sustenance from her was still paramount and even before his perception of her as more than a part object was well organized. His solution was to withdraw to social isolation but in contact with a symbolic object in the form of his mother's fur coat. She did not die but she withdrew from her son, and the substitute caretakers did not supply the experiences of emotional response necessary to change narcissistic libido into object libido. Rochlin emphasizes that withdrawal to the self is not enough when an externally existing object is needed by the immature ego. The needed object is strenuously sought for to prevent disintegration of the self. This may be accomplished at the cost of a rupture with reality (Freud 1924). In *The Ego and the Id* (1923), Freud describes the "reinstatement of the object in the ego" in reaction to loss, and says that this interjection results in a modification of the ego.

In agreement with these and other authors, we felt that the failure to mature was largely due to the absence of a libidinal object whose presence was necessary for the ego's growth towards normal maturation.

In our preliminary report and in this case, it seemed to us that two things had occurred as the immature ego began its work of adaptation to parental death. First, the loss of the love object was experienced by the ego as a danger to itself and reacted to with denial of reality, denial of the absence of the parent, and concomitant repression of affect. The second adaptive mechanism set in motion by this overwhelming situation seemed to result not only in absence of grief but in pathological mourning which could be described as prolonged and still incomplete at the onset of analytic therapy many years after the traumatic loss occurred. These defences of repression and denial of perceptual reality, accompanied by fantasied continuation of the lost relationship, constitute the early stages of a normal mourning process. When prolonged, they absorb the energy necessary for growth and the establishment of new relationships in the present. Pollock (1961) has recently focused on the usual adaptive function of mourning work in bringing about new integrations after the loss of a significant figure. This contrasts with the adaptive function that resistance to mourning serves in the patient under discussion here.

Bowlby, in his recent series of articles on separation anxiety, has described observations of the sequence of behaviour which commonly occurs when children between the ages of about twelve months and four years are removed from the mother figure to whom they are attached and placed in the care of strangers. These behavioural sequences have been termed by Robertson and Bowlby: protest, despair, and detachment. Protest is associated with the problem of separation anxiety, despair with grief and mourning, and detachment with defence and future psychopathology (Bowlby 1960a, 1960b, 1960c, 1961).

These concepts of Bowlby's have aroused controversy as to whether these reactions can properly be termed mourning. The basis of the controversy is whether sufficient structural development has taken place in the still maturing ego for mourning for a lost object to occur, or whether this is simply a separation reaction to loss of a need-satisfying or part object (A. Freud 1960; Schur 1960; Spitz 1960). These questions, of course, must wait further clarification of concepts of ego development and structure before a definitive answer can be reached.

Bowlby has also postulated that the term "mourning" should not be confined only to those cases of successful mourning (Bowlby 1961). Using this broader definition, Bowlby's patients certainly are undergoing a mourning process, but a process which may become interrupted in a particular phase. This interruption may be an arrested state, as where the resistance against the work of detachment was especially demonstrated in our patient. The phase of protest and despair may be successfully managed, but the phase of detachment requires an integrative effort not always possible or in which the mechanisms used result ultimately in some form of pathology.

Our patient gave no evidence of any acute reaction, such as protest or despair, to the loss of her parents. In fact, she reported feeling no grief much as Helene Deutsch's patients did (Deutsch 1937). It would seem that the vigorous and lengthy denial of the loss certainly carries in it "protest." Moreover, upon the activation of mourning, despair was felt by the patient. "I won't see them again. I'll never see them again," and "I must have loved them. I never wanted to look at that."

Freud, in *Mourning and Melancholia,* defines decathexis of the lost object and the freeing of energy for new objects as the essential integrative task. When achieved it brings an end to mourning. Our patient in the light of these definitions must be seen as unable to mourn successfully, but as continuing a pathological mourning process in that she could not accomplish the decathexis of the lost objects. Her failure resulted in incomplete mourning, and confirms the observation of Bowlby that the stage of detachment is difficult to work through. His findings (1961) indicate that serious psycho-pathology may appear during this stage of the mourning process.

Investigation of the mourning process in cases of adults whose loss occurred in childhood many years before coming under observation, offers a fertile field for the study of the normal and pathological aspects of this important experience. It is an experience which confronts the child with demands on his integrative resources that bring those specific stresses and corresponding adaptations into clear focus when observed in the transference repetitions of a psycho-analytic situation. Genetic reconstructions of the childhood vicissitudes of development and a given child's methods of adaptation become possible. The resulting personality structure can be correlated with the childhood trauma and its various dynamics identified. Such information is available otherwise only in long-term studies of a child while living through such an experience over a period of many years. Information from both types of studies should contribute valuable data for metapsychological concepts regarding the function of the object personality development as seen through studies of object loss.

CONCLUSION

The course of an analysis of a 29-year-old woman is presented, which demonstrates a form of pathological mourning; that of the defensive denial of the reality of the parental loss resulting in prolonged mourning and interference with successful maturation. This adaptive equilibrium persisted for fourteen years with a continuation of adolescent developmental conflicts and personality structure. Psycho-analytic treatment was able to penetrate the defensive denial, activate the interrupted mourning work, and help the patient to resume the growth process interrupted at age fifteen, with resolution of adolescent conflicts and new integrations. This complex of prolonged mourning and developmental fixation is discussed in terms of adolescent developmental tasks and in relationship to mourning, growth, and the pathological consequences of unfinished mourning.

NOTES

1. A study being conducted at the Chicago Institute for Psychoanalysis.
2. Pollock, in discussing an earlier presentation of this material before the Chicago Psychoanalytic Society, pointed out that the developing transference neurosis is atypical not only because the patient cannot accept the death but because accepting the death unleashes the guilt and other ambivalent feelings associated with the object that is deceased.

REFERENCES

Benedek, T. (1938). "Adaptation to Reality in Early Infancy." *Psychoanal. Quart.*, 7.
——— (1956). "Toward a Biology of the Depressive Constellation." *J. Amer. Psychoanal. Assoc.*, 4.
Bowlby, J. (1960a). "Separation Anxiety." *Int. J. Psycho-Anal.*, 41.
——— (1960b). "Grief and Mourning in Infancy and Early Childhood." *Psychoanal. Study Child*, 15.
——— (1960c). "Separation Anxiety: A Critical Review of the Literature." *J. Child Psychol. Psychiat.*, 1.
——— (1961). "Processes of Mourning." *Int. J. Psycho-Anal.*, 42.
Deutsch, H. (1937). "Absense of Grief." *Psychoanal. Quart.*, 6.
Fleming, J., *et al.* (1958). "The Influence of Parent-Loss in Childhood on Personality Development." Read at meeting of Amer. Psychoanal. Assoc., May 1958.
Fleming, J. (1963). "Evolution of a Research Project in Psychoanalysis." In H. Gaskill (ed.) *Counterpoint: Libidinal Object and Subject*. New York: International Universities Press.
Freud, A. (1958). "Adolescence." *Psychoanal. Study Child.*, 13.
——— (1960). "Discussion of Dr. John Bowlby's Paper." *Psychoanal. Study Child*, 15.
——— (1962). "Assessment of Childhood Disturbances." *Psychoanal. Study Child*, 17.
Freud, A., and Burlingham, D. (1944). *Infants without Families*. (New York: Int. Univ. Press).
Freud, S. (1917). "Mourning and Melancholia." *S.E.* 14.
——— (1923). *The Ego and the Id. S.E.* 19.
——— (1924). "The Loss of Reality in Neurosis and Psychosis." *S.E.* 19.
Hilgard, J. R., and Newman, M. F. (1959). "Anniversaries in Mental Illness." *Psychiatry*, 22.
Meiss, M. (1952). "The Oedipal Problems of a Fatherless Child." *Psychoanal. Study Child*, 7.
Pollock, G. H. (1961). "Mourning and Adaptation." *Int. J. Psycho-Anal.*, 42.

Rochlin, G. (1953). "Loss and Restitution." *Psychoanal. Study Child*, 8.

Sandler, J. (1960). "On the Concept of Super-ego." *Psychoanal. Study Child*, 15.

Sandler, J., *et al.* (1962). "The Classification of Superego Material in the Hampstead Index." *Psychoanal. Study Child*, 17.

Sandler, J., and Rosenblatt, B. (1962). "The Concept of the Representational World." *Psychoanal. Study Child*, 17.

Schur, M. (1960). "Discussion of Dr. John Bowlby's Paper." *Psychoanal. Study Child*, 15.

Spitz, R. (1957). *No and Yes.* (New York: Int. Univ. Press.)

——— (1960). "Discussion of Dr. John Bowlby's Paper." *Psychoanal. Study Child*, 15.

Introductory Notes to Chapter 17

Rita V. Frankiel

Volkan and his colleagues at the University of Virginia Medical School have been treating and studying "established pathological mourners" since 1966. They have developed a brief psychotherapy technique based on their understanding of the underlying dynamics of chronic involvement with the lost object. They call this treatment "re-grief work," and the present paper briefly describes the technique, the theory on which it is based, and the diagnostic considerations that they feel must determine the kinds of patients who can and cannot be helped with this method.

One significant aspect of this work has been the discovery of what Volkan calls the "linking objects" used by pathological mourners to contain and symbolize their ongoing, dread-filled, loving and hating relationship with their dead object (Volkan 1972). The linking object is a concrete representation to the mourner of the body of the deceased: something that had been worn or owned by the dead one, or something that can be thought to represent him or her (1972, 215–16). Considerable effort is spent in attempting to differentiate the linking object from transitional objects, childhood fetishes, and fetishistic objects used by adults. The linking object is conceived as a device for controlling the lost object. The object that stands in the lost person's stead is under the complete control of the mourner; he/she must at all times know where it is, and becomes distraught when it cannot be safeguarded.

The treatment proceeds as follows: first, a diagnostic interview is conducted to select patients suitable for "re-grief" therapy. It is recommended that the treatment be offered to patients with essentially intact ego functions (except for their use of splitting in coping with their loss): they should be psychologically minded, motivated, and ready to form a therapeutic alliance. Patients with narcissistic pathology are excluded, being regarded as requiring more extensive treatment. Patients are often seen three to four times per week (Volkan 1984–85), although some choose to come less often (Volkan and Josephthal 1980). The treatment first focuses on demarcating similarities and differences between the mourner and the dead one. The patient seems eventually to bring the linking object into the therapy room (with the active support and encouragement of the therapist). Powerful emotions are released. Occasionally, the treatment has been so disturbing that brief psychiatric hospitalization has been necessary. Many of these patients are reported to be able to greatly attenuate their use of the linking object, to face their hatred of the lost one, and finally to say goodbye. Most of these treatments are reported to be completed in four months. A small percentage go on to psychoanalytic treatment after successful re-grief work. Truncated case reports, clinical vignettes, dream sequences, and test-retest findings on the MMPI (Volkan 1972; Volkan, Cillufo, and Sarvay 1975) are offered to support the claims of rapid and remarkable recovery.

If, however, one takes a firmly psychoanalytic stance, it is difficult to feel fully convinced by these reports. Much of what is reported gives the impression of transference manipulation. Insufficient time is allowed the patient to control the direction of his or her work. Since the earliest days of psychoanalysis, we have known that suggestion was the most powerful possible tool in the hands of the analyst or therapist. The patient will do amazing things for love of the therapist and out of motivation to please and be affirmed by the therapist. Not all patients are so obliging, but it is possible to so limit one's treated group that it is composed mainly of obliging patients; gratifying results are then artifacts of the technique rather than genuine or structural alterations in the inner world of the patient. In research like this, the only way to make certain that the experimental condition is accounting for the changes is for the researcher to present a carefully matched, untreated control group or a control group treated by some other method. In the absence of such data, it is necessary to maintain some reserve about this extremely interesting work.

17. The Treatment of Established Pathological Mourners

Vamik D. Volkan and Daniel Josephthal

There is much in the psychiatric literature about the similarities and differences between uncomplicated grief and the reactive depression that follows the death of someone close and important to the mourner. Freud (12) showed long ago how both "mourning and melancholia" may be initiated by such a loss, and how both include painful dejection, a loss of interest in the world outside the self, a decrease in the capacity to love, and the inhibition of any activity not connected with thoughts of the dead. What distinguishes mourning from neurotic depression is the disturbance in self-regard that appears in the latter state. In uncomplicated grief the mourner can loosen his ties to the representation of the dead through the work of mourning, or can form the kind of loving identification with it that promotes his growth. In depression, however, the mourner experiences disruptive identification with it, and the ambivalent relationship he had had with the one now dead becomes an internal process; the yearning to keep the representation and at the same time to destroy it is felt as an issue of one's own—a struggle between cherishing and doing away with one's self.

Further accounts of the complications of grief appear in the literature. For example, the initial absence of a grief reaction is mentioned by Deutsch (7), and the chronicity of what are generally thought of as "normal" grief manifestations by Wahl (48). However, differentiation between varieties of complicated grief and depression over loss by death is not always made, and these diagnostic terms are commonly used interchangeably. The study of adult mourners carried out at the University of Virginia has demonstrated the existence of a type of established pathological grief with a clinical picture and underlying psychodynamics which are unique, persistent, and different

Reprinted by permission of the authors and Brunner/Mazel, Inc., from *Specialized Treatment in Individual Psychotherapy*, edited by T. B. Karasu and L. Bellak, 1980.

from those of either a normal but protracted grief reaction or a neurotic depression. It is, in fact, a common pyschiatric problem.

After the death of someone greatly valued, the grief-stricken relative or friend goes through consecutive phases of mourning. One might anticipate that when the process develops complications these might include fixation in any one of these phases, but clinical research shows that fixation usually occurs at one specific phase—that in which the mourner is in a limbo of uncertainty about the death and yearns to bring the dead to life. The situation is complex inasmuch as along with the longing to restore the dead is a dread of ever seeing him again. These conflicting emotions result in the picture of established pathological grief with its characteristic underlying psychodynamic processes. Once diagnosed, this condition may be successfully treated by a method of brief psychotherapy called re-grief work (39, 41, 46, 47).

THE PHASES OF GRIEVING

The psychological phenomenon involved in the process of grieving over the loss of someone who had been important to one's self is one, the course of which can be represented graphically as though it were the course of a physiologic process seen longitudinally. Indeed, Engel (8), in asking whether or not grief might be called a disease, suggested that it resembled the working-through of a healing wound. Just as a wound can become infected or form keloids, so can the course of grieving become complicated.

It begins when someone is lost, or when his loss is seen as imminent. This external event affects the internal milieu of the mourner, triggering a psychological process. Freud (12) described how this process runs its course over an interval of time. As the work of mourning goes on, memories and expectations connected with the one who died are brought to the mourner's mind one by one. When they are hypercathected and examined, it becomes possible to detach the libido that had been invested in the deceased, and when the mourning is completed the mourner's ego becomes "free and uninhibited again." However, a closer look suggests that the end of the grieving process is not so easy to identify, since the internal image of the lost one remains with us to a certain extent all our lives—and may sometimes be externalized, with a degree of communication with that person continuing. When one is asked to recall a dead relative, for example, his image is usually readily available to the mind's eye; what is more important is that such an image may impress itself on the mourner in moments of need without conscious recall. For example, a woman who has completed the healing of the wound caused by her father's death may find herself preoccupied with his image at the approach of her wedding day, as she longs for his approval of this important step in her life. Nonetheless, the grieving process does terminate for all practical purposes when the image of the dead person is not required in any absolute and exaggerated way to maintain the mourner's internal equilibrium, although it may from time to time be reactivated, as in anniversary reactions (29, 30). The healed wound is, as it were, at least covered over by scar tissue, but it never altogether disappears; the feelings about an internal relationship to the one who is lost continue.

Once initiated, the phrases through which mourning over the death of someone important proceeds are recognizable. Although these have been described somewhat differently by different writers, it is clear that they were all observing similar manifestations. Engel (9) divided grieving into three stages: (1) shock and disbelief; (2) a growing awareness of the loss; and (3) restitution, the work of mourning. Schuster (34) focused further on the stage of shock and disbelief. Bowlby (4) also identified three phrases of grieving, although he and Parkes (5) later worked out a schema with four. They describe the first phase as a brief phase of numbness that may last from a few hours to a week and be interrupted by outbursts of extremely intense anger and distress. The second phase is one "of yearning and searching for the lost figure" that lasts for some months, even years. The third phase is one of disorganization and despair; and the fourth, one in which reorganization appears. Pollock (28, 31) made a special contribution to the psychoanalytic understanding of this reorganization (adaptation) when he went beyond Freud's original notion of the transformation into ego loss that occurs with the loss of a loved object—or even of an ideal—by showing that the ego uses the adaptational process of mourning for its own healing. "Mourning processing, like working through, is internal work to restore psychic balance" (32, 16). Using the term *mourning* in a broad sense to include reaction to losses other than those occasioned by death, he holds that to be able to mourn is to be able to change. People also mourn their *own* impending death; people aware of having incurable cancer, for example, go through similar phases if time allows and they are psychologically capable (17).

This paper refers only to the mourning of *adults,* its complications and therapeutic management. Psychoanalysts debate the possibility that infants or small children faced with loss grieve in the manner of the adult. In his review of children's reactions to the death of someone important to them, Nagera

(23) concludes that such losses interface with development. Our own experience suggests that Wolfenstein (50) was accurate in saying that adolescence constitutes a necessary precondition of the ability to mourn. A painful and gradual decathexis of the living parents is accomplished in adolescence and serves as a model for the adult type of grieving.

As noted, our clinical research (39, 40, 42, 43, 44, 45), which was conducted with a hundred patients during eight years, confirmed our belief that the fixation typical of established pathological mourning occurs mainly in the phase Bowlby and Parkes (5) describe as one of "the yearning to recover the dead" and, to use a term of Kübler-Ross (17), to "bargain" for his return. When such yearning is crystallized, it is inevitably accompanied by dread of such a return. Manifestations of earlier grief stages—denial, numbness, or angry outbursts—may appear also, as well as occasional periods of disorganization usually more typical of a later phase. If the fixation we describe is extended we are, however, justified in diagnosing "established pathological grief."

THE CLINICAL PICTURE OF ESTABLISHED
PATHOLOGICAL GRIEF

Although the pathological mourner has intellectual appreciation of the historical fact of the death, he clings to chronic hope that the lost will return, even after the six months or a year that usually disabuses the normal mourner of any such notion. The pathological mourner's dread of such an eventuality is as strong as his hope. This situation can persist over time without alteration, or the picture may be overlaid by others.

Wistful longing is not abnormal; Parkes (25), for instance, speaks of how a widow yearning for her dead husband may imagine hearing his footfall at coming-home time for a year after his loss, and even "hallucinate" his appearance. In the established pathological mourner, however, longing becomes such a strong preoccupation that it dominates his daily life and keeps him ongoingly involved in the conflict produced by the ambivalence of deciding whether to bring the dead person back or to kill him, i.e., expunge him from consideration. Many pathological mourners become interested in reincarnation (40), the sophisticated sublimating this interest in a related hobby or scientific hypothesis. Some compulsively read obituary notices, betraying not only anxiety over their own death but trying to deny the one they mourn by finding no current mention of his death, while at the same time recalling how such mention as it appeared earlier had the finality of "killing" the lost one. This kind of preoccupation can become extremely morbid, as in the case of one patient who changed his dead wife's burial place three times in as many years, one move taking her coffin some distance away and another bringing her "nearer home." When he came to our attention he was planning a fourth move. His preoccupation with his dead wife's image was ambivalent, clearly reflecting the painful struggle that this religious man had had being faithful to his marriage vows over the many years in which she had been a suffering invalid. He had longed for liberation from her tragic situation, and after her death he went through cycles of trying to draw her close to him and then to put her away.

Some established pathological mourners think they recognize their lost one in someone they see alive. A son pathologically mourning a father dead for years may be struck by a resemblance perceived in some stranger passing by, and rush forward to peer at him over and over to see if this can indeed be his parent. This act represents an effort to return the dead to life; when the illusion is recognized as such it serves the wish to "kill" him. The mourner may make daily reference to death, tombs, and graveyards in ritual ways that obviate painful affect, but it is unusual for such a mourner actually to visit the grave. For example, a twenty-year-old college student still, a year-and-a-half later, mourning the sudden death of a grandfather she described as "the most important person in my life" was surprised when she was asked if she had ever gone to his graveside. Like most people with established pathological mourning, she was quick to find an excuse. She doubted that she could find it in a cemetery as "big" as the one in her small town. Her preoccupation with her grandfather was nonetheless evident in her daydreams about him and her search for him in an affair with a married man thirty years her senior.

The therapist of such a patient gets the impression that the one being mourned is in a sense alive as far as the patient is concerned and still exerts his influence. The patient uses the present tense, stating confidently, "My father likes to go to the movies." One patient joked nervously during our first interviews, cautioning that, "You can't talk much against dead people because if you knock them down they come back."

Certain typical dreams can be expected. They have been classified (40, 41) as:

1. "Frozen" dreams, to use a term many patients use themselves to describe tableaux without motion. One tableau may follow another as though the dreamer were watching the projection of a slide series. One patient used the analogy of watching slices of bread fall out of a package. The patient's associations to each tableau indicate a connection with his complicated mourning and his fixation in the grieving process as though the process had congealed in its course.

2. Dreams in which the dead person is seen alive but engaged in a struggle between life and death. He may be lying in a hospital bed or under the rubble of a collapsed building, or sitting in a burning vehicle. The dreamer tries to save him—or to finish him off. Interestingly, both persons in the dream are usually undisguised. The situation's outcome remains indeterminate because the patient invariably awakens before it is resolved.

3. Dreams of the dead body in which something indicates that death is only an illusion. The body seen in its casket may be sweating, or one long buried may show no sign of decay. Such dreams are not unusual among normal mourners during the months immediately after the death, but these dreams either cease or the appearance of the body begins to change. However, the mourner in pathological grief will dream of the undecayed body many years after death.

Several investigators (28, 41) have spoken of the reporting of dream *series* appropriately parallel to phases of uncomplicated grief in persons either completing their grief work without incident or beginning to re-grieve in normal fashion as the therapy for pathological grief starts taking effect. For example, what is first reported is a view of grass-covered earth in which, in the following area, there is a grave-like excavation. The next dream will include the half-alive body of the lost one lying nearby; the dreamer may next see himself pushing it into the grave. In the final dream of the series, the manifest content of which has been the dreamer's progress toward resolution of his grief, a grave, smoothed over and covered with grass, appears. The established pathological mourner is usually ready enough to disclose to the therapist, when asked about his dream life, the appearance of the kinds of dreams we cite as characteristic of this pathological state. These dreams are usually repeating dreams, and information about them is diagnostically helpful.

The person with established pathological grief can keep in touch with the image of the dead, over which he maintains absolute control. He is able to establish contact with the dead by forming a presence (introject) of the dead person within himself that is perceived, by the patient, as having definite boundaries separating it from the mourner. Most patients, when questioned about it, can give good descriptions of this phenomenon. Volkan (41, 42) and Volkan, Cillufo and Sarvay (46) tell of patients who, during the time of their treatment, would ask the inner presence to get out of their bodies and leave them alone. It is also not ususual for the person with established pathological grief to hold "inner conversations" with the image of the deceased that dwells within him. One patient would hold conversations with his dead brother while driving in his car, and ask business advice from him, feeling that the brother was somehow living within his own breast.

Another sort of contact with the dead, again one under the mourner's absolute control, is maintained by the use of some object contaminated with certain elements, some of which came from the dead while others come from the mourner himself. These have been named "linking objects" (43, 44, 45). They differ from the ordinary keepsake since the mourner invests them with magic capable of linking him with the one he has lost. Typically, he keeps his linking object locked away or located in some place where he can be in touch with it in a way that is consciously or unconsciously ritualized. One patient, still mourning the death of a son from an automobile accident many years earlier, kept his son's shoes, polished except where they were blood-stained, in his own clothes closet. There he could see them daily as he removed and put away his own garments, while all the time never touching them. When he went into full-blown pathological grief after the passage of many years, and was sent by his family physician for consultation, he wore the shoes to the first interview. He was greatly surprised and anxious when the therapist asked if he had kept any special object or objects that had belonged to his dead son, and only then realized what shoes he was wearing.

A great variety of objects may become linking objects. The mourner chooses such an object from among (1) something once used routinely by the dead, perhaps something worn on the person, like a watch ; (2) something the dead person had employed to extend his senses, like a camera (an extension of seeing); (3) a symbolic or realistic representation of the dead person, the simplest example of which is, of course, a photograph; or (4) something at hand when the mourner first learned of the death or when he viewed the body. We have also known patients to cling to something less tangible, such as an elaborate fantasy. For example, the mourner might entertain a certain thought during the burial ceremony and regularly reactivate it to keep controlled contact with the image of the dead.

THE PSYCHODYNAMICS OF ESTABLISHED
PATHOLOGICAL GRIEF

Three major intrapsychic processes underlie the clinical picture described here: splitting, internalization, and externalization. One must identify and understand the defensive use of these mechanisms in order to make definitive diagnosis.

Splitting

The adult patient with established pathological grief uses the mechanism of *splitting* extensively. The term *splitting* refers here not to the "primitive splitting" currently used widely in relation to borderline personality organization—that persistent separation of "all good" self- and object-representations from those seen as "all bad." Here we see splitting on a higher, neurotic level, as a splitting of the ego functions to protect the individual from any global break with reality. Thus the ego's denial of the death can coexist with the ego's knowledge that the death has, in fact, occurred. The pathological mourner's splitting of ego function is selective and concerned only with the issues of the death in question. Freud (13, 14) spoke of this type of splitting in connection with both grief and fetishism. The fetishist does not experience a global break with reality either; he understands that women do not have penises but behaves as though they did. Similarly, the established pathological mourner acknowledges the death but behaves as though it had not occurred. One particular function of his ego has become inconsistent with the rest. He is usually able to identify the point at which splitting began, as when he recalls gazing at the corpse in full knowledge that it was a dead body, and convincing himself that he saw perspiration appearing on its brow as an evidence that life continued in it. Such a notion is not outside the experience of the normal mourner, but he soon sets it aside, whereas it remains a powerful question in the mind of the pathological mourner, militating against the separation/castration anxiety triggered by the death. Two other cogent psychological processes inherent in this condition—internalization and externalization—foster the illusion of continuing contact with the dead and thus support the mechanism of splitting in its defense against anxiety. All three of these mechanisms contribute to the patient's continuing existence in a limbo of uncertainty.

Internalization

Such processes—including introjection and identification—which are involved in both grief and reactive depression, have been known since the original publication of the works of Abraham (1) and Freud (12). When his search for the lost one forces the mourner to test the reality of his disappearance, he uses hundreds of memories to bind him to the one he mourns, and becomes so preoccupied with doing so that he loses interest in the world around him. This painful longing must be worked through piecemeal. Tensions are discharged through weeping, for example. He regresses and resorts to "taking in" the deceased by introjection. Thus, the dead person's representation within the mourner's self becomes hypertrophied and is seen as an introject. As noted earlier, the introject may be perceived by the patient as an inner presence. Although the patient may describe this psychological phenomenon in such a realistic way as to call it "a foreign body in my bosom," it should be remembered that, in actuality, introjects are only code symbols of complicated affective-dynamic psychological processes. Fenichel (11) states that "introjections [introjects] act as a buffer by helping to preserve the relationship with the object while the gradual process of relinquishing it is going on." Our work with established pathological mourners indicates that the gradual process of relinquishing an introject fails to take place. Thus the introject's continued presence does not lead either to disruptive identification, as in reactive depression, or rewarding identification (19) for the enrichment of the patient's psychic system. He is obliged to retain it and, like the introjects of early life representations in psychotic patients, it never evolves further but remains chronically cathected and is continually a party in the yearning/dreading transactions of the patient.

Externalization

The child's transitional object (49), perhaps a teddy bear or a "security blanket," is vitally important to him. Its main function, one universally present, is to cause the infant to develop in response to the ministrations of the "good enough" mother. In it he has created his first "not-me" possession, which falls short nevertheless of being totally "not-me" since it links not-me with mother-me (15). The transitional object provides a bridge over the psychological chasm that opens when the mother and child are apart; the child may need it if he is to sleep, for example. Some children who experience defective child/mother interaction may have such extreme anxiety when separated from the mother that they concentrate unduly on this object and use it in bizarre ways. At this level such objects are called childhood fetishes (37), psychotic fetishes (21), or instant mothers (36). Since the main function of these inanimate objects is to deal with separation anxiety, it is not surprising that the adult suffering a separation, to which he has responded with established pathological grief, may reactivate in his regression this archaic way of dealing with this stress. This would create in a linking object a locus for the meeting of part of his self-representation with the representation of the dead. Thus an externalization—a projection of self- and object-image— is crystallized (43, 45).

Jaffe's (16) emphasis on the dual role played by projection in object relations, and the ambivalence it facilitates, can be applied here. He wrote: "On the one hand of the continuum, the annihilation of the object is predominant, while on the other, the identification with and preservation of the object is paramount" (674–75).

The linking object is completely under the patient's control; he has the unconscious illusion that it makes it possible for him to kill the dead person or bring him back to life. It is contaminated with intense emotion, i.e., the urge to kill, and is nothing that can simply be put to use in the manner of a keepsake. It must be hidden away and perhaps even locked away, or have a ritual for relating to it. For example, one patient had a picture of his father as linking object and developed a ritual concerning it that persisted for many years until he had treatment. He could manage to remain in a room alone with it until, when lost in contemplating the picture, it seemed to him that his father began to move toward him out of the frame. Then he would be so overwhelmed by anxiety that he would rush from the room. He had a strong desire to know at all times where his linking object was. Many mourners are satisfied to keep theirs in a distant place, provided that it is safe and accessible. Another patient used the clothing of his dead brother as a linking object; he kept the garments locked away, but worried constantly that he would grow to "fit" them.

One young woman's psychotherapist committed suicide while she was in the middle of a transference neurosis. When she learned that he had been cremated and his ashes had been placed in an urn, she bought an urn-like vase which she established on the mantel in her living room, depositing her last appointment slip in it as a linking object. Although knowledge of its presence in the vase was necessary to her, she would neither look at it nor throw it away.

No patient we studied reactivated a transitional object in the form of the transitional object or childhood fetish used in his childhood, but patients did employ the same dynamic processes that foster in the infant his illusion of power over the environment. Put into the external world, the linking object also helps the patient externalize the work of mourning and helps him put the work aside for future attention which he keeps on postponing because of the pain it would cause.

DIFFERENTIAL DIAGNOSIS

There is no dearth of observation in psychiatric literature that recognizable mental illness, such as the different neuroses, psychoses, antisocial behavior patterns, psychosomatic conditions, etc., is precipitated by a loss by death (6, 10, 18, 20, 24, 26, 27, 33, 38). In such conditions, while death and loss are precipitating events, these are distinctly different from established pathological grief, the latter state being, as we have stressed, unique in a number of ways. It should be differentiated with care from depression, fetishism, and psychosis.

Depression

Internalization processes are common to both depression and established pathological grief, but in the latter, the introject of the dead does not bring about identification. Thus, the introject does not blend into the patient's self-representation, but it is something he reacts to as an internal presence that has its own discrete boundaries. The mourner's tie to the introject does not loosen. In a reactive depression, however, introjection of the lost objects leads to identification so that the mourner *is* the battleground on which the conflicts, formerly so lively between the patient and the one now dead, continue to be played out. Thus, we see the pathological guilt, and the self-reproachful and self-degrading features of the depression. We agree with Pollock (28) and Smith (35) that in depression, identification tends to be nearly total, with little difference being made between characteristics of the mourner and aspects of the dead he takes in. As Freud (12) indicated: "if the love for the object—a love which cannot be given up—takes refuge in narcissistic identification, then the hate comes into operation on this substitute object, abusing it, debasing it, making it suffer and deriving sadistic satisfaction from its suffering'' (251). To be sure, there are grey areas between pathological grief and a depression that follows a death. One suffering from depression (total identification with the representation of the dead) after a death may, in fact, go into typical established pathological grief with an ambivalently related introject before he is able to respond appropriately to his loss. We have seen situations in which it was hard to determine whether the patient had an introject or identified totally with the dead; since the mourner's behavior resembled on the surface that known to have been characteristic of the deceased, careful scrutiny was required. In any case, the patient who can easily fluctuate psychodynamically between reactive depression and established pathological grief may be a suitable candidate for re-grief therapy. The *fusion* with the image of the deceased that is exhibited by the person in established pathological grief, and which comes and goes, contains manifestations of identification. However, the identification of the reactive depressive is usually different inasmuch as it follows the establishment of an introject before turning into something more clearly identification *per se*.

The pathological mourner may experience feelings of guilt, but with him such feelings are transient, since he maintains the unconscious illusion that he can bring the dead to life again (as well as kill him) if he chooses. Intense guilt is the earmark of depression, which is characterized also by the dominant ego feeling of helplessness (3). In established pathological grief there is *chronic* hope—and dread (40, 42).

Fetishism

High-level splitting occurs in both fetishism and established pathological grief, as does the use of certain objects in magical ways. The differences that distinguish the fetish, the linking object, and the transitional object are described elsewhere in some detail (43, 45). The linking object provides a means for external maintenance of object relationships with the dead. The ambivalence of the wish to annihilate the deceased and to keep him alive is condensed in it so that the painful work of mourning has an external reference and is thus not resolved. The linking object thus deals with separation anxiety, but the classical fetish used by adults serves primarily to deal with castration anxiety and only secondarily with separation anxiety. The literature (2) reports the development of fetishistic behavior in a classical sense after a loss by death, and in this circumstance a grey area between fetish and linking object is evident. If the therapist takes his patient's history with great care and is watchful for any historical loss that might have initiated the appearance of the clinical picture, he is usually able to find clues to the nature of the magical object being used by his patient. One of our patients discovered a pair of women's shoes in the desk of his father after his death, and kept them—primarily fetishistic objects for his father—for his own linking objects.

Psychosis

As noted, a break with reality does in one sense occur in established pathological grief through the use of high-level splitting, but it falls far short of being global, as it would be in a full-blown psychosis. For example, we would not over-diagnose as psychotic a widow who tells of hearing her dead husband's footsteps. If she is suffering from established pathological mourning her experience indicates no more than what might be called "mini-psychosis," since it is focused and reversible by the patient's own capacity for reality-testing.

THE SUITABILITY OF PATIENTS FOR RE-GRIEF THERAPY

There are a number of reasons why an adult may be caught up in established pathological grief. He may not have been prepared for a sudden death, for example, and fall victim to something like traumatic neurosis when a sudden death does occur. His situation may in this case be seen as one of established pathological grief that is a variation of traumatic neurosis, the most suitable variety of pathological grief for re-grief therapy. Or the mourner may have unfinished business with the one who died, and be unconsciously trying to keep him alive for this reason, while at the same time feeling anger toward the dead person that makes him want to "kill" him. Such unfinished business would include uncompleted intrapsychic processes. An example is provided by a young man whose father had died suddenly while the son was courting the girl who was to become his wife. During the boy's puberty his father, a physician, had had some reason to be concerned about his son's genital development and shared these misgivings about what a failure to develop properly might mean to the boy's manhood. So the son, who had a need to prove his virility to his father, accordingly impregnated his fiancée soon after the father died. He had to keep his father's image alive to convey this triumph to him (41).

It is significant whether the death being mourned came about from natural causes or involved violence, as in suicide, accident, or homicide. Violence, unconsciously connected with the mourner's aggressive feelings, fosters guilt that can preclude the expression of natural anger and aggressive reactions. This situation may involve the patient's fixation in established pathological mourning, so that he can avoid feeling aggression and guilt. Such fixation may in some cases be accomplished in the service of so-called secondary gain. When a death brings about such changes in the real world as the blow of losing the family home or having to face a sudden loss of income because of the wage-earner's death, the mourner is more apt to keep the dead one alive and struggle with the wish to "kill" him in order to complete the natural process of grieving.

Any loss, including the death itself, deals a narcissistic blow to the psyche of the one left behind. If the mourner has narcissistic character pathology, brief psychotherapy is unlikely to change this, however closely the clinical picture following the death may resemble that of established pathological grief. He may seem to go through re-grief therapy readily enough but still become symptomatic very easily whenever his narcissistic character organization is threatened. Such patients, while seemingly trying to deal with the lost object, are actually trying to deal, whether in hidden or open ways, with the narcissistic blow itself. For such people to become able to grieve genuinely usually requires more than re-grief therapy by itself can provide. We do not advise taking into re-grief therapy the patient with narcissistic personality organization.

The therapist should ascertain if the individual with the clinical picture indicative of established pathological grief has severe problems that stem from separation/individuation, and has extensively used such primitive defenses as internalization and externalization—that is, if he has moderate-to-severe pathology in his internalized object relations—it is doubtful that he will benefit from "re-griefing." The most suitable patients are those with intact ego functions in all respects other than higher-level splitting, and who are psychologically-minded, motivated, and thus capable of forming a therapeutic alliance. Since "re-griefing" is a process leading to an inner structural change, it is not surprising that candidates suitable for it are those who would be suitable for classical psychoanalysis proper.

It has been demonstrated (46) that the Minnesota Multiphasic Personality Inventory is not only an effective self-rating measurement of change occurring during re-grief therapy, but a promising instrument for the selection of patients for this kind of treatment. It pointed to an underlying personality trait of hysteria and dependence in those patients who received great benefit from re-grief therapy with us. A pilot study suggested that established pathological mourners tended to have an elevation of scales 1, 2, 3, 7 and 8, and, to a lesser extent, of scales 4 and 6 also. Peaks came generally in scales 2 and 7. The data of the pilot study suggest that elevation of scales 2 and 7 to a point in excess of the showing on scale 8 is predictive of maximum benefit from "re-griefing."

A DESCRIPTION OF RE-GRIEF THERAPY

Once the patient has been seen in a diagnostic interview and found suitable for re-grief therapy, he is told that his psychological condition is due to his inability to complete the grieving process, which a brief course of therapy will help him to complete. One of the therapist's first tasks will be to develop a formulation as to the cause of his patient's being "frozen" in the course of his grieving. This requirement makes it necessary for him to have had adequate experience in psychodynamically oriented therapies, and to have developed a high degree of competence in formulating unconscious mental processes. If the patient is capable of really "hearing" at the outset what his reasons are for failing to complete the normal process of mourning, they can be shared with him; otherwise, the therapist may keep his formulation to himself for later use in interpretations when the patient is ready to hear them.

Since the established pathological mourner is in a state of chronic hope that the dead will return—and simultaneously wants to "kill" him in order to complete grieving—he is preoccupied with psychological contact with the introject. During the initial phase of re-grief therapy, after carefully taking a history, we help the patient to distinguish between what is his and what belongs to the representation of the one he has lost, using what have been called (47) demarcation exercises. Demarcating the introject, so to speak, will enable the therapist to help his patient see what he has taken in and thus what he feels about the introject, and which of its aspects he wants to retain in non-disruptive identification and which he wants to reject. It is important here to note again that although the patient employs the kind of physical terms we use in referring to his introject, it is, in actuality, an affective-dynamic *process*. The therapist of such patients should have sufficient experience to keep from engaging in intellectual gymnastics instead of bona fide therapy when he attempts the analytic formulations involved here. The manifest content of the patient's dreams may demonstrate to him how his grieving has been "frozen."

In the initial phase of demarcation, which lasts for several weeks, the therapist does not encourage an outpouring of intense emotions, but helps his patient into a state of *preparedness* for such an outpouring. If the patient senses emotion building up in himself and feels frustrated at being unable to allow himself yet to feel its full impact, the therapist may say, "What is your hurry? We are still trying to learn all about the circumstances of the death and the reasons why you cannot grieve. When the time comes you may allow yourself to grieve."

Following the demarcation exercises and exploration of the reasons why the patient was fixated and unable to work out his grief, the therapist will focus on the linking object. When the linking object is being dealt with, the therapist will make a formulation about its choice from among many possibilities. Meanings condensed in a linking object are discussed elsewhere (43, 45). Because it has physical existence with properties that reach the senses, it has greater impact as "magical" than the introject has. Once the patient grasps how he has been using it to maintain absolutely controlled contact with the image of the dead, as well as to postpone grieving and keep it frozen, he will use it to begin his "re-grieving," and this move will increase his dread. He is asked to bring the linking object to a therapy session, where it is at first avoided. With the patient's permission the therapist may lock it away somewhere in the therapy room, saying that its magical properties exist only in the patient's perception of it. Finally, introduced into therapy, it is placed between patient and therapist long enough for the patient to feel its spell. He is then asked to touch it and explain anything that comes to him from it. We are constantly surprised at what intense emotion is congealed in it, and caution others about this; such emotion serves to unlock the psychological processes contained until now in the linking object itself. Emotional storms so generated may continue for weeks; at first diffuse, they become differentiated, and the therapist, with his patient, can then identify anger, guilt, sadness and so on. The linking object will then at last lose its power, whether the patient chooses to discard it altogether or not.

A graft of secondary process thought is needed to help heal the wound that this experience has torn open. During the weeks that follow, patient and therapist go over in piecemeal fashion memories of how news of the death came; recognition of when splitting began; the funeral; the attempts to keep the dead alive, etc. Although this review may make the patient highly emotional at some point, he can now observe what is happening to him, and disorganization no longer frightens him. Many patients spontaneously plan some kind of memorial ritual. For example, one went, without advice from us, to the synagogue from which his father had been buried and to the grave in which he lay, making a photographic record of it all. Many patients consult their priests, ministers, or rabbis for religious consolation as they begin to accept the death toward the conclusion of re-griefing. With suitable patients, we were successful in using, toward the end of their therapy, the manifest content of their serial dreams to indicate where they were in their re-griefing (41). Patients then have a sense of the introject's leaving them in peace, and they are often able to visit the grave to say "goodbye." They feel free, even excited with the lifting of their burden, and begin to look for new objects of their love. Re-griefing is over. Our experience has been that it can be completed in about four months, with sessions occurring at least three times a week.

TRANSFERENCE: THERAPEUTIC EFFICACY

In re-grief therapy the transference relationship becomes the vehicle whereby insight into ambivalence and the conflict between longing and dread may be gained, and resolution effected. A truly supportive approach is required, as in all other therapies whether psychoanalytic or not. The therapist must convey his non-exploitative desire to heal, and encourage his patient to express himself directly without any fear of hostile, punitive, engulfing, or abandoning responses. The therapist should actively, directly, and instructively oppose any initial shame or excessive control with which the patient may conceal the complications of his grief, and encourage his head-on exploration of feelings and fantasies about the person he has lost and the internal and external relationship he has with him. Through his activity the therapist offers himself as a new object for the patient's consideration, aiming, as in psychoanalytic therapy, to develop a therapeutic alliance without encouraging an *infantile* transference neurosis. Transference—but not transference neurosis—is inevitable, and may be therapeutic by providing close and intimate contact within the therapeutic setting as conflicts are understood. At times the patient may relate to his therapist as he had related to the one he mourns, and thus make it possible to work through in a focal way the conflicts he had had with him. The fresh grief caused by separation as therapy terminates can be put to appropriate use.

Although re-grief therapy is brief, lasting for some months rather than for years, it is intense, intimate, and certainly not superficial. It can be likened to a "mini-focal analysis" since it leads to the activating of certain areas of intrapsychic process, however focalized, and effects intrapsychic change in areas under treatment by means of "working-through." Thus, it is not recommended for therapists inexperienced in listening to the flow of unconscious process. It requires adherence to a therapeutic position and expert handling of transference and countertransference.

A CASE REPORT

A thirty-year-old, well-respected, and highly competent female lawyer sought treatment from one of us (Josephthal) for the trouble she was having in resolving her grief reaction to her husband's death in an airplane accident six months earlier. Although she showed some manifestations of what could be understood as prolonged "normal grief," her case history revealed a basic picture of established pathological grief with typical psychodynamics underlying it. She continued unable to control the tears and weeping that came whenever she thought of him, and she was ashamed over so losing her self-control and dismayed that the situation seemed not to improve as time went on. Her tears were accompanied by sad and poignant longing for her husband and for her own death to come in order that they might be together again. She reported being especially upset on the tenth and twelfth of each month; she had had to identify the body on the tenth of the month in which he died, and to make arrangements for the cremation two days after.

Her history indicated no significant psychological, developmental trauma, nor deprivation, overindulgence, or difficulties with object relations. She grew up in a farm family in which self-reliance was a virtue, and she rejected any sign of dependency within herself. Her social, educational, sexual, and vocational development progressed smoothly, and when she was twenty-four she married a dynamic, successful, and glamorous lawyer who was also a real-estate investor, and she spoke of having had a full and exciting life with him. The couple traveled extensively and had many friends. She felt that her relationship to her husband, which was deep, rich, and intimate, had only one flaw—his engagement in several transient extramarital affairs while on business trips. Although she tried to condone this as unimportant in the contemporary climate of openness and enlightenment, and felt that he did not, in fact, have any real emotional involvement with the women in question, she was inwardly upset and felt that her husband had shown less than total commitment to their marriage. She tried to feel accepting and liberated, and not to be controlling, but, however she questioned her objections intellectually, emotionally she continued to resent his affairs. This was an unresolved issue at the time of his death, but otherwise she felt hers had been a very happy marriage. The couple had chosen to delay having children, but the patient was making plans for a child when her husband lost his life in the crash of a private plane while on a business trip abroad.

In the first few sessions she recounted her experiences immediately after being notified of her husband's death. She had felt shock and disbelief at first, and continued to hope against hope that the news was in error until she identified the body two days after the accident in the country where the plane had crashed. The identification had been very traumatic for her; she saw to her horror that his face had suffered severe mutilation. Part of his jaw was gone, and the tissue that remained was bloated and discolored. His mutilated face kept appearing in her mind's eye in what she called a "flash," but it was interesting to hear that as time went on it began to return to its normal appearance without volition on her part; the missing area was filling in, and the swelling was subsiding. Such gradual fading of horror was reminiscent of what happens in the recurring dreams of traumatic neurosis.

The patient kept her husband's ashes in her bedroom in a wooden box. Although she had made plans to dispose of them in several places meaningful in terms of their shared experiences, she found that she kept procrastinating. She had never been able to open the box and examine the ashes but she could not dispose of them. When she happened to see the Tutankhamen exhibit which was touring the country, she had what she described as a "weird experience." In reading the dates of the excavation of the Tutankhamen tomb and doing some mathematical calculations concerning her husband's birthdate, his age at death, his age at the excavation dates, etc., she had a sudden flash of insight that momentarily persuaded her that her husband had been the king's reincarnation. She quickly saw the absurdity of this and understood that it indicated a wish that her husband could return through reincarnation. This insight was replaced by a search for meaning. Being of a philosophical turn of mind and well-read in Eastern philosophy, she began trying to understand what lessons or meaning her husband's death would reveal to her.

She came weekly for therapy, except for one week during which the box of her husband's ashes was in the therapist's office, where she opened it in his presence; then she came on four consecutive days. She began treatment with a well-developed capacity for the alliance and unusual insight and psychological-mindedness, and she seemed at each session to bring in fresh and absorbing material, showing deep and appropriate affect. She had shared her grief response with no one and seemed eager to unburden herself and to work on some of her difficulties. She very quickly began to work through her problems while the therapist encouraged her and acted as an auxiliary super-ego to help her overcome her initial resistance based on shame and fear over being what she thought of as weak, dependent, and vulnerable. After the first few visits she had fewer episodes of crying; now they seemed to occur chiefly during her sessions in therapy. Shortly after beginning treatment she took a previously arranged trip which included a plane flight. This was preceded by a dream:

> Five pterodactyls fly over my property. I hide. One of them seems to have a man's body. He swoops down and carries me off. It felt pleasant.

Her immediate associations were that there had been five people in the plane crash, that the pterodactyl was her husband, and that this was a dream of reunion. The therapist offered that her husband has mastered what killed him by being able to fly, and she immediately added "and thus be immortal." She then reported a recurring thought, a quotation from T. S. Eliot's *Quartos:* "After all our searchings we return to the same place and see it for the first time."

She then suggested—as the therapist had been about to do—that it might be therapeutic to open the box of ashes in the therapist's office. Her wish for reunion, seen in the dream, along with the attendant dread, was experienced and worked through in the following way. She brought the box to her therapist's office and left it there in his safekeeping while together they explored all her fantasies about it. These included what she called her "terrible imaginings"; she had not opened the box because she was afraid she would be impelled to smear the ashes over her face and hug herself if she did so. Although clearly pointing to images of merger, the opening of the box also meant the final separation from her fantasized reunion, and thus an act of "killing" her husband.

On the day she opened the box she was dressed completely in black without realizing the meaning of this, and wore a necklace of seashells. When she opened the box, trembling and with great trepidation, she gasped at unexpectedly seeing chips of bone. She likened these to seashells—she and her husband had enjoyed sailing and spent considerable time at the seashore. She sifted through the ashes in an almost caressing manner, then unconsciously patted the side of her jaw. When this gesture was called to her attention, she immediately realized that she was trying to "fix him." She then realized and examined the ashes with a more detached interest. After that session she took the ashes home with her and went on to dispose of most of them, keeping some in the box. She would occasionally pat it as she walked out of the room, and engage in fond reminiscence as she did so. The box of ashes continued to be a linking object, but further exploration disclosed that it no longer evoked anxiety and dread, but held a new meaning. At first she said, "I'd rather keep it and not think about it." She explained that if she thought about it she was afraid that she "would think angry thoughts and lose the fond memories." She also thought, "I'm keeping him in the box," and this came to mean that she was holding him as she had been unable to do completely when he was alive. She was somewhat ashamed to realize that she was acting this fantasy out, but her shame gave way to greater interest in her motivation. She began to work with more integration on the ambivalence she felt, trying to sort out and reconcile the anger she had been denying and the affectionate feelings that had contained an over-idealization of her husband. At this point, "further unfinished business" came up when she described in greater detail her experience of mourning the death of her father when she had been in her early twenties. He had died of metastatic cancer and until the end so used denial that she had been unable to discuss his impending death with him. Any approach to the subject disturbed him and with tears in her eyes she would begin talking of something more hopeful. She felt that she had never had "the chance to say goodbye," and she realized that this had been true also with her husband.

After six months, reference was made to terminating her treatment. She was reluctant to terminate, recognizing spontaneously that this would involve yet another separation and experience of grief that she would have to resolve. She recognized also that the positive feelings and the closeness and intimacy that she had invested in her treatment had served at some level as a replacement for the loss of closeness and sharing with her husband. She reported what she called a termination dream. In this she was a schoolgirl painting with great care and in considerable detail the portrait of a girl. She was unable to finish the portrait in the time allotted because when she applied the brush to one eye and one side of the mouth no color resulted although the rest of the face had been colored without difficulty. She thought, ''Oh well, I can always come back and finish it later; besides, what I've done is beautiful.'' She saw the incomplete eye as evidence that there was more to see about herself, and the incomplete mouth as testimony that there was more to say.

The therapist offered the interpretation that the lack of color around the eye represented her tears, and wondered about the incomplete mouth as representing her husband's jaw. This made her tearful and she said ''I thought I had gotten over identifying with him.'' She went on to describe her feeling that a piece of her had died with him. Delineating a small square space with her hands, she spoke of ''this space in me where he resides.'' However, there was now a boundary around her and the dream, and the dream face, although a fusion of herself with her husband, was also separate from her, the dreamer. The suggestion in the dream that she could ''finish the portrait later'' represented her thinking that she might like to be analyzed at some future time since some characterological issues—some obsessional and superego features, and her concerns about dependency—had come into discussion. Agreement had been reached that analysis might await fuller resolution of her grief. The feeling that the rest of the painting was beautiful had to do, she surmised, with her feeling of being otherwise fairly hopeful and optimistic about herself and her life. Thus a termination date was planned for a short time after the first anniversary of her husband's death.

During the termination period she presented what she called a ''healing dream.'' It was introduced in association with her mention of a man she had been seeing toward whom she now felt it possible that she might come to respond deeply; she had until then been judging men as, first, not her husband, and then, not like him.

I was running in a marathon, a peculiar kind with a lot of obstacles, over a gorge. It was 26.2 miles. My husband was there encouraging me. In the first part of the dream it was as if I were running in a slow motion. I thought I'd never do it. It got dark. I didn't want to stop but I was afraid I'd trip in the dark. My husband went into a store, bought me a flashlight, and gave it to me. I was able to run easily. The next morning I had finished the race. Getting the light was a great relief. At the finish, where I placed or what my time was didn't matter—it was a notable finish.

She immediately connected this dream with her experience in therapy and the past year of dealing with her husband's death—how hard it had been, how slow and painful. In association to getting the light she felt that her husband's death had made her aware of troubles previously warded off, and that the therapist had given her light of the therapeutic process to guide her way. She began that session with a radiant smile which reflected her relief and well-being—her delight at finishing the race after dreaming heretofore of incompleteness. She had not finished grieving, but the obstacles and complications of her grief were gone. The obstacle of the gorge or chasm with an unfathomable black bottom represented her wish for union with her husband in death. She had gotten over that obstacle, hand over hand, in therapy. The finish of the race, which came in the morning in the dream, transformed *mourning* into *morning;* she associated to this by saying that she had once again begun to enjoy the morning sunrise on her way to work. She wept as she said that although she had been eager to tell her therapist this dream, it also made her very sad because it was so evident that she was ready to leave him. He had appeared as her husband in the dream as she lived again through the loss of her husband with him. She felt that if she could set a date for terminating therapy she could prepare herself for losing the therapist, and feel some control over the loss as she had been unable to do when she lost her husband so unexpectedly. She was wearing a black dress, but a white blouse and grey jacket with it, and she commented that she realized after dressing so that she had finally become able to blend white and black.

REFERENCES

1. Abraham, K. (1924). A short study of the development of the libido, viewed in the light of mental disorders. In: *Selected Papers in Psycho-Analysis.* London: Hogarth Press, 1927, pp. 418–501.
2. Bak, R. C. Fetishism. *J. Amer. Psychoanal. Assoc.,* 1953, 1:285–298.
3. Bibring, E. The mechanism of depression. In: P. Greenacre (Ed.), *Affective Disorders.* New York: International Universities Press, 1953.
4. Bowlby, J. Process of mourning. *Int. J. Psycho-Anal.,* 1961, 42:317–340.
5. Bowlby, J. and Parkes, C. M. Separation and loss within the family. In: E. J. Anthony and Cyrille Koupernik (Eds.) *The Child in His Family,* vol. I. New York: Wiley Interscience, 1970.
6. Brown, F. and Epps, P. Childhood bereavement and subsequent crime. *Brit. J. Psychiat.,* 1966, 112:1043–1048.

7. Deutsch, H. Absence of grief. *Psychoanal. Quart.*, 1937, 6:12–23.
8. Engel, G. L. Is grief a disease? A challenge for medical research. *Psychosom. Med.*, 1961, 23:18–22.
9. Engel, G. L. *Psychological Development in Health and Disease.* Philadelphia: W. B. Saunders, 1962.
10. Evans, P. and Liggett, J. Loss and bereavement as factors in agoraphobia: Implications for therapy. *Brit. J. Med. Psychol.*, 1971, 44:149–154.
11. Fenichel, O. *The Psychoanalytic Theory of Neurosis.* New York: Norton, 1945.
12. Freud, S. (1917). *Mourning and Melancholia.* In: J. Strachey (Ed.), *The Complete Psychological Works of Sigmund Freud, Standard Edition.* London: Hogarth Press, 1957, 14:237–258.
13. Freud, S. (1927). *Fetishism.* In: J. Strachey (Ed.), *The Complete Psychological Works of Sigmund Freud, Standard Edition.* London: Hogarth Press, 1961, 21:149–157.
14. Freud, S. (1940). *Splitting of the Ego in the Process of Defense.* In: J. Strachey (Ed.), *The Complete Psychological Works of Sigmund Freud,* London: Hogarth Press, 1964, 23:271–278.
15. Greenacre, P. The fetish and the transitional object. *Psychoanal. Study Child,* 1969, 24:144–164.
16. Jaffe, D. S. The mechanism of projection: Its dual role in object relations. *Int. J. Psycho-Anal.*, 1968, 49:662–667.
17. Kübler-Ross, E. *On Death and Dying.* New York: The Macmillan Company, 1969.
18. Lehrman, S. R. Reactions to untimely death. *Psychiat. Quart.*, 1956, 30:565–579.
19. Loewald, H. Internalization, separation, mourning and the superego. *Psychoanal. Quart.*, 1962, 31:483–504.
20. Lidz, T. Emotional factors in the etiology of hyperthyroidism. *Psychosom. Med.*, 1949, 11:2–9.
21. Mahler, M. S. *On Human Symbiosis and the Vicissitudes of Individuation.* New York: International Universities Press, 1968.
22. McDermott, N. T. and Cobb, S. A psychiatric survey of fifty cases of bronchial asthma. *Psychosom. Med.*, 1939, 1:203–245.
23. Nagera, H. Children's reactions to the death of important objects, a developmental approach. *Psychoanal. Study Child,* 1970, 25:360–400.
24. Parkes, C. M. Recent bereavement as a cause of mental illness. *Brit. J. Psychiat.*, 1964, 110:198–205.
25. Parkes, C. M. *Bereavement, Studies of Grief in Adult Life.* New York: International Universities Press, 1972.
26. Parkes, C. M. and Brown, R. J. Health after bereavement: A controlled study of young Boston widows and widowers, *Psychosom. Med.*, 1972, 34:449–461.
27. Peck, M. W. Notes on identification in a case of depressive reaction to the death of a love object. *Psychoanal. Quart.*, 1939, 8:1–18.
28. Pollock, G. Mourning and adaptation. *Int. J. Psycho-Anal.*, 1961, 42:341–361.
29. Pollock, G. Anniversary reactions, trauma and mourning. *Psychoanal. Quart.*, 1970, 39:347–371.
30. Pollock, G. Temporal anniversary manifestations: hour, day, holiday. *Psychoanal. Quart.*, 1971, 40:123–131.
31. Pollock, G. On mourning, immortality, and Utopia. *J. Amer. Psychoanal. Assoc.* 1975, 23:334–362.
32. Pollock, G. The mourning process and creative organization. *J. Amer. Psychoanal. Assoc.*, 1977, 25:3–34.

33. Schmale, A. H. Relationship of separation and depression to disease. I. A Report on a hospitalized medical population, *Psychosom. Med.,* 1958, 20:259–275.

34. Schuster, D. B. A note on grief. *Bulletin of the Philadelphia Association for Psychoanalysis,* 1969, 19:87–90.

35. Smith, J. H. Identificatory styles in depression and grief. *Int. J. Psycho-Anal.,* 1971, 52:259–266.

36. Speers, R. W. and Lansing, C. *Group Therapy in Childhood Psychosis.* Chapel Hill, North Carolina: University of North Carolina Press, 1965.

37. Sperling, M. Fetishism in children. *Psychoanal. Quart.,* 1963, 32:374–392.

38. Volkan, V. D. The observation of the "little man" phenomenon in a case of anorexia nervosa. *Brit. J. Med. Psychol.,* 1965, 38:299–311.

39. Volkan, V. D. Normal and pathological grief reactions—A guide for the family physician. *Virginia Medical Monthly,* 1966, 93:651–656.

40. Volkan, V. D. Typical findings in pathological grief. *Psychiat. Quart,* 1970, 44:231–250.

41. Volkan, V. D. A study of a patient's re-grief work through dreams, psychological tests and psychoanalysis. *Psychiat. Quart.,* 1971, 45:255–273.

42. Volkan, V. D. The recognition and prevention of pathological grief. *Virginia Medical Monthly,* 1972a, 99:535–540.

43. Volkan, V. D. The linking objects of pathological mourners. *Arch. Gen. Psychiat.,* 1972b, 27:215–221.

44. Volkan, V. D. Death, divorce and the physician. In: D. W. Abse, E. M. Nash, and L. M. R. Louden (Eds.), *Marital and Sexual Counseling in Medical Practice.* Harper & Row, 1974, pp. 446–462.

45. Volkan, V. D. *Primitive Internalized Object Relations.* New York: International Universities Press, 1976.

46. Volkan, V. D., Cillufo, A. F., and Sarvay, T. L. Re-grief therapy and the function of the linking object as a key to stimulate emotionality. In: P. T. Olson (Ed.), *Emotional Flooding.* New York: Human Sciences Press, 1975, pp. 179–224.

47. Volkan, V. D. and Showalter, C. R. Known object loss, disturbances in reality testing, and "re-griefing" work as a method of brief psychotherapy. *Psychiat. Quart.,* 1968, 42:358–374.

48. Wahl, C. W. The differential diagnosis of normal and neurotic grief following bereavement. *Psychosomatics,* 1970, 11:104–106.

49. Winnicott, D. W. Transitional objects and transitional phenomena. *Int. J. Psycho-Anal.,* 1953, 34:89–97.

50. Wolfenstein, M. How is mourning possible? *Psychoanal. Study Child,* 1966, 21:93–123.

PART V

MOURNING IN CHILDHOOD

PART V

MEANING IN CHILDHOOD

Introductory Notes to Chapters 18, 19, 20, 21, and 22: Do Children Mourn? A Controversy

Rita V. Frankiel

In no aspect of the literature on object loss is there more confusion, contradiction, and uncertainty than exists around the questions of whether, how, and when, after the death of a parent, children can come to a meaningful resolution of their feelings, healing of their blasted inner worlds, and a resumption of healthy development. One aspect of the confusion has to do with the use of the word "mourning." The answer to the question, "Do children mourn?" depends on what one means by the word "mourn." A second aspect of the confusion revolves around the questions, "Is recovery from object loss possible before adolescence? If so, under what conditions? And to what extent?" A third aspect of the confusion is the consequence of vastly differing ideas about what constitutes reliable evidence in support of a set of ideas or a theoretical position; conjecture and opinion, while of use when expressed by a seasoned expert, can be misleading when used in the place of carefully and objectively accumulated data, and should be recognized for what they are. The clarification of these areas of confusion, even when the status of current knowledge does not permit resolution, is important in understanding prognosis in child treatment and in planning how to maximize chances for recovery, most particularly in situations of traumatic loss.

In "Mourning and Melancholia," Freud spelled out the process of mourning in the adult in almost schematic form: the gradual painful decathexis of the many mental representations of the lost object is accomplished by remembering each aspect of the object and the relationship, and reminding oneself each time that the object of love is gone. Time and time again, with intense affect, the bereaved person must confront the realization that reality requires accepting the idea that the loved one no longer exists; if life is to go on in reality, the bereaved one must acknowledge the loss. This process is time limited and accomplished in a state of intermittent and at times almost complete withdrawal of interest from the surrounding world, especially from other persons.

If this definition of mourning is the one accepted, some influential researchers and writers agree that children cannot be said to be equipped to mourn before the later stages of adolescence (Wolfenstein 1966, 1969; Nagera 1970). The need for nourishing interaction and care, appropriate to their developmental level, is so central to the survival of young children that the withdrawal necessary for adult mourning is simply not possible. However, this claim that mourning is not possible before late adolescence flies in the face of the clinical and research experience of many who have studied and worked intensively with bereaved preoedipal, oedipal, latency-age, and preadolescent children, these investigators having provided convincing reports of their children's grief and profound movement toward resolution of their grief (E. Furman 1974, 1981; R. Furman 1964a, 1964b; Lopez and Kliman 1979; Barnes 1964; McCann 1974; Winnicott 1965). The key issue seems to be how to define mourning so that it is consistent with the clinical experience and understanding of those who have found that processes quite reminiscent of those observed in adults can occur in children, even if in a different form, specifically, a form appropriate to their developmental level.

In their descriptions of infants and toddlers in nursery care during World War II, Burlingham and Freud (1942) describe emotional reactions to separation and loss that are extremely intense but do not persist. The young children seen at the Hampstead Nurseries accepted sustenance and care from relative strangers rather quickly. They were thought to have withdrawn cathexis from the mother and invested it in a friendly newcomer, under the pressure of need. According to Anna Freud, before object constancy is achieved, this is how it must be, because the infant or toddler is under the influence of infantile narcissism. This conclusion is in marked contrast with the inferences drawn from their own observations by Bowlby (1960, 1961, 1963, 1980) and Bowlby, Robertson, and Rosenbluth (1952). Although Anna Freud notes (1960, 53) that there is little difference between the observations collected during the war by the Hampstead Nursery team with regard to separated children and the observations made later in Bowlby's study (from the Tavistock Institute) of separation anxiety with hospitalized children, there emerged from these two different centers two very different sets of inferences based on similar and at times identical observational data.

For Bowlby, rooted in ethology, direct observation, and strict attention to external reality, sometimes to the neglect of the inner world (according to some analysts), his early work showed that when removed from their mothers, even very young children grieve; further, the ones who have a healthy outcome do not quickly move on to new attachments even if their creature needs are satisfied by a substitute caregiver. In fact, even an infant as young as six months forms an attachment to particular objects, and grieves when removed from that object. In the research that led to both the scientific paper and the film, "A Two-Year-Old Goes to the Hospital," Bowlby, Robertson, and Rosenbluth (1952) demonstrate that Laura, the two-year-old in question, was indeed depressed, preoccupied with her absent mother, and very angry at her. Nurses approaching her were responded to superficially or rebuffed. When they were reunited at the end of her hospital stay, Laura was withdrawn from mother and unresponsive, although she related to her father as usual. Some time later, when the team came to Laura's home to show her parents the film after her bedtime, Laura awoke, entered the room and reproached her mother tearfully, "Where was you, Mommy? Where was you?" Later research work by Robertson and Robertson (1971) confirms the observations of Anna Freud (1960) and Nagera (1970) that the responses of children who are removed from their customary caretaker and familiar surroundings and possessions are much more extreme and disturbed than the responses of children in their own homes.

On the subject of the cathexis and decathexis of the lost parent, Erna Furman, who recently reported that she and her colleagues have by now treated fifty-three children who have lost a parent by death (Furman and Furman 1989), has said "We have found considerable variations in the course of decathexis among bereaved toddlers, depending on differences in personality growth, circumstances, and nature of the lost relationship. Our experience suggests that object cathexes may be maintained for several years, and decathexis may occur slowly and painfully in bereaved children from as early as sixteen months on" (E. Furman 1974, 253). In another publication, Robert Furman has observed "To withdraw a feeling investment from a mental image of a lost loved one, to decathect the internal representative of the lost object, a child must first have a stable internal representative that can survive and endure after the vast majority of loving investment has been removed" (1973, 227). Furman argues that the phallic-oedipal stage must have been reached for object constancy of this level to have been attained. It seems to me and to others as well (Sekaer 1987; Bowlby 1980; E. Furman 1974; Miller 1971) that whether or not one recognizes that decathexis in childhood may follow a different pathway than decathexis in adult life is at the heart of the differences of opinion about whether mourning is possible before adolescence.

Bowlby's claim has been the most extreme; he has asserted that mourning can be observed in children between the ages of six months and four years (1960) that is, even before stable object constancy is likely to have been established. This claim was later revised, and its revision represents a greater accommodation to the "consensus psychoanalytic position" (Miller 1971), namely, "The mourning responses that are commonly seen in infancy and early childhood bear many of the features which are the hallmark of pathological mourning in the adult" (Bowlby 1963, 504). However, Bowlby's definition of healthy mourning is persistent, protracted, unconcealed yearning and an angry effort to retrieve the lost object. His is a phenomenological theory of attachment and loss, based in ethology and observational research; decathexis is not an issue for him. His data are focused on finding and seeing the overt similarities between childhood and adult mourning, and the collection of vast quantities of data about observable patterns of grief in children of all ages and adults. Anna Freud (1960), Schur (1960), Spitz (1960), Wolfenstein (1966, 1969), and Nagera (1970) are in basic disagreement with him.

Wolfenstein's work has been most influential and calls for extensive discussion here. In her studies, she concluded that mourning, defined as decathexis, is not possible before adolescence. In an extremely influential paper that has been cited extensively, Wolfenstein (1966) describes her data as coming from a project that studied forty-two cases of children and adolescents who lost a parent by death. She does not, however, specify the form of treatment these children got, whether they were in fact treated, or, if so, how intensively. Although two youngsters are described, only one of the two was a patient. It is not made clear on what basis the information on the nonpatient was obtained. She gives no information about the population of patients included in the total study other than their ages on coming under observation or entering treatment. We learn nothing about their presenting complaints or the nature and timing of their losses. More modern understanding of the etiology of pathological mourning emphasizes that it is based in pathological defenses in operation at the time of the loss. In contrast, Wolfenstein assumes that object loss itself produces psychopathology: pathogenic hypercathexis, a lingering expectation that the lost parent is about to return, and reluctance or inability to tolerate painful affects such as would be expected in decathecting the dead parent, and a host of other emergency defenses. She argues further than the withdrawal of cathexis from the parents that occurs as a normal developmental step in adolescence "constitutes the necessary precondition for being later able to mourn . . . [it] serves as an initiation in how to mourn. . . . In circumstances of later loss he is able to recapitulate the process" (113). We must note, however, that normally the major love object continues to be present in reality, whatever detachment is going on in the inner world of the adolescent. Thus, the task is really quite different psychically; in normal adolescence, the present object must be decathected and a new, nonincentuous object must be chosen. The decathexis is really a displacement, or what Anny Katan (1937) has called "object removal." It surely is a very different process from that which follows the total absence of the parent following death. Wolfenstein's analogy to adolescence is not well chosen.

In a subsequent publication (1969), Wolfenstein provides an extensive report of a treatment she herself conducted, along with four case vignettes of psychotherapies conducted by others. In neither paper do we learn what we have come to know is essential for understanding the nature of a child or an adolescent's response to an object loss. Before developing intrapsychic explanations, those who have worked closely with bereaved children have come to pay strict and close attention to environmental factors, both around and after the loss, and to intrapsychic factors, especially as relating to the child's relationship with both the dead parent and the surviving parent beforehand. The core of the difference is not that those who take the environment into account exclude intrapsychic factors; both Furmans are psychoanalysts, and trainers and teachers of psychoanalysis. Rather, analysts now understand more fully how childhood mourning can easily turn into a pathological process if there is insufficient support for emotional expressiveness and an absence of a suitable supportive replacement object.

The Furmans (R. Furman 1973; E. Furman 1974) and Bowlby (1980) concur. Bowlby has observed, "the closer in time to the loss that a patient, adolescent or child, has been studied and the larger the number of cases that a clinician has seen the more likely is he not only to describe environmental factors but to implicate them when explaining outcome. Among the many who now lay emphasis on environmental factors, especially the influence of the surviving parent are the clinicians R. Furman (1964), E. Furman (1974), Kliman (1965), Becker and Margolin (1967) and Anthony (1973) . . ." (Bowlby 1980, 318).

With particular reference to one of the two cases reported in Wolfenstein's

1966 paper, Bowlby observes that the patient Ruth's emotional situation prior to her mother's death was such that treatment had been sought even before the loss was an issue. In contrast to Wolfenstein's view that the loss created the pathological defenses of euphoria and depersonalization, Bowlby argued that Ruth's responses, rather than being typical of adolescent mourning, are a "pathological variant" based on her earlier relationship with her mother. He conjectures from the data offered that the mother had been brusquely unsympathetic with distress and anxiety about her own absences and unsympathetic toward Ruth's desire for love and care. Ruth then would have grown up knowing that sorrow and tears are rewarded not with comfort but with reprimands, that to be unhappy when mother is busy with everything but herself is held to be babyish, silly, or senseless, and that she was expected to be bright and happy. "Brought up this way, a child will naturally come to fear responding to a loss with sorrow, yearning and tears" (1980, 374).

About this same case, Robert Furman (1968) develops some very important points parallel with Bowlby's about the prerequisites for mourning in the young: in the absence of a climate in which the bereaved youngster can feel that there is a reasonable expectation that his or her realistic needs will be met, there will be a development of pathological defenses, and *these* will interfere with the young person's ability to mourn. In R. Furman's words, as cited by E. Furman (1974, 282), "We are left with the impression [in Wolfenstein's article] that Ruth's inability to mourn produced these defensive responses. It would seem to me quite the contrary: that it was her pathological defenses that made her unable to mourn."

Bowlby was convinced that early separations and losses have powerful and long-lasting consequences "unfavorable to future personality development" (1960, 10); they render the person vulnerable to pathological grief and separation reactions later in life and, in more severe circumstances, vulnerable to serious psychiatric and sociopathic deviations. He began to demonstrate this with assemblages of research reports from all over the world (1944, 1951). Later, he reasoned that those theoretical formulations commonly used in psychoanalytic theories of object loss that emphasize primary narcissism, identification and introjection, part-object strivings and satisfactions (reactions to weaning and the early depressive position) obscure rather than illuminate the meaning and significance of behaviors that follow separation and loss, and they also obscure those sequelae of earlier traumatizing separations and minor losses that involve a propensity to respond with pathological mourning to later losses.

In the third volume of his trilogy on attachment, separation, and loss, specifically the one devoted to loss, Bowlby carefully reconsiders these factors in a number of cases in the psychoanalytic literature that report serious psychopathology subsequent to object loss. Case reports by Winnicott (1965), Shambaugh (1961), Scharl (1961), McCann (1974, also in this volume), E. Furman (1974), Wolfenstein (1966, also in this volume), and Root (1957) are among those he reexamines. He uses them to illustrate his thesis that for "childhood mourning to follow a favorable course: the child should have enjoyed a reasonably secure relationship with his parents prior to the loss; secondly, that he be given prompt and accurate information about the death and be allowed to ask questions and participate in family grieving; thirdly, that he has the comforting presence of his surviving parent or of a known and trusted substitute" (Bowlby 1980, 320). Erna Furman similarly reviews on a case-by-case basis many of the reports of child psychotherapy and child analyses dealing with loss of parents (1974, 277–90). Her pithy and clear comments on the cases, which draw on her very extensive experience, provide a significant review of other clinician's observations and conclusions.

What is absent from this controversial literature is evidence that one might consider an adequate basis for drawing more definitive conclusions on the matter of childhood mourning. Followup data are absent. Until we know more about the later lives of the children treated after childhood losses, we must remain in the grip of conjecture and incomplete clinical evidence. The opinions of such seasoned and well-grounded psychoanalytic thinkers as the Furmans are compelling; to me they are as convincing as such material can be. In my opinion, what would be even more convincing would be data drawn from an examination of the later lives of some of those children thought to have been able to bring their mourning to a more or less satisfactory conclusion. A comparison of these children's outcomes with those of a group whose mourning could not be so well resolved would begin to bring this controversy to a more satisfactory conclusion. That conclusion would be of great value in the clinical work of child therapists and analysts.

The papers that follow have been selected to illustrate the various issues in this controversy so that the reader can form his or her own opinion on the current status of our knowledge.

18. How Is Mourning Possible?

Martha Wolfenstein

I

The ability to form, and also, when necessary, to dissolve, object relations is essential to the development of every human being. At present we know more about the progress and vicissitudes of developing object relations than we do about reactions to their being broken off in different phases of life. In "Mourning and Melancholia" (1917), Freud described the phenomenon of mourning as it occurs in adults in reaction to the death of a loved person. There is a painful and protracted struggle to acknowledge the reality of the loss, which is opposed by a strong unwillingness to abandon the libidinal attachment to the lost object. "Normally, respect for reality gains the day. Nevertheless its orders cannot be obeyed at once. They are carried out bit by bit, at great expense of time and cathectic energy, and in the meantime the existence of the lost object is psychically prolonged. Each single one of the memories and expectations in which the libido is bound to the object is brought up and hypercathected, and detachment of the libido is accomplished in respect of it" (244–45). The lost object is thus gradually decathected, by a process of remembering and reality testing, separating memory from hope. The mourner convinces himself of the irrevocable pastness of what he remembers: this will not come again, and this will not come again. That the decathexis of the lost object is accomplished in a piecemeal way serves an important defensive function, protecting the mourner from the too sudden influx of traumatic quantities of freed libido. Painful as it is to endure, mourning serves an invaluable adaptive function, since by this process the mourner frees major amounts of libido which were bound to the lost object, which he can utilize for other relations and sublimated activities in the world of the living (Pollock, 1961).[1]

Reprinted by permission of International Universities Press, Inc., from *Psychoanalytic Study of the Child*, vol. 21, 1966, 93–123.

When in the sequence of development does an individual become capable of responding to a major object loss in this adaptive way? Bowlby, in a series of recent papers (1960, 1961a, 1961b, 1963), has been exploring reactions to separation and loss in young children. He has stressed the persistence of the demand, on a more or less conscious level, for the return of the lost object, the inability to renounce it, which he finds also characterizes nonadaptive reactions to loss in adults. Bowlby (1961a) raises the question: "At what stage of development and by means of what processes does the individual arrive at a state which enables him thereafter to respond to loss in a favourable manner?" And he adds his impression that "an early dating of this phase of development . . . is open to much doubt" (323). Investigators who have reported on adult patients who lost a parent in childhood or adolescence have confirmed that expressions of grief, acceptance of the reality of the loss, and decathexis of the lost parent have not occurred. Helene Deutsch (1937) spoke of "absence of grief" in an adult patient whose mother had died when he was five, and whose inhibition of sad feelings had extended to all affects. Fleming and Altschul (1963) have reported cases in which the patients suffered the loss of parents in adolescence but had never mourned and continued covertly to deny the reality of the loss. Jacobson (1965), speaking of related cases, recounted persistent fantasies of finding the lost parents again.

In contrast to these observations, Robert Furman (1964a) has advanced the view that mourning can occur in quite early childhood. He specifies as its preconditions the acquisition of a concept of death and the attainment of the stage of object constancy, both of which are possible by the age of four. I would suggest that these may well be necessary conditions, but they may be far from sufficient to enable the immature individual to tolerate the work of mourning. We need more empirical observations of how children in various phases of development actually do react to the loss of a major love object. Robert Furman (1964b) has reported the case of a six-year-old patient whose mother died while he was in analysis, and whose reactions Furman characterizes as "mourning." However, the main manifestation was that the boy painfully missed his mother in many circumstances where formerly she was with him. The expression of such feelings is no doubt useful in helping the patient to avoid the pathological affectlessness which developed in Helene Deutsch's patient. But the evidence remains inconclusive as to whether a mourning process, in the sense of decathecting the lost object, was under way. We can miss and long for someone we still hope to see again.

In the psychoanalytic literature there have been many contributions on adult reactions to loss, particularly those which take a pathological course, eventuating in one or another form of depressive illness. In recent years there have also appeared an increasing number of observations on reactions of very young children to separation from their mothers (notably A. Freud and Burlingham 1943, 1944; Spitz and Wolf 1946; Robertson 1958; Bowlby 1960, 1961a, 1961b, 1963). However, relatively little has been reported on reactions to loss of a major love object of children in the age range from the beginning of latency into adolescence.[2]

In this paper I shall draw on research data on children within this age range who have lost a parent by death.[3] Our subjects are children and adolescents in treatment in a child guidance clinic (and some cases from private practice). The clinical material has also been supplemented by observations of nonpatient subjects. The age at which our subjects suffered the death of a parent varied from earliest childhood to well into adolescence. The time of their coming under our observation also varied. In some instances our acquaintance with the child antedated the parent's death; in others, it began only years afterwards. However, as compared with efforts to reconstruct the effects of such a loss in adult analysis, we were in most instances much closer in time to the event. We were observing still immature individuals who had experienced a major object loss in the course of growing up, and we could see some of the more immediate reactions and the consequences for further development.

When we began our investigation we were aware that persons who have lost a parent in childhood more often succumb to mental illness in adulthood than those who have not suffered such a loss (Barry 1949; Brown 1961). From a therapeutic point of view we hoped that relatively early intervention might help to forestall such pathological effects. At the same time we did not know in what ways the vulnerability to later mental illness might manifest itself earlier in life. Also, since not everyone who has lost a parent in childhood shows later severe disturbances, we were alert to the possibilities of various adaptive reactions.

As our observations accumulated we were increasingly struck by the fact that mourning as described by Freud did not occur. Sad feelings were curtailed; there was little weeping. Immersion in the activities of everyday life continued. There was no withdrawal into preoccupation with thoughts of the lost parent. Gradually the fact emerged that overtly or covertly the child was denying the finality of the loss. The painful process of decathexis of the lost parent was put off, with the more or less conscious expectation of his return. Where depressed moods emerged, especially in adolescence, they were isolated from thoughts of the death of the parent, to which reality testing was not yet applied. Thus we gained the definite impression that the representation of the lost object was not decathected, indeed that it became invested with an intensified cathexis.

It might be supposed that the nonoccurrence of mourning in our subjects indicates only some limitation in their selection. However, from our observations an increasingly strong impression emerged that there was a developmental unreadiness in these children and adolescents for the work of mourning. It is the purpose of this paper to explore this unreadiness and to offer a hypothesis concerning the developmental preconditions for being able to mourn. What I have said does not preclude an adaptive reaction to major object loss in childhood. Only, as I shall try to show, such a reaction follows a course different from mourning.

II

The following case of a young adolescent girl illustrates many of the reactions which we observed in our subjects following the death of a parent. The patient had been in treatment for half a year before the sudden death of her mother, so that it was possible to have some impression of the antecedent emotional situation. I shall focus on two mutually involved aspects of her reactions to the mother's death: the denial of the finality of the loss, and the defenses against the related affects.

Ruth was just fifteen when her mother died of a brain hemorrhage. In the months preceding the mother's death, Ruth had shown much ambivalence toward her. She shrank from her mother's demonstrations of affection and was intensely irritated by her little mannerisms. On the occasion of her mother's last birthday, she had left the present she had made for her at a friend's house and then had rushed to retrieve it at the last moment. At that time Ruth appeared to be in an incipient phase of adolescent detachment from and devaluation of her mother. Almost immediately following the mother's death, Ruth began to idealize her. She said repeatedly that she was just beginning to realize what a remarkable woman her mother was. While this in part echoed what was being said in the family circle, it also expressed an effort to purify her feelings and her image of her mother of the ambivalence which had been so noticeable previously. In remembering her mother,

Ruth reverted many times to an episode just before she had started treatment, when she had been greatly distressed and her mother had been very sympathetic and understanding. This incident became archetypal of her relation with the mother, who now appeared always to have been a comforter and protector. She tended to gloss over the many real difficulties and frustrations in her life with her mother. Periods of her childhood took on an aura of enveloping emotional warmth, though she knew that her diaries from those years told of much unhappiness.

What happened here was a reversal of the adolescent process of detachment from the mother. There was instead an intensified cathexis of the image of the mother, with a strong regressive pull toward a more childish and dependent relation, seen now in a highly idealized light. Freud (1926) said that there is a tendency toward hypercathexis of a lost object, just as toward a diseased body part. We can view this tendency as an effort to deny the possibility of loss of something so essential to the self.

Ruth had repeated fantasies of finding again mother substitutes from the past, a former therapist, a beloved teacher, neither of whom she had seen for many years. It was as if by a displacement from the dead to the absent she were saying: those I have lost can be found again. There was also an intensified attachment to a camp counselor, which was characterized by feelings of disappointment when they were together and desperate longing for the counselor when the were apart.

Expectations of the mother's return emerged gradually. In the second year following her mother's death, Ruth began a stringent course of dieting. She had had long-standing problems of overeating and being overweight, and her mother had repeatedly urged and encouraged her to diet. Now Ruth succeeded over a period of months in becoming surprisingly slim. She received many compliments on her improved appearance, to which she reacted paradoxically in a rather disappointed way. However, as it appeared later, these were not the compliments she was seeking, which would have had to come from her mother. On the eve of her birthday, Ruth went for a long ramble by herself through springtime fields and experienced a dreamy euphoria, a kind of oceanic feeling. When on her return home she tried to describe this experience to her father and felt he failed to understand it, her good mood began to dissolve into disappointment. The night of her birthday she started on an uncontrolled eating binge which continued for many weeks thereafter. Subsequent analysis disclosed that the sacrifice of delightful food represented a kind of bargain with fate, like a vow, in exchange for which she expected the return of her mother on her birthday. The oceanic feeling of oneness with nature may be taken as a symbolic realization of the wish to be reunited with mother, and was perhaps experienced as a portent of imminent reunion. Being confronted at home with her still grieving father precipitated the feeling that the wish was not coming true. The bargain with fate was vitiated and the self-imposed renunciation was abandoned.

Not quite three years after her mother's death, Ruth's father married again. Ruth was filled with emotional confusion, feeling as if her father had become discontented with her mother and thrown her out or as though he were committing adultery. While the father had gone through a period of concentrated mourning, following which he could turn to a new love object, the daughter was still unable to detach her feelings from the mother. She felt as though the mother's place should be kept open for her possible return. Thus father and daughter were out of phase with one another in their tempos of giving up the lost love object.[4] Ruth reported with grim satisfaction a dream in which her mother confronted her father and his new wife in their bedroom. It was as if she felt they deserved being called to account by the wronged wife. Before the father's remarriage she had had fantasies of her mother's return in which she imagined herself frustrated by her father's again asserting his greater claim to the mother. After her father's remarriage, she imagined her mother's returning and mother and herself going off together, leaving behind the strange new ménage.

Ruth repeatedly slipped into the present tense in speaking of her mother. Three years after her mother's death she admitted that she kept in her room a plant which had been dead for a considerable time but which she continued to water. At times when I had occasion to remind Ruth that her mother was dead, she had a pained, offended feeling as if I should not say this to her.[5] At other times she forced herself to think of her mother's body decaying underground, but such thoughts remained isolated from the persisting fantasies of her mother's return. She said that there should be an arrangement for people to be dead for five years and then to come back again. She felt as though she was constantly waiting for something. Gradually she acknowledged thoughts of wishing the therapist could be her mother, but such thoughts occasioned feelings of painful compunction, as if they implied disloyalty to her mother.

Four years after her mother's death Ruth was facing a decisive separation from her therapist (she was about to start further analysis in the city where she was going to college). During the summer vacation Ruth wrote about a cantata in which she was participating, in which the chorus voiced the desperate feelings of drowning children. She quoted verses in which the children cry: "Mother, dear Mother, where are your arms to hold me? Where is your voice to scold the storm away. . . ? Is there no one here to help me? . . . Can you hear me, Mother?" And she said that the author of these lines had expressed for her what she felt.

I should like to elaborate further on the affective manifestations which accompanied this struggle to deny the finality of loss. Shortly after her mother's funeral Ruth found herself no longer able to cry. She felt an inner emptiness, and as if a glass wall separated her from what was going on around her. She was distressed by this affectlessness, and was subsequently relieved when, comparing notes with a friend whose father had died some time earlier, she learned that the other girl had had a similar reaction. The interference with affect was overdetermined by a fear of sharing her father's grief. Shortly after the mother's death, Ruth reported a dream in which her grandfather (standing with her father) leaned close to her and said: "Let us mingle our tears." This dream aroused feelings of intense horror in her: the sharing of such strong emotion was frought with libidinal overtones and the incest taboo was invoked.

In the week following her mother's death Ruth said: "I guess it will be pretty bad this week." Thus she expressed her intolerance of the prospect of protracted suffering, her expectation of early relief. In the time that followed there were many alternations of mood, each good mood being hailed as the end of her distress. This illustrates what I have called the "short sadness span" in children, the desperate effort to recapture pleasurable feelings in whatever circumstances (Wolfenstein 1965). Good moods are the affective counterpart of denial and help to reinforce it: if one does not feel bad, then nothing bad has happened.

Shortly after her mother's death Ruth appeared for her session in an exuberant mood. She had written a successful humorous composition, in which she congratulated herself on getting through her first year of high school with only minor mishaps. She explained this surprising statement by saying that she referred only to events at school, and proceeded to detail various embarrassing predicaments she had got into, which she turned to comic effect. Such denials, accompanied by euphoric moods, tended to be countered by catastrophic dreams, in which, for example, she and her father were taking flight from a disaster-stricken city, then turning back to try to rescue the dying and the dead. Conversely, sad moods were relieved by gratifying dreams.

Several months after her mother's death, upon returning to school in the fall, Ruth went through a phase of depression. She complained that nothing gave her pleasure any longer, not being with friends, not listening to music; everything she had formerly enjoyed had lost its savor. She felt she had nothing to look forward to, wished only to stay in bed, often felt like crying, and that any effort such as that involved in schoolwork was too much for her. Such feelings of sadness, loss of all zest for life, withdrawal and depletion are familiar components of mourning. What was striking in this instance was that these feelings were not consciously associated with the fact of the mother's death or with thoughts about the mother. Rather, Ruth berated herself for the senselessness of her distress. At other times she blamed her unhappiness on her difficulty in ever feeling at ease with her schoolmates. This had been a long-standing complaint, but according to her now distorted view, she had felt much happier with her friends the year before, when in fact she had spoken constantly of the same malaise. Thus a strenuous effort was maintained to keep the feelings of sadness and despair isolated from thoughts of the mother's death. When the therapist repeatedly attempted to connect these feelings with the loss which the patient had suffered, the connection was accepted only on an intellectual level, and again the struggle to recapture pleasurable moods was resumed.

A major maneuver for achieving euphoric moods consisted in transitory identifications with her mother. Ruth would briefly engage in some activity which her mother had pursued and would feel extraordinarily well. Such incidents should be distinguished from the more stable perpetuation of characteristics of the lost love object which typically follows mourning. What Ruth was doing resembled more the play of a young child who, when mother is away, plays at being Mommy. This creates the illusion: Mother is not away, she is here, I am Mother. It operates in the interest of denial of a painful reality.

Other incidents exemplify the effort to keep painful longings and regrets isolated from thoughts of the mother. Sometimes in bed at night Ruth suffered confused feelings of desperate frustration, rage, and yearning. She tore the bedclothes off the bed, rolled them into the shape of a human body, and embraced them. She was quite uncertain and doubtful whether it was her mother she so longed to embrace. Walking through the different rooms of her house she reflected with regret how everything was changed from the time when she was a child. The furniture and drapes had all been changed through the years. She herself occupied a different room from that of her childhood. When she went back to the old room, it no longer was the way it had been. With all this there was no conscious thought that the great change which had occurred and which made home so different from what it had been was her mother's death. Ruth spoke of feeling at times when she was talking to me or other people that she was not really addressing the person before her. When asked to whom she was speaking, she replied that she might say it was to her mother. But this was a kind of detached speculation, carrying no conviction. When she became able to say that the song of drowning children crying for their mothers expressed her own feelings, the isolation between painful affects and awareness that mother was not there was beginning to break down.

At times of separation or impending separation from the therapist, Ruth was impelled toward trial reality testing of the loss of her mother. On one such occasion she said: "If my mother were really dead, I would be all alone"; and at another time: "If I would admit to myself that my mother is dead, I would be terribly scared." Thus we see incipient reality testing and alarmed retreat. The fears of what the finality of her loss would mean maintained the denial and persistent clinging to the love object, which continued to live in her imagination. We may consider that what is feared is the emergence of an unbearable panic state, in which inner and outer dangers are maximized. In the outer world there would no longer be any source of gratification or protection ("I would be all alone"). Within there would be a release of traumatic quantities of objectless libido.

It goes beyond the scope of this paper to consider the ways in which therapy may help an immature individual to give up a lost love object. However, there are a few points on which I should like to remark briefly. We have seen how the warding off of painful affects supports the denial that anything bad has happened. In therapy the child or adolescent can be helped to achieve a greater tolerance for painful feelings. One of the fears that children have of such feelings is that they may continue without letup and increase to intolerable intensity.[6] The therapist can help to insure that painful affects are released at a rate which the immature individual is unable to control independently.

In the case of Ruth, as in the case reported by Fleming and Altschul (1963), separations from the therapist repeatedly had the effect of initiating trial reality testing in regard to the loss of the parent. The current separation, for which the patient has been prepared, may serve as a practice exercise in parting. The fact that the patient can tolerate separating from the therapist may suggest to him that he may be able to bear the more final separation from the lost parent. In Ruth's case it was a decisive separation from the therapist which precipitated the desperate cry for the lost mother. In being able to bring together her feelings of desperate longing with the thought of her mother, in abandoning the defensive isolation previously maintained, she had taken one step toward acknowledging that her mother was really dead.

There were other instances in which Ruth underwent a trial giving up of lesser objects of attachment. I have spoken about her prolonged dieting. During that time she literally mourned the wonderful food which she had formerly enjoyed, remembering it with longing and sadness, which was quite different from her way of remembering her mother. This trial mourning did not at that time serve to advance her toward giving up her mother. There was an implicit *quid pro quo* in it, an expectation that through this ordeal of renunciation she would get her mother back. When this expectation was not fulfilled, the capacity for renunciation became for a time drastically reduced. A later trial giving up consisted in her decision not to return to the camp which she had attended for many years. After this decision was made, there was much regret and longing for beloved counselors and camp mates with whom she would not again enjoy the same close companionship as in the past. It would seem that the giving up of a major love object lost in childhood or adolescence requires many preparatory stages.

III

What we have seen in the case of Ruth was observed repeatedly in other children and adolescents whom we studied. Sad affects were warded off. When they broke through, they were isolated from thoughts of the lost parent. Denial of the finality of the loss was overtly or covertly maintained. Bowlby (1961a) has spoken of the importance of expressing what he calls "protest" in reaction to loss, that is, a vehement demand for the return of the lost object and strenuous efforts to regain it. He considers the full expression of such feelings and strivings essential to attaining the conviction that the object is in fact irretrievable.[7] "Protest" involves a painful awareness of the absence of the object, an awareness which may be for long postponed. The emergence of painful longings and crying for someone who does not come is a step toward reality testing and eventual tolerance for giving up the lost object.

Our subjects gave many indications that they denied that the dead parent was irretrievably lost to them. They frequently slipped into the present tense in speaking of the dead parent. They reported seeing someone on the street whom they fleetingly mistook for the lost parent. There was intolerance of any reminder that the parent was dead. Memories of the dead parent were not fraught with the painful feelings of the mourner who is in the process of realizing that these things will not come again. Where sad feelings emerged in relation to the lost parent, there was an effort to get away from them as quickly as possible. For example, a ten-year-old girl, whose father had died when she was seven, was moved to tears when her therapist said sympathetically that she must often miss her father. After being briefly downcast she proposed, "Let's change the subject," and was soon chatting in a cheerful and animated way about events at school. The intimate relation between tolerance for sad affects and reality testing appears throughout our material.

Fantasies of the dead parent's return often appeared in disguised form. Thus a ten-year-old boy, whose father had died when he was three, had a fantasy of a robot who would come out of the wall and teach him all he needed to know, so that he would not have to go to school. The robot (something both dead and alive) no doubt represented the omniscient father who could transmit his powers to his son. Perhaps the amount of distortion here is related to the age of the child at the time of the parent's death. We may recall Helen Deutsch's (1937) case of the patient who had lost his mother when he was five, and who remembered the childhood fantasy of a big mother dog coming into his room at night and showing him affection. Our material suggests that fantasies of the parent's return are either more clearly conscious or more readily admitted in adolescence than at earlier ages. It seems likely that the fantasy of the parent's return may be a more closely guarded secret in younger children. A readiness to admit the fantasy, thus risking confrontation with reality, may represent one of the many steps toward giving up the lost parent.

The denial of the parent's death coexists with a correct conscious acknowledgment of what has really happened. All our subjects could state that the parent was in fact dead, and could recall circumstances related to the death such as the funeral. Yet this superficial deference to facts remained isolated from the persistence on another level of expectations of the parent's return.[8] What we see here is a splitting of the ego in the defensive process.

Freud (1927) observed the use of this mechanism in relation to the loss of a parent in childhood. He reported that two young men patients, one of whom had lost his father in his second year, the other in his tenth year, both had denied the reality of the father's death. They could feel and behave as if the father still existed. But this denial represented only one sector of their mental life. There was another sector in which the death of the father was acknowledged. In speaking of this defense against accepting an unbearable piece of reality, Freud remarked: "I also began to suspect that similar occurrences in childhood are by no means rare" (156).

Following the death of a parent a child's image of him and feelings toward him undergo a change. It is not the parent as he last knew him in life, but the glorified parent of early childhood who is perpetuated in his fantasy. This, for a child in the age range we are considering, represents a regression. I may note parenthetically that a major loss suffered at any age precipitates some regression. The adult mourner becomes for a time "an infant crying in the night." The loss of a loved person evokes feelings of terrible help-lessness, like those of a deprived infant who is powerless to relieve his distress. Children seem to respond to this predicament by conjuring up the fantasy of an ideally good and loving parent who can do everything for them. Their own feelings toward the lost parent also become, for a time, ideally loving. This is partly an attempt at posthumous undoing of bad feelings or wishes previously directed toward the lost parent.

Bowlby (1961b, 1963) has pointed out that young children express raging reproach against the mother who goes away and leaves them. In older children whose reactions to the death of a parent we have observed, there seems to be a strenuous effort to divert such feelings from the image of the lost parent. Similarly, the negative sector of the ambivalence formerly felt toward the parent is split off. These hostile feelings are directed toward others in the child's environment, notably the surviving parent. Thus, far from being able to turn to substitute objects, the bereaved child often feels more at odds with those around him and alienates them by his angry behav-ior. His fantasied relation with the idealized dead parent is maintained at great cost. It seems to absorb most of his libidinal energies and involves a diversion of hostile feelings toward those who could help and befriend him.[9] With time, perhaps particularly in adolescence, reproachful feelings toward the abandoning parent emerge. Thus a twenty-year-old patient, whose father had died when she was fourteen, spoke of having idealized him following his death. Now, however, she was bitterly reproachful toward him, blaming his death, which had left her in such hard straits, on his reckless disregard of doctor's orders. The return of ambivalence toward the lost parent, like the ability to associate sad feelings with his loss, represents one step toward reality testing.

We have observed then that instead of decathecting a lost love object, which is what happens in mourning, children and adolescents tend to develop a hypercathexis of the lost object. Why do they cling in this way to a lost parent, unable to give him up? To understand this, we must consider what object relations mean in different phases of development. What happens when an object relation is externally served gives us crucial clues as to what the relation meant to the individual who suffers this loss. Spitz and Wolf (1946) demonstrated dramatically that infants in the second half of the first year become radically retarded in all areas of development when they are separated from their mothers (and when no adequate mother substitute is provided). Recently Fleming and Altschul (1963) have presented strikingly similar observations about adult patients who experienced the loss of a parent as late as adolescence. They found that these patients had remained arrested in their development at the stage in which they were at the time of the parent's death. If the parent, or parents, had been lost when the patient was an adolescent, the patient was still, years later, living emotionally like an adolescent. These findings suggest that, despite the impressive development in so many areas which can be observed between infancy and adolescence, something in the child's relation to the parents persists throughout this time. The child needs the continuing relation with the parents in order to advance in his development.

I shall consider some of the indispensable prerequisites for the child's growth which the parents provide. While parents do not, in the normal course of development, remain exclusively need-gratifying objects, they do continue to provide for the child's needs until he is able to make his own way in the world. Apart from material needs, they are sources of narcissistic supplies. While with the infant and young child the mother provides support for his body narcissism, with the schoolchild the parents give essential support to his pride in his growing accomplishments. The parents also retain external ego and superego roles. With the infant and young child they mediate wholly between him and reality, for instance, guarding him from dangers of which he is not yet aware. They act as an external superego from the time they utter the first "No, no" when the toddler approaches some forbidden object. As the child develops internal ego and superego functions, these functions remain for a long time far from autonomous, dependent on external support from the parents.

To illustrate what happens when this manifold support is lost: we have observed repeatedly that some children and adolescents begin to decline in their school performance following the death of a parent. Other children begin to behave badly in school. In yet other instances, truancy and stealing begin after a parent has died. We may suppose that the child who in this way declines in his accomplishments or deviates from previous good behavior is suffering from the loss of narcissistic rewards and external ego and superego support. These disturbances are no doubt overdetermined. These children may be in part criminals out of a sense of guilt, seeking punishment for the guilt they feel for the parent's death (Bonnard 1961). Another factor which may be operative is that the child's previous good behavior may have been predicated on a kind of bargain with fate. He was being good to insure that nothing bad would happen. When his parent died, the bargain with fate was abrogated. Such a sequence could be reconstructed in the case of the twenty-year-old girl, mentioned before, whose father died when she was fourteen. The father had had a heart attack when she was eight. Following this the girl had developed compulsive rituals and many scruples about bad thoughts and bad words, the unconscious purpose of which was presumably to prevent anything bad from happening to her father. When he died, of a second heart attack, it was as if fate had failed to keep the bargain and she was released from her part of it. Immediately following her father's death, her school-work, which had been excellent, declined. In adolescence she became promiscuous, and on starting treatment at nineteen she presented a picture of an impulse-ridden character.

I have tried to indicate in the case of Ruth that her clinging to her lost mother was motivated by incipient panic at the thought of letting go: "If I would admit to myself that my mother is dead, I would be terribly scared." I should now like to explore the factors which make for this overwhelming fear of acknowledging that the dead parent is irretrievably lost. One such factor has already been indicated in the discussion of the external ego and superego support that the child needs from the parents: without this the child fears the disintegration of the psychic structure he has achieved. On the most primitive level he fears annihilation: he could not survive if the parent were not still there. Ruth's saying, "If my mother were really dead, I would be all alone," expresses this. There would be no one to care for her, no one to gratify any of her needs, she would be abandoned in an alien world. This apprehension of annihilation in a child of Ruth's age is related to the evocation of a much more infantile image of the mother than that of the mother whom she recently knew. It corresponds to the sense of acute helplessness provoked by the loss of the parent.

A related fear is that of the breakthrough of massive amounts of objectless libido, of traumatic intensity. In mourning there is a gradual decathexis of the lost object, and this gradualness protects the mourner from a traumatic release of more unbound libido than he can cope with. I would like to suggest that children and young adolescents lack the capacity for this kind of dosage in emotional letting go. We know that in the sphere of action there is a gradual progression in being able to postpone action and to substitute the trial action of thought, in which smaller quantities of energy are involved. It would seem that there is a similar slow or late development of the capacity to release affective energies in any gradual way (Fenichel 1945, 393). Children operate on an all-or-none basis. A tentative trial of what it would mean to let go of a lost parent thus evokes the threat of being overwhelmed and they revert to defensive denial.

Another factor contributing to the fear of acknowledging such a grievous loss is that the child still conceives of the parent as a part of himself. Jacobson (1965) has recently pointed this out, and has compared the desperate striving of a child to recover a lost parent with the little girl's longing to recover her lost penis.[10] That the parent is felt to be a part of the child, or an inalienable possession without which he is incomplete, helps to account for our repeated finding that children are deeply ashamed of having lost a parent. They often try to conceal this fact, or feel chagrined when it is revealed. The bereaved child feels a painful inferiority to children who have an intact family. Sometimes this feeling is displaced to material possessions.[11] For instance, the ten-year-old boy mentioned earlier, whose father had died when he was three, was particularly occupied with cars because his father had had such an impressive big car. He was keen on collecting toy model cars and became distressed when he saw another boy with a larger collection than his. He characterized the feeling evoked by the comparison of himself with such a more fortunate boy as "jealancholy," a term he coined as a condensation of "jealousy" and "melancholy." This boy was deeply ashamed of lacking a father and tried to conceal this fact from his schoolmates.

There is one further fear I would mention which reinforces the child's denial of the loss of a parent; that is the fear of regression. Repeatedly, children and adolescents have reported that they were unable to cry following the parent's death or that an inhibition of crying set in after a brief period of time. So, for instance, a thirteen-year-old boy said he felt nauseated on the trip back from his father's funeral and attributed this to the fact that he had swallowed his tears. Adolescents often feel distressed, uneasy, and self-accusing at this inhibition of crying, as we saw in the case of Ruth. We have to do here with an insufficiently explored topic: the relation of crying to different phases of development. Young children cry readily at any frustration, deprivation, disappointment or hurt. In latency there is normally a marked inhibition of crying and conscious repudiation of it as babyish. We are probably justified in suspecting that there is something amiss with a child in this phase who continues to cry easily. The inhibition of crying seems to extend well into adolescence. There is of course also a sex-typing in this regard in our culture: it is more shameful for boys to cry than it is for girls. However, in response to a major loss adults of both sexes cry more freely than children or adolescents.[12] The crying of adults in grief, if it is not indefinitely protracted, appears as a normal regression. Children and adolescents seem to hold back from such a regression, perhaps out of fear that once under way it would have no bounds and precipitate them to total infantility.

I should now like to consider a question which probably has already occurred to the reader: the child who has lost one parent still has a parent—why is the surviving parent not an adequate support for the child, an object to whom the child can transfer the feelings he had for the parent who has died? According to our observations, the child's relations with the surviving parent regularly become more difficult (Neubauer 1960). There are many reasons for this, which I shall indicate here only in part. When a parent has died, the child is confronted with a widowed parent, afflicted, grief-stricken, withdrawn in mourning, sometimes otherwise disturbed. Whether the widowed parent is of the same or opposite sex, the child's incestuous strivings toward him are stimulated from seeing him now alone. But the parent seems to take little comfort from the child's presence; he is lost in grief. It is as if the child wished to say, ''Don't you see me? I am here.'' And the parent replied, ''You are no help.'' The child thus experiences anew the oedipal chagrin, the sense of his inadequacy in comparison with an adult marital partner. At the same time there is a futile but desperate urge on the part of both the child and the widowed parent to put the child in the place of the missing parent. One of our most repeated findings is that, following the death of a parent, a child shares the bedroom and sometimes the bed of the widowed parent. Many rationalizations are given for this arrangement: the parent is lonely, the child is frightened at night, the family has moved to smaller living quarters. One boy told us that he had to go to his mother's bed because he was cold. When the warm weather came he still had to go there because there was a fan in her room. Evidently behind such trivial justifications there are deep needs on both sides. Even when the child is not sharing the parent's bedroom, incestuous impulses are intensified and arouse alarm. In struggling to ward off these impulses, the child becomes withdrawn or antagonistic toward the widowed parent.

There is also the child's tendency, as previously noted, to concentrate intensified positive feelings on the lost parent. The negative sector of the ambivalence formerly felt toward the lost parent is split off, and its most available target is the remaining parent. As the lost parent is idealized, the surviving parent is devalued. Often there is the conscious wish that he (or she) had died instead. Jacobson (1965) has pointed out that on a deeper level the child blames the surviving parent for the loss he has suffered. In the child's fantasy this parent has destroyed the other or been deserted because of his unworthiness. Thus for a child who has lost a parent, relations with both parents become distorted. As to the narcissistic supplies and ego and superego support which the child so needs, a parent withdrawn in grief is little able to provide them. The child often feels and reacts as though he has lost both parents.

IV

I have tried to show that there is a developmental unreadiness in children for the work of mourning. I should now like to turn to the question: what are the developmental preconditions which make mourning possible? Adolescence has been repeatedly likened to mourning (A. Freud 1958; Lampl-de Groot 1960; Jacobson 1961, 1964). In adolescence there is normally a protracted and painful decathexis of those who have until then been the major love objects, the parents. The hypothesis which I wish to propose is this: not only does adolescence resemble mourning, it constitutes the necessary precondition for being later able to mourn. The painful and gradual decathexis of the beloved parents which the adolescent is forced to perform serves as an initiation into how to mourn. The individual who has passed through this decisive experience has learned how to give up a major love object. In circumstances of later loss he is able to recapitulate the process.

It is not until adolescence that the individual is forced to give up a major love object. We have seen how little external loss enforces such a decathexis. The conflicts of the oedipal phase, as Anna Freud (1958) has pointed out, lead to a change in the quality of the child's love for his parents, making it love with an inhibited aim. But the parents remain the major love objects. It is only in adolescence that developmental exigencies require a radical decathexis of the parents. With sexual maturity, the adolescent is powerfully impelled to seek a sexual object. The images of the parents become relibidinized, but there the incest barrier stands in the way. The adolescent is confronted with the dilemma: to withdraw libidinal cathexis from the parents or to renounce sexual fulfillment. This may be likened to the dilemma of the mourner as Freud described it. The mourner is bound to the beloved object, no longer available; at the same time he is attached to life and all it may still have to offer. Eventually the decision is in favor of ongoing life and the renunciation of the past which this requires. The adolescent, impelled forward by his sexual urges, is similarly constrained to detach himself from his beloved parents and his childhood past.

We know that the struggle of the adolescent to achieve this detachment is a long and difficult one. Forward movement often alternates with regression. The adolescent has many possibilities, both in terms of opportunity and of his newly developing capacities for diverting freed libido into new love relations, friendships, and sublimated activities. But these newfound interests are often unstable; new relationships prove transient and disappointing. Libido reverts again to the old objects or becomes absorbed in the self and the work of inner reorganization. To the extent that freed libido remains objectless, depressed moods occur. Abraham (1911, 1924) has pointed out that depression is experienced not only when an object is lost externally, but when there is an inability to love someone formerly loved. This is what happens with the adolescent as his capacity to love his parents declines. Jacobson (1961, 1964) has said that the adolescent experiences an intensity of grief unknown in previous phases of life.

Freud has stressed the crucial role of remembering in mourning and the reality testing by means of which memories are consigned to the irrevocable past. I should like to suggest that we find an analogue of this too in adolescence, that in adolescence a new feeling about the past emerges. There is a nostalgia for a lost past, a combined yearning and sense of irrevocability. The ways of remembering one's own past in different phases of development remain incompletely explored. We may consider, however, certain earlier phenomena in this area. The young child may yearn for the past, but he does not consider it irrevocable. He has not yet grasped the irreversibility of time. If he wishes to be a baby again, we will see him crawling on all fours and saying "da, da." He becomes a baby. In the latency period, with the repression which follows the oedipal phase, the attitude toward the past changes. It becomes one of repudiation. When his parents recall amusing and endearing things he used to do when he was little, the latency period child is inclined to disclaim these babyish things with some contempt. He puts his past behind him and prides himself on his new skills and accomplishments.

It is in adolescence that the sense of a longed-for past develops with the conviction that it can never come again. The past assumes a mythical aura. Fantasies of a golden age of the personal and the historic past probably have their inception in this time of life. Let me cite an early "memory" which a thirteen-year-old girl said had recently come to mind and which seemed to her very real. She recalled being wheeled in a baby carriage, in which she was cozily and contentedly ensconced, while her mother and father walked behind. She attributed to her infant self the thought, "Too bad this can't last." We would recognize this as a screen memory, in which memories and fantasies have been condensed. This girl had been the eldest child in her family and no doubt had envied the younger siblings whom she had seen replacing herself in the baby carriage, as they had in her parents' affections. In this memory she was again in sole possession of the parents. By ascribing to her past self the awareness that this could not last she was attempting to undo the traumatic surprise at the arrival of the next sibling. At the same time the sense of transience, of past pleasures having to be renounced, which pertained to her adolescent state, became part of the content of her childhood memory.

Probably nostalgic memories generally preserve something from very early childhood, antedating the oedipal troubles so painfully revived in adolescence. The theme of such memories, more or less disguised, is of the self as a greatly loved small child. As Wordsworth says, in his great nostalgic poem on recollections of early childhood: "Heaven lay about us in our infancy." The adolescent, in the enforced giving up of his parents, feels a sense of all he is losing. He conjures up regressively the most ideal aspects of being a child encompassed by parental love. We know that few real memories survive from the earliest years. Yet most individuals possess a history of themselves starting from birth, which is based on their parents' reminiscences. The parents themselves have felt nostalgic when they recalled to the older child the happenings of his first years. They have suffered some sense of loss as the confiding and affectionate small child seemed to grow away from them into greater independence. I would suggest that the adolescent, in his nostalgia for the past, identifies with his parents nostalgically recalling his early years.

The sense of the irrevocability of the past appears in many ways in adolescence. There may be an acute awareness of the transience of present pleasure, that every moment is slipping into the past, that life itself is ephemeral. Adolescents often find in their preferred poetry expression of those moods. A. E. Housman's poems, for instance, express an adolescent longing for a lost past, never wholly renounced. "That is the land of lost content, / I see it shining plain, / The happy highways where I went / And cannot come again." It has been said that Housman's poems are best appreciated by adolescents. Similarly, adolescent girls weep over songs of unhappy love, of partings and longing for an absent lover. Their conscious thoughts may be of a boy who has recently disappointed them. But the intensity of their grief is for the loss of a much greater love, the waning of their love for their parents, and the renunciation of their childhood.

In comparing adolescence with mourning we should also consider the ways in which they differ. The mourner is well aware that he is sad because of the loss of a beloved person and his mind is dominated by thoughts of the lost object. The adolescent does not know why he is sad or depressed and does not attribute these feelings to the loss of his capacity to feel love for his parents. Where the mourner has suffered an external loss, the adolescent undergoes an enforced renunciation because of internal conflicts. Whether the adolescent's renunciation is experienced as more active and voluntary than that of the mourner varies with the individual. This probably depends in large part on the relative strength of the forward impulsion and the regressive pull. The objects from which the adolescent is freeing himself are still there. Aggression can be directed toward them with some impunity since, in a reassuring way, they continue to survive. This is in contrast to the tendency to divert aggression from objects lost by death. While the mourner thinks of the object he has lost in a loving and idealizing way, the adolescent is devaluing the objects he is in the process of giving up. When the adolescent's struggle to withdraw from the parents becomes too difficult, he can still turn to them again, and, not without mixed feelings, derive gratification and support from their presence. In mourning a major amount of the libidinal attachment to the lost object is dissolved and the mourner is released from his painful, incessant preoccupation with the lost object. Yet he retains loving feelings for the one he has lost. Even more in adolescence, the decathexis of the parents is incomplete. Normally a positive attachment to them continues, though the feelings for them are no longer of such intensity or pre-eminence as those of earlier years.

The likeness of the adolescent process to mourning appears in the very considerable decathexis of major love objects, occurring over a period of time, accompanied by painful feelings, and with reality testing affirming the irrevocability of the past. The exigencies of adolescence which enforce this renunciation are without precedent in the child's antecedent life. Until he has undergone what we may call the trial mourning of adolescence, he is unable to mourn. Once he has lived through the painful, protracted decathecting of the first love objects, he can repeat the process when circumstances of external loss require a similar renunciation. When such loss occurs, we may picture the individual who has been initiated into mourning through adolescence confronting himself with the preconscious question: "Can I bear to give up someone I love so much?" The answer follows: "Yes, I can bear it—I have been through it once before." Before the trial mourning of adolescence has been undergone, a child making the same tentative beginning of reality testing in regard to a major object loss is threatened with the prospect of overwhelming panic and retreats into defensive denial in the way we have observed.

We have seen that the younger child's panic at the prospect of having to give up a lost parent is related to the characteristics of the object relation. The parent is felt to be an indispensable source of material and narcissistic supplies, an auxiliary ego and superego, a part of the self. The renunciation of the parents in adolescence entails a giving up to a considerable extent of the kind of relationship which the child has had with them heretofore. Where the giving up of the child-parent relationship is not accomplished, the individual may merely turn away from his parents to seek others who will fulfill the same functions. Where in this way the work of adolescence has remained uncompleted, the adult remains unable to accomplish the work of mourning in response to loss.

V

We have considered the struggle of children and adolescents to deny the finality of the loss of a parent and their unreadiness to decathect the lost object through the work of mourning as we know it in adults. The question arises whether there is an alternative way for the immature individual to decathect a lost parent without undergoing the process of mourning. Such an adaptive alternative may not be available to our child patients, handicapped as they usually are by disturbances in development which antedate the parent's death. To assess the range of possibilities it is important for us to supplement our clinical data with observations of children whose development has been relatively unimpeded up to the time of the parent's death. I shall now turn to an instance of this sort, in which we can see an adaptive reaction to the loss of a parent in childhood, and at the same time contrast this reaction with that of mourning.

Walter, whose life course I have been able to follow from infancy to young manhood, lost his mother at the age of ten. The mother died of cancer after a period of progressive debilitation. During her last illness both she and the boy were cared for by the young woman's mother, who had great love and understanding for them both. Little by little, as the mother declined and became unable to satisfy the boy's needs, he transferred his affections to the grandmother. She was there, providing for his material wants, attentive to his accounts of his school days, appreciative of his accomplishments, involved with everything that concerned him. It was no doubt important that the grandmother was no newcomer in the boy's life. He had known her well before, and for a period of time she had cared for him in his mother's absence. Thus it was not a question of forming a new attachment, but of transferring a greater amount of feeling to someone already loved. What I believe happened here was that there was a piecemeal transfer of libido, detached from the mother, to an immediately available and acceptable mother substitute. This began while the mother was dying, and the boy turned gradually from her, withdrawn as she was in her illness, toward the grandmother. The process continued after the mother's death, when the grandmother devoted herself to Walter's care and upbringing.

Walter showed some of the same emotional inhibitions in reaction to his mother's death which appeared in the child patients we have discussed. He did not cry, and made strenuous efforts to deny and ward off feelings of distress. When his mother died he was sent to spend the day with friends of the family. In thanking these friends for their hospitality Walter laid exaggerated stress on what a happy day this had been for him. Unlike the adult mourner, he showed no diminution in his interest in usual activities. He was anxious to return to school at once and to carry on as if nothing had happened. In his spare time he began to immerse himself in incessant reading. We may suppose that partly this served to exclude painful thoughts and feelings. Partly his involvement with fictional heroes helped him to experience vicariously emotions which he could not acknowledge more directly. It was in relation to fictional characters that he experienced a belated breakthrough of his inhibited grief. Three years after his mother's death, when he came to the end of the series of books about the Three Musketeers, he wept profusely, saying, "My three favorite characters died today." I have characterized this phenomenon elsewhere as "mourning at a distance" (Wolfenstein 1965).

The angry feelings in reaction to loss, which we have observed repeatedly, were not absent here. Following his mother's death, Walter was diffusely irritable and quick to anger. In an altercation with his grandmother, intolerant of her rebuke, he said he was leaving home and stormed out into the night. When he returned, his grandmother said that they would have to talk about how bad they both were feeling because of his mother's death. She told him of the efforts that had been made to save his mother's life, that drugs had been flown in from other cities, and how sad it was that medical science was not yet sufficiently advanced to cure the terrible illness which she had had. Walter then was moved to confess that he blamed himself for his mother's death. Two years before she died she had had a breast operation and had returned from the hospital very weak. Nevertheless she had got up in the mornings to prepare Walter's breakfast before he went to school. He now felt that if she had not had to get up to get his breakfast, she would not have died. The grandmother assured him that this was not the cause of his mother's death, and that his mother's love for him and interest in him helped to keep her alive as long as possible. Their discussion went on far into the night, and at the end the boy, greatly relieved, and with the intolerance for prolonged distress characteristic of his age, exclaimed, "I feel great!"

While his mother was dying and for a considerable time after her death, Walter was insatiably hungry. He consumed great amounts of food and was particularly greedy for sweets. In this intensification of oral needs we may see a manifestation of the bereaved child's regressive longing for the all-fulfilling parent of earliest years. In this instance the regression remained circumscribed. The child's libido did not remain overly bound to the fantasy image of an idealized lost parent. The regressive greediness expressed only that part of the libido which was not yet transferred to the grandmother. But the greater part of the child's needs were being fulfilled in reality by the grandmother, who was able to supply material and narcissistic gratifications and to give ego and superego support.

In adolescence Walter showed strong feeling for and interest in friends, and developed an increasing capacity for sublimation in intellectual pursuits. At twenty-five he is married, with two beloved young children, and is progressing his chosen career with pleasure and accomplishment.

Such an outcome requires a combination of favorable external and subjective conditions. The major external condition is the availability of an adequate parent substitute. Our culture generally makes little provision for such substitutes. The nuclear family, consisting of young parents and their growing children, entails an exclusiveness of attachment of children to their parents. Margaret Mead (1965) has pointed out that the nuclear family is especially well adapted to life in a rapidly changing culture. There is minimal boundness to old ways and customs. However, such a family is very little adapted to changes in its own personnel. In times and places where children have been raised in an extended family, there is a greater possibility of finding immediately available and acceptable substitutes if a parent dies (Volkart and Michael 1957). In the context of our culture, the case of Walter is relatively exceptional in that a good mother substitute was immediately available to the bereaved child. The preexisting mutual attachment of grandmother and grandson and his previous experience of living with her in his mother's absence facilitated the transition. Moreover, the collaborative, noncompetitive way in which mother and grandmother had shared the boy's care probably lessened what feelings he may have had of being disloyal to his mother in turning to his grandmother.

The subjective factors favoring a major shift of object cathexis in childhood require further exploration. I can allude to them here only in a preliminary way.[13] We know that the fate of feeling toward a lost object is related to the ambivalence with which the object was regarded. Paradoxically the more ambivalent the relation has been, the harder it is to give it up. Where there has been strong ambivalence toward the object, its loss is likely to precipitate the protracted reproachful demands for its return which Bowlby has described. In the case of Walter, ambivalence toward his mother, whose only child he was, appears to have been of moderate intensity.

Freud stressed that no libidinal position is abandoned without great reluctance. More recent observations of children, however, have also made us aware of an opposite tendency, a developmental push which impels them toward more advanced levels of functioning. There are probably great individual differences in the balance between the tendency to cling to early libidinal positions and the impulsion to move forward. In the readiness to welcome persons other than the mother, we can observe marked individual differences among children in the first years of life. Walter was one of those children who very early in life showed a great eagerness toward people. Thus a facility for forming object relations was probably another condition favoring his successful shift from mother to grandmother.

In the case of Walter, we have seen an adaptive reaction to the loss of a parent in childhood, in which apparently a major decathexis of the lost parent was accomplished. However, the process here differs markedly from that of adult mourning. There was no protracted sadness or withdrawal into painful preoccupation with memories of the lost object. In the gradual decathexis of the mother, while she was dying and after her death, Walter was able to transfer freed libido immediately to an already present mother substitute. If we imagined an analogue to this in an adult, we would have to picture a widower, let us say, having at his side a new wife, even one who had been an auxiliary wife before, to whom he could transfer at once the libido he was detaching from the wife he had lost. This is not adult mourning as we know it. The adult mourner can transfer his feelings to a new object, if one is found, only after a period of time in which he is emotionally occupied with detaching libido from the lost object. There is a hiatus here which the child is unable to tolerate.

VI

This paper has been concerned with determining the developmental preconditions for mourning. Observations of children in the age range from latency into adolescence, who have suffered the death of a parent, have shown that they are unable to mourn. In many instances, instead of a decathexis of the lost object, we find an intensified cathexis, with an overt or covert denial of the irrevocability of the loss. In the favorable instance of an adaptive reaction to such a loss, the process differed from that of mourning. There was an immediate transfer of freed libido to an available substitute parent. I have considered the factors making for the developmental unreadiness to mourn in children and young adolescents, in terms of the nature of the object relation to the parents. The hypothesis has been advanced that adolescence constitutes the necessary developmental condition for being able to mourn. Adolescence has been likened to a trial mourning, in which there is a gradual decathexis of the first love objects, accompanied by sad and painful feelings, with reality testing of memories confirming the irrevocability of the childhood past. It is only after this initiation into mourning has been undergone that the individual becomes able to perform the work of mourning in response to later losses.

NOTES

1. There has been some confusion in discussions of whether or not children mourn, because the discussants have attached different meanings to the term "mourning." I shall use the term "mourning" in the sense in which Freud used it in "Mourning and Melancholia," to mean that reaction to loss in which the lost object is gradually decathected by the painful and prolonged work of remembering and reality testing. Bowlby (1960, 1961a, 1961b, 1963) has extended the term "mourning" to include a wider range of reactions to loss. Those reactions in which the demand for the return of the lost object persists then become "pathological mourning." Bowlby feels that, in order to establish the relations between reactions to loss in early childhood and in later life, it is necessary to bring them under a common rubric. There is no logical necessity for this. All relations, whether of cause or similarity, can be established among distinct phenomena whether we call them by the same or different names. It seems to be in the interest of clarity to confine the meaning of a term to a distinct phenomenon rather than extend it to a range of differing phenomena.

2. Some observations of beginning latency period children who had suffered the loss of a parent may be found in Scharl (1961) and Shambaugh (1961).

3. The research project, some findings of which I am reporting here, has been conducted in the Division of Child Psychiatry at the Albert Einstein College of Medicine. Forty-two cases of children and adolescents who have lost a parent by death have been observed or are currently under observation. At the time of entering treatment the patients ranged in age from three and a half to nineteen years, the majority being in adolescence. We have had one child under six, eleven between the ages of six and eleven, eighteen between twelve and fifteen, and twelve between sixteen and nineteen. Sixteen of the patients came under observation within a year of the parent's death; eight within two or three years; eighteen from four to fourteen years later.

   The following have participated in this project: Drs. Raymond Bernick, Peter Bokat, Betty Buchsbaum, Richard Evans, Daniel Feinberg, Karl Fossum, Lester Friedman, Paul Gabriel, Charles Goodstein, Phyllis Harrison, Leonard Hollander, Allan Jong, Saul Kapel, Dr. and Mrs. Gilbert Kliman, Drs. Sally Kove, William Lewit, Donald Marcuse, Manuel Martinez, Eli Messinger, James Pessin, Judy Roheim, Rita Reuben, Edward Sperling, Eva Sperling, Sherwood Waldron, Alex Weintrob.

4. The different tempos of reaction to loss in children and their widowed parents, which put them out of phase with one another, are generally a cause of much mutual misunderstanding.

5. Bowlby (1961a, 1963) has pointed out how much the bereaved person resents those who speak of his loss as a *fait accompli*. Hated are the comforters.

6. A nine-year-old boy vividly evoked the awful prospect of unstoppable grief that would

overwhelm children if they were not able to "forget" about a painful loss: "They would cry and cry. They would cry for a month and not forget it. They would cry every night and dream about it, and the tears would roll down their eyes and they wouldn't know it. And they would be thinking about it and tears just running down their eyes at night while they were dreaming" (from an interview by Dr. Gilbert Kliman on children's reactions to the death of President Kennedy).

7. According to Bowlby (1961a), a bereaved individual gives up a lost object when prolonged expressions of "protest" (clamorous demands and strivings for the return of the object) are seen to bring no result. These strivings then "gradually drop away or, in terms of learning theory, become extinguished" (334). However, observation suggests that clamoring for the return of a lost object can continue indefinitely despite lack of response from the external world as long as the internal representation of the lost object is not decathected.

8. Furman (1964a) takes the verbal acknowledgment of a young child that his parent is dead and not coming back as indicating a readiness to mourn. What is overlooked is the defensive splitting of the ego as a result of which the death is at the same time denied and the attachment to the lost parent perpetuated.

9. Lindemann (1944) called attention to the occurrence of rage in bereavement. Bowlby (1961a, 1961b, 1963) has stressed what he considers the omnipresence of rage in reaction to loss. He has also pointed out that, while its main object is the lost person, who is reproached for his abandonment, it is frequently displaced to others.

10. In discussing the splitting of the ego as a defense against unbearable aspects of reality, Freud (1927, 1940) cited two main instances in which this defense was invoked: in relation to the castration complex, and in relation to the death of a parent.

11. Robertson (1958) has pointed out how young children, in prolonged separation from their parents, shift from longing for their presence to increasing demands for material gifts.

12. Studies of reactions to the death of President Kennedy showed that adults wept more than did children or adolescents (Sheatsley and Feldman 1964; Sigel 1965).

13. We would expect a child's readiness to accept a substitute object to be related to the phase of development in which he was when he experienced the loss of a major object. Thus we would hypothesize that when a child is still almost wholly dependent on a need-gratifying object, he will be most ready to transfer his affections to someone who is able to provide for his needs (A. Freud and D. Burlingham 1943, 1944).

BIBLIOGRAPHY

Abraham, K. (1911), Notes on the Psycho-Analytical Investigation and Treatment of Manic-Depressive Insanity and Allied Conditions. *Selected Papers on Psycho-Analysis*. London: Hogarth Press, 1942, pp. 137–156.

———— (1924), A Short Study of the Development of the Libido, Viewed in the Light of Mental Disorders. *Selected Papers on Psycho-Analysis*. London: Hogarth Press, 1942, pp. 418–501.

Barry, H. (1949), Significance of Maternal Bereavement before the Age of Eight in Psychiatric Patients. *Arch. Neurol. & Psychiat.*, 62:630–637.

Bonnard, A. (1961), Truancy and Pilfering Associated with Bereavement. In: *Adolescents: A Psychoanalytic Approach to Problems and Therapy*, ed. S. Lorand & H. I. Schneer, New York: Hoeber, pp. 152–179.

Bowlby, J. (1960), Grief and Mourning in Infancy and Early Childhood. *Psychoanal. Study Child*, 15:9–52.

———— (1961a), Processes of Mourning, *Int. J. Psa.*, 42:317–340.

——— (1961b), Childhood Mourning and Its Implications for Psychiatry. *Amer. J. Psychiat.*, 118:481–498.

——— (1963), Pathological Mourning and Childhood Mourning. *J. Amer. Psa. Assn.*, 11:500–541.

Brown, F. (1961), Depression and Childhood Bereavement. *J. Ment. Sci.*, 107:754–777.

Deutsch, H. (1937), Absence of Grief. *Neuroses and Character Types.* New York: International Universities Press, 1965, pp. 226–236.

Fenichel, O. (1945), *The Psychoanalytic Theory of Neurosis.* New York: Norton.

Fleming, J. & Altschul, S. (1963), Activation of Mourning and Growth by Psycho-Analysis. *Int. J. Psa.*, 44:419–431.

Freud, A. (1958), Adolescence. *Psychoanal. Study Child*, 13:255–278.

——— & Burlingham, D. (1943), *War and Children.* New York: International Universities Press.

——— ——— (1944), *Infants Without Families*, New York: International Universities Press.

Freud, S. (1917), Mourning and Melancholia. *Standard Edition*, 14:237–260. London: Hogarth Press, 1957.

——— (1926), Inhibitions, Symptoms and Anxiety. *Standard Edition*, 20:77–175. London: Hogarth Press, 1959.

——— (1927), Fetishism. *Standard Edition*, 21:149–157. London: Hogarth Press, 1961.

——— (1940), Splitting of the Ego in the Process of Defence. *Standard Edition*, 23:271–278. London: Hogarth Press, 1964.

Furman, R. A. (1964a), Death and the Young Child. *Psychoanal. Study Child*, 19:321–333.

——— (1964b), Death of a Six-year-old's Mother during His Analysis. *Psychoanal. Study Child*, 19:377–397.

Jacobson, E. (1961), Adolescent Moods and the Remodeling of Psychic Structures in Adolescence. Psychoanal. Study Child, 16:164–183.

——— (1964), *The Self and the Object World.* New York: International Universities Press.

——— (1965), The Return of the Lost Parent. In: *Drives, Affects, Behavior*, ed. M. Schur. New York: International Universities Press, 2:193–211.

Lampl-de Groot, J. (1960), On Adolescence. *Psychoanal. Study Child*, 15:95–103.

Lindemann, E. (1944), Symptomatology and Management of Acute Grief. *Amer. J. Psychiat.*, 101:141–148.

Mead, M. (1965), Paper presented at Ciba Foundation Conference on Transcultural Psychiatry, London.

Neubauer, P. B. (1960), The One-Parent Child and His Oedipal Development. *Psychoanal. Study Child*, 15:286–309.

Pollock, G. H. (1961), Mourning and Adaptation, *Int. J. Psa.*, 42:341–361.

Robertson, J. (1958), *Young Children in Hospitals.* New York: Basic Books.

Scharl, A. E. (1961); Regression and Restitution in Object Loss: Clinical Observations. *Psychoanal. Study Child*, 16:471–480.

Shambaugh, B. (1961), A Study of Loss Reactions in a Seven-year-old. *Psychoanal. Study Child*, 16:510–522.

Sheatsley, P. B. & Feldman, J. J. (1964), The Assassination of President Kennedy: A Preliminary Report on Public Reactions. *Pub. Opinion Quart.*, 28:189–215.

Sigel, R. S. (1965), An Exploration into Some Aspects of Political Socialization: School Children's Reactions to the Death of a President. In: *Children and the Death of a President*, ed. M. Wolfenstein & G. Kliman. New York: Doubleday, pp. 30–61.

Spitz, R. A. & Wolf, K. M. (1946), Anaclitic Depression. *Psychoanal. Study Child*, 2:313–342.

Volkart, E. H. & Michael, S. T. (1957), Bereavement and Mental Health. In: *Death and Identity*, ed. R. Fulton. New York: Wiley, 1965, pp. 272–293.

Wolfenstein, M. (1965), Death of a Parent and Death of a President: Children's Reaction to Two Kinds of Loss. In: *Children and the Death of a President*, ed. M. Wolfenstein & G. Kliman. New York: Doubleday, pp. 62–79.

19. Additional Remarks on Mourning and the Young Child

Robert A. Furman

Recent papers by Wolfenstein (1965, 1966) have presented thoughts about mourning in childhood which seem somewhat at variance with those I have described (1964). A review of these papers has stimulated thinking in a number of directions. In discriminating between areas of disagreement and those in which Wolfenstein has apparently misunderstood me, it has seemed possible to discern ways of presenting my ideas more clearly. In delineating the areas of disagreement, it has been possible to explore more clearly the significance of these disagreements. And in considering the sources, the origins of these areas of divergence, certain clarifying concepts have emerged about psychoanalytic research.

I shall begin with a brief restatement and recapitulation of my ideas on mourning and the young child. These are detailed in the papers referred to above.

After a child has started acquiring a reality comprehension of death, and I agree with Anna Freud (1943) that this is possible for him from age two on; and after he has reached the object-centered phallic phase of relationships and acquired the concomitant level of maturation of ego functions, presumably possible at three and a half to four years of age, the child then has the potentiality or capability of mourning. This does not mean he will spontaneously mourn after he has suffered a severe loss, but it does mean that he can mourn if he is given the proper support and is in the proper milieu.

By "proper milieu" I mean a milieu that realistically assures him fulfillment of his age appropriate needs. By proper support I mean the understanding willingness of those responsible for his care to seek as well as accept his affective responses. In Wolfenstein's most recent paper (1966) Walter's

Reprinted by permission of the Philadelphia Association for Psychoanalysis from *Bulletin of the Philadelphia Association for Psychoanalysis* 18 (1968): 51–64.

grandmother offers an excellent example of what I mean by proper support. In approaching the ten-year-old boy after his first emotional upset after his mother's death, she told him "that they would have to talk about how bad they both were feeling."

I believe these thoughts about a child's capability of mourning are important because if they are correct, they have three significant practical implications. (1) It is sound prophylactic mental health work to encourage the parents of two-, three- and four-year-olds to educate their children about the reality of death. (2) It is equally sound to supply professional assistance to a surviving parent to support him in doing what Walter's grandmother apparently could spontaneously do in enabling the child to fulfill the requirements of the mourning task. (3) It is also sound analytic technique not to interrupt a treatment because of a young patient's severe loss, assuming his reality needs can be met by his environment, but rather to continue the analysis, to assist and support him in completing the requirements of the mourning task.

It is not necessary to dwell on why it is important for a child or for any person to fulfill the requirements of the mourning task. In "Mourning and Melancholia" Freud (1917) says, "We rely on its [mourning] being overcome after a certain lapse of time, and we look upon any interference with it as useless or even harmful." Clinical examples of the consequences of an incompleted or absent mourning are available from many sources. In "Absence of Grief" Helene Deutsch (1937) presented four brief case reports illustrating some vicissitudes of emotional development that ensued when mourning was not successful. Her thesis was that the absent grief would find expression in otherwise inexplicable periods of sadness or depression or else its warding off would be accomplished only at the cost of warding off all affects. In her four cases, regardless of the outcome of the struggle with the apparently absent grief, all had most serious impediments in forming any meaningful object relationships.

Next I want to describe the source of my ideas. They came from the analytic work with little Billy, a case that I have reported previously (1964b). To my surprise this neurotic little boy was able to accept the painful reality of the loss of his mother and was able to respond affectively to this loss. In addition he proceeded to a recurrent sorrowful remembering and missing of his mother in what seemed like every situation in which he ordinarily would have been aware of her presence. This process I felt differed in no essential way from that which we observe in an adult who is mourning and which we accept as indicating his preoccupation with the painful mental task of decathecting the inner representation of the lost object which is the essence of mourning. This process involved Billy primarily for about a year and had passed its high point when he said to his father months after his mother's death, "Is it all right that I don't think about mother all the time? Sometimes now when I play, I just play and don't think about her. I used to [think about her] all the time."

After this analytic experience I wondered how it had been possible for him to have accomplished this task. I approached this question, I believe, in an analytic way by considering the structuralization and personality maturation that would be necessary for a child to be able to mourn (1964b). This led me to the conclusion that by the age of three and one half or four a child would be capable of mourning if, and again I repeat *if,* he is given the proper support and has the proper milieu in which to approach this task.

I started with this capsule summary for two reasons. First I want to point out that my theoretical thinking was stimulated by and evolved from the understanding which became available in the course of an analysis; an analysis in which I could utilize fully all the technical tools the child analyst has at his disposal. Second, I want to correct two misunderstandings which appear in Wolfenstein's (1966) paper. In a footnote she states that I take "the verbal acknowledgment of a young child that his parent is dead as indicating a readiness to mourn." This is incorrect. I have always stressed that the comprehension of the reality of death is but one of a number of attributes that must be at the young child's disposal to give him the capability of mourning. In what I call the second misunderstanding Wolfenstein attributes to me a child's achieving object constancy as one of the prerequisites for being able to mourn. This does not appear in my published paper, although it was in an earlier version which I believe she may have read. Anna Freud in her unpublished lectures in New York (1960) used the term "object constancy" to refer to what she now calls the object-centered phallic level of object relationships. Object constancy is used now to describe a much earlier level of relationships. In my published paper I adopted the more current terminology to describe the level of object relationship necessary for the ability to mourn, a level well beyond that connoted by the expression object constancy.

I shall now discuss Wolfenstein's papers, particularly her most recent one, her theoretical formulations, the case of Ruth, and return later to her report on Walter.

I regard mourning as she does "in the sense in which Freud used it in

"Mourning and Melancholia" to mean that reaction to loss in which the object is gradually decathected by the painful and prolonged work of remembering and reality testing." This decathexis is not a simple phenomenon, and I will discuss it later. Continuing on, and again I quote from Wolfenstein's paper, she discussed this "invaluable adaptive function of mourning . . . which frees major amounts of libido . . . [to be utilized] for other relations and sublimated activities in the world of the living."

In his description of mourning, Freud says, "Reality testing has shown that the loved object no longer exists, and it proceeds to demand that all libido shall be withdrawn from its attachments to that object. This demand arouses understandable opposition . . . it is a matter of general observation that people never willingly abandon a libidinal position, not even, indeed, when a substitute is already beckoning to them. . . . Normally respect for reality gains the day. Nevertheless its orders cannot be obeyed at once. They are carried out bit by bit, at great expense of time and cathectic energy, and in the meantime the lost object is psychically prolonged. Each single one of the memories and expectations in which the libido is bound to the object is brought up and hypercathected, and detachment of the libido is accomplished in respect to it. . . . The fact is, however, that when the work of mourning is completed the ego becomes free and uninhibited again."

Freud's remarks on mourning seem to me to describe the process I observed in Billy. His statement about people's unwillingness to abandon a libidinal position "even when a substitute is already beckoning to them" is most germane to our topic. Wolfenstein has postulated that "in the favorable instance of an adaptive reaction to such a loss . . . there was an immediate transfer of freed libido to an available substitute parent." I do not think that such an immediate transfer of libido is possible. A child turns to a substitute parent for fulfillment of the needs he cannot fulfill for himself and begins a relationship that will be based on the fulfillment of those needs. Rather than representing the immediate transfer of freed libido, which I think is indicative of the abandonment of a libidinal position, I believe the turning to the substitute parent is on the basis of need fulfillment, and carries with it not only the transfer of relatively small amounts of libido, but constitutes the first step towards the creation of the situation in which the child of four years or older can begin the mourning process that would truly free the major portion of his libido.

To return to Wolfenstein's definition of mourning, with which I find myself in basic agreement, I believe that if a bereaved person has fulfilled the requirements of his mourning task he will, if a child, incur no arrest in his development which will then be able to continue in a progressive manner and he will, if an adult, ultimately return to full activities in the world of the living, for a young adult, perhaps even marrying or remarrying as the case might be. There is nothing in this dynamic concept of mourning that says how the unfolding of this internal mental process should appear externally to any observer of the mourner's behavior. We would not expect a child as evidence of successful completion of the mourning task to marry, as this is not in harmony with the nature of childhood. Similarly we would not expect a child in his mourning to evidence to an outside observer the behavioral characteristics of the adult, the protracted weeping, for example. This too may not be in harmony with the nature of childhood. To insist on a conformity in external manifestations of mourning in an adult and in a child is to focus on descriptive observation which in this instance leads us away from metapsychological understanding.

Spiegel (1966) speaks to this point in the section of his paper "Affects in Relation to Self and Object" that deals with the question of mourning in childhood and adolescence. He says, "In addition to the distinction between pain and grief, it is also useful to distinguish between the *state* of mourning as a clinical fact and the *work* of mourning as the cause of the state. . . . In childhood and adolescence the grieving state of mourning is usually not observed. However, this does not permit us to infer the absence of the *work of mourning*." It is interesting in this connection to note Strachey's first footnote to the text on "Mourning and Melancholia": "(The German 'traurer,' like the English 'mourning' can mean both the affect of grief and its outward manifestation.)"

Wolfenstein (1965) has described a child's resistance to crying and inability to cry fully, referring to it as "the short sadness span" of childhood (68). She has quoted (1966) in a footnote (103 n. 6) the nice example from Kliman of a child's expression of the fear of the strength of his feeling. This fear is met in four-year-olds as well as forty-year-olds and is amenable to therapeutic intervention not on the basis of age but rather on the basis of internal economic considerations. In a case to be reported in "The Therapeutic Nursery School" I describe a four-year-old girl with enuresis expressing the exact same fear but then, with reassurance by her mother, losing her inhibition to crying and simultaneously regaining control of her urine at night.

If, when Wolfenstein sets the completion of adolescence as the earliest time a person can mourn, she refers to fully independent mourning which can occur regardless of external support or milieu, I would probably concur. But I believe, although I cannot be certain, that she feels that only after completion of adolescence is true mourning possible. After completion of adolescence, adulthood is reached, albeit young adulthood. Once adulthood is reached, the mourning process will, of course, appear externally to any observer as usual adult mourning. I think that it is the external observable phenomena of mourning, not the internal dynamic factors, that may have in part influenced Wolfenstein's selection of the completion of adolescence as the time when mourning is possible.

If I qualify Wolfenstein's thinking about the relationship between adolescence and mourning as referring to completely independent mourning, then I find wide agreement in the theoretical considerations which she has developed. In her recent paper she has added the postadolescent's independence from the parental fulfillment of needs as of crucial significance and has with great insight described the persistence of these needs through adolescence. I would tend to emphasize this as more important for the preparation for independent mourning than the usually concomitant adolescent decathexis of parents. It seems important to emphasize that this decathexis is a partial one as are most decathexes, even those of successful mourning. The internal representation is never completely abolished in either. I believe partial decathexes occur from earliest infancy on, of the mother who nurses, the mother who trains, the phallic mother, the oedipal mother or father, etc. We see young children's capabilities to decathect in their response to moves, changes of school, neighborhood, loss of friends.

Before turning to the case of Ruth I would like to say a few words about defense mechanisms, focusing on what might be called their adaptive use in the service of the ego as opposed to their pathological use to ward off neurotic anxiety. When someone is faced by a realistic external danger, the anxiety about which might preclude any effective action to protect himself, denial of the danger becomes an adaptive defense. If the denial persists after the danger is passed, it has become a pathological defense mechanism. Soldiers in wartime danger who denied tremendous threats to their survival to preserve their ability actively to defend or protect themselves were responding adaptively. Persistence of this denial after the danger has passed would indicate it had become pathological. This distinction has recently been elaborated regarding the successive layers of denial in the formation of the fetish by M. Katan (1964).

The early latency child whose mother has died and who denies her death because his reality needs are not being met will be responding adaptively if, by his denial, he wards off an anxiety about his survival that might paralyze his own efforts to seek fulfillment of these needs. And foremost among these needs is the acceptance of his feelings. Once these reality needs are being met, persistence of his denial would indicate that his denial had become pathological. Pathological defense mechanisms require interpretation; adaptive defense mechanisms should not be interpreted, or should be interpreted most judiciously. Where the mechanisms seem basically adaptive, all efforts should be directed to removal of the external threat in the situation of a child losing a parent, to seeking ways of insuring fulfillment of all the child's needs. In this context the denial that is integral to the split in the ego in the defensive process should not be interpreted and analyzed if it is adaptive, but should be interpreted and analyzed if it is pathological.[1]

We turn now to Wolfenstein's description of the case of Ruth. There is a beautiful description of this girl's defensive activity and its consequences as well as many suggestive clues to its origins. The mechanism used most extensively by Ruth after her mother's death was denial. This apparently was supported by isolation and regression, regressing to times of her life before her mother's death. When her feelings about her loss broke through into consciousness, the denial and isolation were maintained by displacement or reversal. My impression was that her euphoria represented a reversal of affect. The idealization of her mother seems quite properly described as a defense against the recognition of her aggression to her mother. The screen memory about which this idealization was focused primarily is not elucidated for us. Prominent in the consequences of all this defensive activity is the disorder of her reality testing that led to the expectation of her mother's return and to a marked impairment of her affective freedom. In a late adolescent these severe interferences with normal functioning with a father and later with a stepmother enable us to feel quite safe in assuming that her defenses were primarily not adaptive, and not in the service of her ego.

But we are given a description of her defenses with little exposition of any analysis of them. This would be a necessary first step to seeking and then analyzing the anxiety beneath these defenses. We could really understand Ruth only through analysis of her pathological defenses and the neurotic conflicts and anxieties they warded off, provided there was any reasonable semblance of the fulfillment of her reality needs. We are left with the impression that Ruth's inability to mourn produced these defensive responses. It would seem to me quite the contrary: that it was her pathological defenses that made her unable to mourn. Her inability to mourn was, as it is with many adults from whom she would differ in no way, a consequence of this defensive activity.

Ruth says, "If I would admit to myself that my mother is dead, I would be terribly scared." In other words, she is saying "my denial wards off my anxiety." We can see some of the sources of her anxiety. Her idealization of her mother tells us of her dread of her aggression toward her mother and indicates the existence of superego anxiety. The adolescent who dreads being alone, as Ruth did, tells us possibly of her masturbatory conflict and its associated superego and objective anxiety. Her dream of mingling her tears with her grandfather tells us of the acute reactivation of her oedipal conflict and its neurotic involvement with the tragic death of her mother. I think we are correct in inferring that Ruth dreaded an intolerable intensity of her feelings, the very common anxiety we recognize in children, adolescents and adults as a fear of being overwhelmed by the strength of instincts or affects.

But all these anxieties are most familiar to us and would require analysis with Ruth as with any other patient, child or adult. Only by analysis of *Ruth's defenses, underlying anxieties and associated conflicts to the genetic* origin of these conflicts and defenses could we gain true insight into Ruth's capability of mourning. Only with such analysis could it be said whether or not Ruth could mourn. At this juncture it could only be said that the reason Ruth could not mourn her lost love object was because her neurotic anxiety demanded the pathological defensive use of denial of this loss.

I believe that her defenses precluded her mourning and that it was not an inability to mourn that in some way evoked these defenses. My belief is based on my analytic work with Billy. I have described the second eight-months' period of his analysis in a paper given at the mid-winter meeting of the American Psychoanalytic Association in 1964. It has since been published in *The Child Analyst at Work,* edited by Dr. Geleerd (1967).

During this period of work Billy's recurrent painful missing of his mother, which ultimately touched almost all the places of his original contacts with her, began to have periods of interruption when it would disappear for many days. He wanted to take walks with me again and finally it became clear that it was because he hoped he might see his mother. I pointed out to him this would be possible only if she still were alive and wondered why he had to pretend in one part of him something another part of him knew was not true. In response to this interpretation of his denial, which was repeatedly offered to him, his behavior, talk and play in the sessions took a new turn. He became angry with me over minute frustrations, trying to provoke me. He asked anxiously about angry feelings. His play battles between soldiers became battles between children and parents. Then he told me his fear; that his anger had made mother angry and her anger caused her death. That is, that he had wished her dead.

With this guilt-laden fear now conscious and in words, his denial stopped and his mommy-missing returned slightly less intensely, as it had by now passed its high point. Needless to say, we reworked this material many times, in many forms, including within the transference. The denial returned intensely a month or so later and then stubbornly refused to yield to the old interpretations. Finally I asked him why he had to persist in thinking he had caused mother's death. His immediate response was an airplane battle with an American plane, which we knew from prior work stood for mother, shot down by a sneaky German plane. I asked if the German plane was Billy. It was not. Was it his brother? No, but I was closer. Was it father? Yes!

We understood that his fear he had killed his mother hid the dread that his father had. The relation of this material to primal scene exposure, his oedipal conflicts, the relation of the German plane to me in the transference cannot now be pursued. Suffice to say that analysis of this anxiety resulted in a disappearance of his denial and a return of his mommy-missing. What is important for our purpose is that analysis of his defense to the anxiety beneath led to the inactivation of the defense and its interference with his mourning which then resumed its course.

With Ruth we have a beautiful description of her pathological defenses. To the child analyst, description is but the first step to be followed by defense analysis to the conflicts beneath, present-day ones, and via the transference, to the genetic origin of these conflicts. Without this analytic work, it is not possible to know what actually exists in the inner mental life, essential knowledge if we are to gain insight or dynamic understanding.

This difference between descriptive phenomena and the material that becomes available after the arduous work that is psychoanalysis underlines the great difficulties inherent in theoretical formulations that are not based on psychoanalytically derived data. From situations where such data is unavailable, in the pre-verbal infant, in analytic biography (to name but two), most significant contributions to psychoanalysis have emerged. M. Katan (1966) points out in discussing Henry James and "The Turn of the Screw" that constructions differ from speculations in such analytic work when they fit within a coherent whole covering all the data available. Further, it could be said that basic formulations derived in such research methodologies would ultimately have to fit within the framework of psychoanalytic psychology and derive confirmation in psychoanalytic clinical experience.

The barrier to understanding the child which his defenses impose enabled me to understand more of the questionnaire studies of children or the studies utilizing topic-directed themes children are asked to write. Studies like these try to bypass the child's defenses through creating apparently impersonal, neutral situations which might minimize defensive activity. These studies are often stated to be well controlled because the subjects involved are derived from balanced groups. But what is totally uncontrolled is any understanding of which children are able to set aside which defenses and why, and the investigator is thus left with no way of being able to gain insight into the children's internal psychic functioning.

In the context of formulations fitting within the whole of available data I turn briefly to Wolfenstein's description of Walter, the ten-year-old who lost his mother. He fortunately had turned gradually from her to his grandmother before the mother's death, and was getting mother's approval, tacitly at least, for turning away or withdrawing from her. Anna Freud, in discussing this question in Cleveland (1964), described this as the optimal situation for the young child in such a crisis. As was mentioned before, Walter's grandmother's ability to fulfill his needs, facilitated by the reality situation of her gradual assumption of this role, and her active acceptance of his feelings created the circumstances in which one would expect him to be able to mourn. Wolfenstein felt that "a major decathexis of the lost parent was accomplished," although she does not give us any direct evidence of this process in action. She describes from her reports of his adolescence and young adulthood that no significant arrest of his development occurred as a consequence of his mother's death. Despite her feeling that the significant decathexis occurred and despite the evidence that he achieved the results we associate with successful completion of the mourning task, she feels this was an adaptive reaction and not mourning. Her reasons are that there was "no protracted sadness or withdrawal into painful preoccupation with memories of the lost object." I would add, visible to any observer of his manifest behavior. But as analysts we can draw no conclusion from the description of his manifest behavior that he was never sad or painfully preoccupied. As analysts we are concerned not with what appeared externally but rather with what transpired internally. I reported about Billy that his most painful mommy-missing which he shared with me, to which he affectively responded with his father, was never visible in his behavior to any outside observer. I can add here that an analytic colleague, a close friend of the family, saw him frequently in this period and was not aware of the child's mourning.

Although our information is limited, it seems likely that Walter successfully accomplished the "invaluable adaptive function of mourning" (Wolfenstein) and that because this work was completed his "ego (became) free and uninhibited again" (Freud). And this despite the fact the external manifestations of this process in Walter might quite logically not have conformed to the picture of the mourning adult. What I believe quite probably to be the successful mourning of this latency boy was achieved in the manner and for the reasons I have described that enabled the young child to be assisted and sustained to mourn.

It might be asked: What difference does it make what words are used to describe what Billy and probably Walter accomplished? Is it of any importance if this is a true mourning or an adaptive reaction that is not mourning? Is there any difference between the two? The latter is not an illogical question, particularly as early in her paper Wolfenstein (1966) describes mourning as "responding to a major object loss in [an] adaptive way." On general scientific principle we should be as precise and accurate as our current psychoanalytic psychology and our own understanding allow us to be. Only through the struggle to achieve this accuracy can specific problems be mastered, insights be gained that may have broader applicability and the way be demarcated to further problems.

In this particular instance it would seem important to distinguish between formulations derived from descriptive data and those based on material derived from the deeper understanding available only through clinical analysis. It is not that formulations derived from the one source will invariably be more accurate than those from the other. It would seem, however, that metapsychological thinking is more difficult to maintain with descriptive data, so many vital factors remaining unavailable. In addition and perhaps more important, a preference for descriptive data may herald a turning towards statistical type studies or empirical observation, as Wolfenstein puts it, for further elucidation of a metapsychological problem, instead of awaiting the slow evolution of the appropriate psychoanalytic case material. Such a development (turning towards empiric studies) seems unwise as well as unfair. It seeks of these studies answers that by their very structure they cannot supply. It ignores the limitations inherent in these studies, limitations of which the analyst is otherwise fully aware. And it accords such studies a scientific validity the analyst can find only in clinical psychoanalytic work.

A second significance of the words used to describe these processes could derive if the dictum becomes established that a child cannot mourn. I believe both Wolfenstein and I would agree there are two steps involved in assisting a child who has suffered a severe loss. The first concerns the arduous task of making certain that a child's reality needs are being met and the second concerns the equally arduous task of helping him with his feeling responses to the loss. It is with the understanding and technical handling of this second step that it seems Wolfenstein and I may enter a disagreement. Both these steps are most difficult to effect and are trying and painful to the one seeking to aid the bereaved child. My fear is that should it become established that a child could not mourn very few therapists would long persevere with the second of these laborious and exhausting tasks.

For many adults a child's grief is so poignant they prefer for their own sake to deny its existence. The dictum that a child cannot mourn could only support this unfortunate attitude. One example might be pertinent here. In a followup of graduates of our Therapeutic Nursery School a mother was interviewed whose husband had been murdered during the previous year. At first she described an affectless response in all her children, but, as she continued, she recognized the many clues she had missed and ultimately realized she had missed these because of her own inability to mourn. She sought psychiatric help then for herself. When the male teacher of her thirteen-year-old son was interviewed, he described how the boy had returned to school after the tragedy apparently without feeling, acting as if nothing had happened, never once referring to his father's death. When the boy was interviewed and the therapist asked about his father, offering an appropriate sympathy for his loss, he burst into tears. The therapist later asked the boy if his mother knew of his intense feeling. He replied that he had tried to tell her but that she could not listen . . . ''she just couldn't.'' When the therapist asked about the teacher, the boy told her bitterly how disappointed he had been because this teacher had not been able to say one word to him about his father's death. Again it could be verified that the boy was absolutely correct. Examples of this nature are so tragically and repetitively available that it is difficult to avoid the comparison between the adult's denial of a child's ability to mourn and the more familiar adult denial of a child's sexuality. When our clinical work so often pinpoints the basic difficulty in the adults' denial of the child's capacity to feel deeply, then it seems crucial to scrutinize most carefully and scientifically the dictum that a child cannot mourn.

I realize full well that experiences such as this thirteen-year-old endured have no scientific validity in considering whether or not a child is capable of mourning before completing adolescence. I realize that Wolfenstein would neither advocate nor support the mother's and teacher's unfortunate inhibition of a human response to a tragedy. My point is that the question of a young child's capability of mourning may have wide and significant practical importance in addition to the scientific or metapsychological factors involved.

NOTES

1. Even the phrase "splitting of the ego in the defensive process" may be one that is descriptively accurate and yet metapsychologically unsound. See M. Katan (1964).

BIBLIOGRAPHY

Deutsch, H. (1937), Absence of grief. *Psychoanal. Quart.*, 6:12–22.

Furman, R. (1964a), Death and the young child: some preliminary considerations. *Psychoanalytic Study of the Child*, 19:321–333. New York: International Universities Press.

—— (1964b), Death of a six-year-old's mother during his analysis. *Psychoanalytic Study of the Child*, 19:377–397. New York: International Universities Press.

—— (1967), A technical problem: the child who has difficulty in controlling his behavior in analytic sessions. In: *The Child Analyst at Work*, ed. E. R. Geleerd. New York: International Universities Press, pp. 59–84.

—— (1969), Case report: Sally. In: *The Therapeutic Nursery School*, ed. R. A. Furman. New York: International Universities Press.

Freud, A. & Burlingham, D. (1943), *War and Children*. New York: International Universities Press.

—— (1960), Unpublished Lectures given in New York City.

—— (1964), Unpublished Lectures given in Cleveland, Ohio.

Freud, S. (1917), Mourning and melancholia. *Standard Edition*, 14:239–258. London: Hogarth Press, 1957.

Katan, M. (1964), Fetishism, splitting of the ego and denial. *Int. J. Psycho-Anal.*, 45:237–245.

—— (1966), The origin of "The Turn of the Screw." *Psychoanalytic Study of the Child*, 21:583–635. New York: International Universities Press.

Spiegel, L. (1966), Affects in relation to self and object: a model for the derivation of desire, longing, pain, anxiety, humiliation and shame. *Psychoanalytic Study of the Child*, 21:69–92. New York: International Universities Press.

Wolfenstein, M. (1965), Death of a parent and death of a president: children's reactions to two kinds of loss. In: *Children and the Death of a President*, ed. M. Wolfenstein & G. Kliman. New York: Doubleday, pp. 62–79.

—— (1966), How is mourning possible? *Psychoanalytic Study of the Child*, 21:93–123. New York: International Universities Press.

20. A Child's Capacity for Mourning

Robert A. Furman

I have been asked to present here a brief summary of my thoughts about a child's capacity for mourning, the factors that can interfere with the utilization of this capacity, and the consequences for the child who fails to fulfill the requirements of the mourning task. My thoughts on this were first presented in 1964 (1, 2), parts of which were disputed by Wolfenstein in 1965 (3) and 1966 (4) and by Nagera in 1970 (5). I attempted to deal with some of these criticisms in papers in 1968 (6) and 1970 (7).

I mention these differences of opinion at the outset to make certain the reader is aware that the thoughts I will present are not universally accepted and to offer the necessary references for those who might wish to pursue these questions further. In essence, I have felt a child usually has the capacity for mourning, under proper circumstances, from somewhere around age four, whereas Wolfenstein and Nagera feel that a child cannot mourn until the termination of adolescence. This would mean, to me, until young adulthood is reached. In other words, I believe a child from about age four on has the capacity for completing the requirements of the mourning task; and they believe, if I understand them correctly, that no child can complete this task.

Attempting to understand scientific disagreement can be both stimulating and helpful. I believe one of the difficulties lies in the utilization of certain manifestly grieving adults as the model for mourning. This seems unfortunate as the focus is then apt to be placed on what Spiegel (8) described as the "grieving state of mourning" as opposed to "the work of mourning [which is] the cause of that state." In *Mourning and Melancholia,* Freud's description of this work of mourning is of an adaptive or reparative response to loss that is characterized by the gradual decathexis of the internal mental

Reprinted by permission of John Wiley & Sons, Inc., from *The Child in His Family: Impact of Disease and Death. Yearbook of the International Association for Child Psychiatry,* edited by E. J. Anthony and C. Koupernik, vol. 2, 1973.

representative of the lost object, the withdrawal of the feeling investment in the mental image of the lost loved one. This is accomplished through recurrent remembering of the object and then the painful acceptance of its permanent absence. In 1923 in *The Ego and the Id,* Freud (10) added that "It may be that an identification is the sole condition under which the id can give up its object." It is these psychological tasks that are to me the essence of mourning. When these are completed, feeling investments will have been freed and made available for new object relationships in the reality world of the living. The child's lack of an externally visible grief reaction similar to that of an adult has to my mind no more bearing on his internal capacity for mourning than his apparent sexual innocence would indicate the absence of his sexual feelings and fantasy life.

Many factors complicate for everyone a consideration of a child's mourning. The child's apparently helpless fragility at a time of grave loss has a poignancy that evokes from all a great depth of feeling and a recall of one's own past losses. All of us who have worked with bereaved children either directly or through their surviving parent have been so impressed with the personal emotional strain of such work that no one wants to take on more than one such case at a time. The reader should be prepared that in considering doing any supportive work in this area an emotional response of his own cannot be avoided.

In addition, at the heart of the question about mourning is that of death. This means the topic will also immediately involve us with questions of aggression and our comfort or discomfort with this aspect of our own psychological makeup. What has always been striking to me is the adult's usual need to deny the small child's ability to understand the concept of death, something the child can comprehend from somewhere around age two on. A colleague described for me the situation of coming upon a dead bird while on a walk with some friends and his children, including a two-and-a-half-year old. One of the friends was about to remove and hide the bird "so the little one won't be upset" when the little boy spied the bird himself. He came over, picked it up and said, "The poor birdie is dead. I'll put it back into the woods, O.K. Daddy?" A. Freud (11) states that adults deny the child's capability to understand death to protect themselves from the child's sadism. I doubt if she would object to the addition "that recalls for them their own conflicts over sadism."

I pursue these points at the outset because I believe the reader should be prepared for the difficulties inherent in this topic and because I want to put central the question of the work of mourning to enable us to examine the attributes a child must have acquired to manage this psychological task.

To begin with he must have the concept of death and its finality. If this is realistically taught the small child, he can readily accept it. If his parents avoid or deny the reality of death, the child will accept his parents' prohibition and denial. No prelatency child can cope with the abstractions involved in the concept of heaven and will comprehend it only as a reality place where people go and exist and hence are not dead. The explanation of death as the absence of life is best offered the child when he first encounters it with insects and animals. Without such a reality concept of the death, no child can cope with its feeling consequences.

To withdraw a feeling investment from a mental image of a lost loved one, to decathect the internal representative of the lost object, a child must first have a stable internal representative that can survive and endure after the vast majority of loving investment has been removed. Our theoretical knowledge and clinical experience would indicate to us that this is possible after the achievement of object constancy dominance and a mastery of the ambivalence conflicts of the anal sadistic phase of development. In an otherwise emotionally healthy child it is reasonable to anticipate this level of development sometime around age four. The ability to form adequately mature ego identifications is to be anticipated at about the same age.

It is in proceeding with the internal psychological work of mourning that difficulties arise for many, children and adults. There must be a healthy availability of feeling, not an unwarranted degree of suppression of feeling by neurotic defenses. There must be a fluidity, a flexibility of personality structure, not a rigid character unable to adapt to change. It is with these personality attributes that many children and adults fall short of having the capacity for successful mourning and would need psychological treatment to attain the mental health necessary successfully to complete the mourning task. In underlining a child's inability to mourn, it has seemed to me as if some have idealized adult mourning which would mean a denial of the inability of so many adults fully to master the demands of mourning.

But to do this painful work a child has some special requirements that do not exist for the adult who has attained the maturity and independence that should accompany the successful completion of his adolescent development. A child has physical and emotional needs that must be met for his survival and if his loss is that of a parent, he must be certain, before he loosens his attachment to his internal representative of the lost one, that these needs will be met. In response to his bereaved son's question as to who would take mother's place, one father said simply, "No one can ever take Mother's place, but I can see to it that all her jobs are done." This is an enormously difficult task, even in the best of circumstances, calling for the most resourceful family and often community effort. If the physical needs can be met and the child has been consistently shown that they are being met, he will then be in the position of being able to begin the decathexis of the internal representative. The child's ability to continue his psychological development in the absence of one parent will depend on two factors. First, he must decathect the image of the lost parent to free his feelings for growth through investment in new objects. Second, there must be available to him some consistently interested adult of the proper sex, grandparent or close family friend, for example, in whom these feelings can be invested sufficiently for their growth and maturation.

But a child will need even more to be able to utilize his capacity to do the mourning work. He will need the acceptance of his feelings, fears, and reality evaluations as he is able to put them into words. One little bereaved girl with whom I was working to help her accomplish, somewhat belatedly, her mourning of her mother, received a terrible setback in this work when her father and stepmother had to deny quite strongly some of her reality observations about some of her dead mother's quite human shortcomings. At times a child may need the judicious interpretation of the defenses he might employ to avoid his pain. One father replied in such a situation, "We both know Mother is not alive any more. Maybe sometimes we want to pretend it isn't so because it makes us so unhappy." Some surviving parents, in the midst of their own mourning, may need support to make such a statement. In one instance I know of it came from another sibling. A younger child was concerned that mother was cold in the grave and the father was explaining that despite the fact it was winter, the casket would keep mother from being cold. The older sister said, "But Daddy, you know Mother is dead and can't feel any more."

And yet there is one more difficulty that a child will face. The losses he endures of parents or siblings are always premature and untimely, either because of illness or accident. The manner in which these premature deaths have occurred has a tremendous potential as a trauma in and of itself. The child who has lost a sibling through illness will, for a very long time indeed, have a tremendous dread of even the most minor illnesses in himself and all others. The child who has witnessed a violent death, such as in a car accident, or has been aware of or seen the results of extensive surgical procedures, such as a mastectomy, will have these most difficult realities facing him whenever he begins to cope with his loss. Deaths of grandparents at an advanced age are always so much easier because the unnatural and so often terrifying aspects mentioned above are absent. These potential traumata in the premature losses must be taken into account in helping a child achieve some degree of freedom from untoward anxiety before he can utilize his capacity to mourn.

I hope that by now I have sufficiently sketched why I believe a young child has the capacity to mourn as well as the factors that can readily interfere to preclude his utilization of this capacity. Specifically, I am referring to the need to present death realistically, meet a bereaved child's needs consistently, accept his feelings, support his reality testing, judiciously interpret his defenses, and assist him with mastering the inevitably terrifying reality which caused his premature loss. These are all most difficult tasks, sometimes impossible to accomplish. But this should not preclude our making the maximum effort we can, for success is possible and its rewards very great indeed.

A loss in childhood that is unmourned, unmastered stays active in the personality and, through the defenses utilized to ward off its awareness, influences all aspects of dealing with feelings and the making of lasting object relationships. In addition, if the feelings stay invested and attached to a deceased parent or sibling, they are unavailable for growth and maturation and this will inevitably lead to varying degrees of arrest at that stage of development when the loss occurred. The absence of conscious awareness of such losses or their meaning is exactly what enables them silently and unimpeded to exert such influence. In this regard, Helene Deutsch's (12) 1937 paper, "Absence of Grief," remains a classic. She presents four such case examples in which the unmastered loss caused either inexplicable periods of recurrent sadness and depression or else the warding off of such feelings was accomplished only by the suppression of all feeling. Needless to remark, in part because of these difficulties with feelings, all four of her patients had serious impediments to forming meaningful adult object relationships.

The ideas presented here have been refined through two years of study with the Bereavement Research Group of the Cleveland Center for Research in Child Development headed by Mrs. Erna Furman.

BIBLIOGRAPHY

1. Furman, R., Death and the young child: some preliminary considerations, *Psychoanalytic Study of the Child*, 19 (1964), 321–333.
2. Furman, R., Death of a six-year-old's mother during his analysis, *Psychoanalytic Study of the Child*, 19 (1964), 377–397.
3. Wolfenstein, M., Death of a parent and death of a president: children's reactions to two kinds of loss, in *Children and the Death of a President*, edited by M. Wolfenstein and G. Kliman, Eds., Doubleday, New York: (1965), 62–79.
4. Wolfenstein, M., How is mourning possible?, *Psychoanalytic Study of the Child*, 21 (1966), 93–123.
5. Nagera, H., Children's reactions to the death of important objects: a developmental approach, *Psychoanalytic Study of the Child*, 25 (1970), 360–400.
6. Furman, R., Additional remarks on mourning and the young child, *Bulletin of the Philadelphia Association for Psychoanalysis*, 18 (1968), 51–64.
7. Furman, R., The child's reaction to death, in *Loss and Grief: Psychological Management in Medical Practice*, B. Schoenberg, A. Carr, D. Peretz, and A. Kutscher, Eds., Columbia University Press, New York, (1970), 70–86.
8. Spiegel, L., Affects in relation to self and object: a model for the derivation of desire, longing, pain, anxiety, humiliation and shame. *Psychoanalytic Study of the Child*, 21 (1966), 69–92.
9. Freud, S., *Mourning and Melancholia*, Standard Ed., 14 (1917), Hogarth Press, London, 1957.
10. Freud, S., *The Ego and the Id*, Standard Ed., 19 (1923), 3–66, Hogarth Press, London, 1961.
11. Freud, A., see footnote in Children's reactions to death of important objects: a developmental approach, *Psychoanalytic Study of the Child*, 25 (1970), 379.
12. Deutsch, H., Absence of grief, *Psychoanalytic Quart.*, 6 (1937), 12–22.

21. Some Effects of the Parent's Death on the Child's Personality Development

Erna Furman

SHORT- AND LONG-TERM EFFECTS OF A PARENT'S DEATH

When a loved person dies, the bereaved has a threefold task—to cope with the immediate impact of the circumstances, to mourn, and to resume and continue his emotional life in harmony with his level of maturity. None of these tasks is completed within a circumscribed period of time. Depending on internal and external factors, each task may present ongoing difficulties for the bereaved or it may be resolved in such a way as to impede functioning in later years. Within the personality, these psychic processes are interrelated and mutually influential, but there is merit also in recognizing the differences between them. Our clinical and theoretical understanding profited from examining them separately and in their interaction. Our understanding of these processes was gained through work with patients at the time of the parent's death or from treatment at a later period in their development.

We found that in some instances a child's difficulties stemmed primarily from his inability to cope with the impact of the circumstances of the parent's death. We include here the stresses connected with the form of death or those arising from major interference with the bodily and psychological need fulfillment following the death. In other cases the child's problem related especially to some aspect of the mourning process, for example failure to understand death, inability to tolerate sadness or anger, or pathological identifications. With a number of children the trouble lay predominantly in the establishment of new relationships and continuation of emotional development. In this phase the problem sometimes focused on conflicts with

Reprinted by permission of Yale University Press from *A Child's Parent Dies: Studies in Childhood Bereavement*, 1974.

the stepparent. Inevitably, difficulties in one area overlapped with and affected those in another area. It proved clinically important to trace the patient's conflicts to their specific causes, and it helped our theoretical understanding to distinguish difficulties with mourning from other problems related to the parent's death.

The immediate stressful impact of the parent's death has been discussed—fear of death, difficulty in appropriate differentiation from the dead, anxieties related to the way in which the death occurred, concern with bodily and psychological need fulfillment. Some developmental differences in experiencing these concerns were emphasized, as well as the fact that the bereaved person's capacity to master them depends on internal and external factors—personality makeup, nature of actual experiences, extent of support from surviving loved ones. The individual variations and interrelations of these factors are infinite in number. Intensive psychoanalytic observation and exploration enabled us to come close to the necessary understanding in individual cases. Even using this approach, at the time of bereavement or through later reconstruction, there were inevitable limitations.

By comparing our data from many cases we come to feel certain that the circumstances of the loved one's death and the life situation in which it places the bereaved constitute an important set of events. Their impact on the individual and his means of dealing with them are a mental task separate from mourning. We found that some persons began their mourning while they still coped with their reactions to the immediate situation. With others the mourning process was delayed until they had come to terms with these anxieties. There were some whose mourning was jeopardized altogether because they could not master the stressful circumstances. No instance was observed in which mourning could appropriately proceed and be completed unless a person had first dealt adequately with immediate concerns and anxieties. It sometimes appeared that a patient had difficulty in mourning; closer study revealed that the patient's difficulty lay primarily in coping with his anxieties about the circumstances surrounding the death, which his mind could not master and his environment failed to allay.

The stress of the circumstances is usually greater for the younger child. This is due to his limited ability to test reality and to master anxiety, as well as to his bodily and psychological dependence on the adult. In some cases, however, the circumstances are so upsetting that even latency-aged and older children cannot cope with them adequately. Unmastered conflicts and anxieties may result in behavior difficulties and symptoms at the time of the initial stress or at a later date when additional hardships have produced a cumulative effect on the personality. They may also affect a child "silently"; that is, he may adopt defense measures or characterological solutions which at first appear adaptive but which later impede growth and adjustment because they are too rigid or extensive. The unmastered stress of the circumstances surrounding the parent's death also interferes with the child's ability to mourn, which further jeopardizes his chances of healthy development.

Geraldine was almost eight years old at the time of her mother's death (see chapter 24, this volume). She had experienced years of her mother's hospitalizations, operations and bodily disintegration. In the absence of realistic explanations, she linked her mother's illness with the parents' violence and sexuality, which she had repeatedly witnessed. After the mother's death Geraldine lived for one and a half years in the homes of relative strangers who barely met her bodily needs and did not intend to keep her. She used a number of defenses in order to maintain herself in the face of these stresses. She denied and repressed what she had seen, repudiated all aspects of sexuality and aggression in herself and others, and functioned like a "good" schoolgirl who made diligent intellectual efforts. In spite of lapses this adaptation served her well for some years. It ingratiated her well enough with her wardens so that they continued to care for her and it staved off her conflicts around her earlier experiences. Her strong defenses, however, contributed to her inability to mourn, prevented her from forming appropriate new relationships later, and jeopardized her adolescent development. At a later time of additional stress, her defenses proved inadequate and she developed severe hysterical symptoms.

After mastering the stressful circumstances surrounding the death, the bereaved person's next task is to adapt psychologically to the loss of the loved one. Mourning, as defined earlier, is the best means of accomplishing this adaptation because it paves the way for a continued healthy mental life. Through mourning, a bereaved person frees himself for establishing new relationships and enriches his personality with selected new identifications. Failure in mourning may present an obstacle to the individual's future growth and adjustment. This is particularly important with children at all stages of development when their parent dies. The child's maturation is not complete and, at least before late adolescence, he must invest his love in a parent figure in order to progress. Therefore the child is especially handicapped in his mourning for a parent, since he needs a parent's help with this task.

Under favorable circumstances the surviving love objects can fill these gaps sufficiently to create a milieu in which a child can utilize his capacity for mourning and in which his efforts receive the necessary support.

For the purpose of the present discussion, the child's internal difficulties in mourning his parent are not separated from those that stem from external sources, such as the failure of his environment to extend sufficient help. In clinical work such a differentiation is important to understand the child's problems and to assist him in resolving them. In the following assessment of the effect on the child of an incomplete or pathological mourning, only the outcome of the combined internal and external factors will be considered.

At the stage of achieving object constancy and during the toddler period, the death of the parent, especially the mother, may deplete the infant's personality to the extent that the functions necessary for the mourning process may not be maintained. This not only prevents mourning but also seriously affects the child's functioning in some or all areas and manifests itself in immediately discernible pathology. Among some of our patients in this age group we observed loss of such recently acquired ego functions as walking and talking, failure of affective response, regression in object relationships, and impoverishment of the libidinal cathexis of the self-representation. Recovery of these aspects of the personality was a painfully slow and laborious effort. Even when educational and therapeutic help was available at once it had to extend over many years. Many studies by others show that such damage cannot be repaired fully at a later period in the person's life (Bowlby 1951; Gyomroi 1963).

In other toddlers, in older preschoolers and latency children, the death of the parent did not interfere with the child's functioning. The continued absence of the parent, however, led to the child's inadequate investment of new functions and activities in some instances. With many of our patients, even those at the toddler level, basic personality functioning was not affected by the death of the parent. Although they had reached different developmental stages at the time of their bereavement, the mental functions necessary for the mourning process were sufficiently developed and maintained. They encountered numerous difficulties, however, with different aspects of the mourning process so that they either could not complete it or did so in a pathological manner. Some of their symptoms and maladjustments resulted directly from their impeded mourning; others were caused by their inability to progress in their emotional development, an indirect outcome of the same difficulty.

Some could not master the initial steps in mourning, that is, understanding and accepting death and differentiating themselves from the dead parent. The children's difficulty in understanding and accepting death was intensified by inaccurate information conveyed by the adults. In time the children usually acquired some realistic knowledge through their own efforts at observation and exploration, but this sometimes brought them into conflict with the expectations and views of those on whom they depended. They then either rejected their own evidence and interrupted their quest for knowledge so that they never attained a coherent concept, or they guiltily maintained their ideas side by side with the adults' story. Death became linked to instinctual conflicts instead of being mastered intellectually and emotionally. Since these solutions were for the most part not arrived at consciously, the children's defensive struggles tended to lead to symptom formation.

Addie, aged four years, lived with her grandparents during her mother's terminal hospitalization. She was not told of her mother's death and was expected not to know about it. She later learned the sad reality from a peer who had visited the funeral home and who initiated Addie into the forbidden knowledge of the concrete aspects of death. At first Addie managed to ward off her anxious thoughts and feelings, but a year later she developed a hysterical stiffness of the neck. She also became very hyperactive. In her analysis the stiffness of the neck was found to be related to the stiffness of the dead body, and the hyperactivity was seen to ward off the motionlessness of death.

The need to differentiate themselves from the dead was a special developmental difficulty for the youngest children, who were still in the process of delineating and stabilizing their object and self-representations, especially in relation to the parent. The experience of death overtaking a beloved person sometimes constituted a great threat to themselves, endangered their feeling of personal safety and colored their later developmental concerns, for example castration anxiety at the phallic level.

Danny was only eleven months old when his father died of a viral infection. Danny himself was hospitalized at the time and survived an infection of the type that took his father's life. Danny learned about death and the circumstances of his father's death from his mother and older sibling. His ideas about his father were closely linked to his feelings about himself because he had not only barely escaped his father's fate but bore his name and resembled him physically. During his phallic phase Danny was terrified of illness both in himself and in others. He always expected illness to be followed by death. Sometimes he warded off his anxiety by scaring others, at other times he denied injury to himself.

Many children of all ages encountered difficulties with aspects of the mourning proper. Among the causes were inappropriate defenses against affects, conflicts over ambivalence, inability to detach love from the deceased parent, undue proportion of identification, or identifications which were too primitive or pathological. The resulting symptoms and behavior problems encompassed a wide range. On the surface they did not appear to be related to the parent's death. There were hysterical symptoms such as amnesia; phobias, fears, and bad dreams; disturbances of ego functions such as restriction of motility or hyperactivity; difficulties in relationships with adults and peers, in learning, in frustration tolerance and self-control; apathy, truancy, stealing, accident proneness, and self-injury. For the most part these problems did not arise at once but tended to follow a long period of relatively appropriate functioning, marked by controlled behavior, subdued affective response, and little reference to the parent's death. The adults in the child's environment tended to regard this quiescent period as a sign of good adjustment, and even those who were concerned or puzzled at the child's apparent lack of reaction often welcomed it and hesitated to interfere by bringing up the subject of the dead parent. It was therefore striking that with the children who were referred for help some time after the parent's death the family usually did not relate their presenting problems to the bereavement.

Most frequently the child's maladjustment became manifest when his mourning difficulty interfered in his progressive development. In some instances the child remained arrested at the level he had reached at the time of the parent's death, in others he could not cope with the conflicts of the next maturational phase. This led to a pathological exaggeration of phase-adequate conflicts or to regression in some areas. In a number of cases such problems arose around the adjustment to a new parent, which highlighted the developmental failure and made it impossible for the child to resume his place in a normally constituted family.

A different problem arose for those children who were consciously grappling with their mourning but whose struggles were prolonged, intensified, and distorted because no new parent figure of the same sex as the deceased was available to them at the appropriate time. The further structuralization of their personality depended on two parents being available. In some cases this real lack led to a prolonged hypercathexis of the deceased. These children utilized every resource to maintain their image of the dead parent—such concrete reminders as photographs and belongings; and stories told them about the parent, describing his appearance, qualities, interests, and incidents in his life. They also modeled their ideas on observations of other children's parents and on their own fantasies, wishes, conflicts, and anxieties.

For the prelatency children this hypercathexis was particularly important and contributed to their chances of maintaining emotional health. It exposed them, however, to constant frustrations, anger, pain, and disappointment, as in many daily situations they were faced with the contrast between inner and outer reality and had to compare their hardship to the good fortune of peers. At the same time their relationship with the surviving parent was burdened. The libidinal attachment was intensified and insufficiently limited or frustrated by reality. Aggressive feelings against the surviving parent were also complicated. The children tended to direct their anger at the dead parent against the living one so that the latter would receive more than double the amount of anger. Yet the children's intense dependency on the only living parent made it particularly difficult for them to tolerate any anger against this parent. These complications placed a special burden on the child and on the parent-child relationship. They sometimes impeded the child's ability to resolve phase-appropriate conflicts and left their mark on the development of his character. Our experience suggests that the danger is especially great for the prelatency child whose oedipal experiences are affected and consequently imperil the formation of the super ego. Some children in that age group could nevertheless be helped to mature adequately.

The child's ability to continue a healthy emotional life depends on his mastery of the previous tasks—coping with the stress of the circumstances surrounding the parent's death and mourning. It also depends on whether a new parent or parent figure is available at the appropriate time to provide, in Winnicott's words (1949), a "good enough" relationship.

When an adult is ready to reinvest his love he can actively seek a new person. The child cannot do that, particularly when he wants a new parent. The decision rests with the adults in his environment. The child under five years of age is quite helpless in this respect. Latency children can more easily procure for themselves helpful relationships with adults who fulfill a partial parental role. This differs from a defensive search for a parent substitute. Children in analysis, or those who were treated via the parent, usually assigned this role first to the therapist if he was the sex of the dead parent. Work with the patient showed to what extent healthy or defensive reasons predominated. It showed too whether the defenses helped or impeded the treatment process and the child's development at any given time.

Hank was four and a half years old when his father died suddenly. Hank coped with his mourning with the help of treatment-via-the-parent and progressed into latency. At six and a half years of age he left kindergarten but independently maintained contact with the male analyst who had worked with his mother and whom Hank had gotten to know well. Hank wrote him many letters and the analyst replied to them briefly, feeling that this contact was important and meaningful to the boy. Hank also became interested in woodwork, found a neighbor who shared his interest, and enrolled this neighbor as an advisor and older friend in regard to this hobby.

Jerry, Hank's older brother by one year, was close to six years at the time of the father's death. Jerry's more advanced personality structure and his set defensive patterns made it impossible for his mother to work with him at the time when she could still be helped to assist Hank. Jerry could not mourn, but repeatedly sought out father substitutes in order to ward off his longing and sadness. Invariably his contacts with these people proved disappointing and were interrupted by Jerry. For example, Jerry insisted on joining a father-son social group and enrolled a neighbor to accompany him. Jerry behaved very poorly in the group. It did not work out and he soon gave it up.

The adolescent is at a greater advantage. His need for a parent is less and he is more able to find new love objects. He is helped by his tendency toward object removal and by living more independently in the wider community with its opportunity for meeting a variety of people.

In some cases the main difficulty for the child arose from the unsuitability of a new parent and from the circumstances associated with such a change in the family's way of life.

Bobby's mother had died when he was two and a half years old. His grandparents had cared for him in their home following the mother's death and he had been close to them in spite of some difficulties. The father remarried after a brief courtship when Bobby was six years old. The family moved into a small apartment where Bobby shared the parental bedroom. The stepmother insisted on breaking off all contact with the grandparents and demanded Bobby's exclusive love. When he developed behavior problems she was appalled and alternately attacked Bobby and withdrew from him. Her mental condition deteriorated to the point where she was unable to care for Bobby.

Not all situations were so extreme, but several were serious enough to jeopardize the chances of a normal parent-child relationship, to cause new maladjustments in the children, and to reinforce their previous problems.

For some children the difficulty in continuing their emotional lives lay neither with their current environment nor with their pathological resolution of the tie to the dead parent. Rather, it stemmed from personality difficulties which had preceded the loss of the parent and had not interfered with the child's mourning but handicapped his maturation.

Ken, aged thirteen, had been in analysis for some time when his father died suddenly. Thanks in part to analytic work he had already accomplished in relation to other losses, Ken could cope well with the circumstances of the father's death and mourned for about eighteen months. Ken's bisexual conflicts had mainly caused the symptoms for which he had come to treatment. These conflicts were not significantly affected by the father's death and did not interfere with Ken's reaction to it, but they continued to affect his personality in the later phase of adolescence.

This does not imply that the death of a parent is ever a negligible event in the child's life. In some instances a child can be helped to cope with the tragedy of his loss and to mourn adequately. In others he may be so young that the parent was not yet a major love object for him and he was not affected by the stress of the immediate circumstances. In either case the child's life is from then on shadowed by the death of the parent. A parent who was well known and loved will forever be missed to some extent with each new developmental step, be it a new emotional phase or an important event, a period of personal distress or a time of special pleasure to be shared. A parent who was hardly known accompanies the child through life differently but remains as meaningful. What was my parent like and would he have liked me? Shall I be like him and would I have liked him? Am I glad that he died or am I angry that he is not with me? Above all the death of a parent faces the child with an early excess of helplessness at the hands of fate, a need to accept the utterly unacceptable at a time when his mental resources are not yet equipped for doing so. Some may be better able to cope with this tragedy than others; for all it becomes a lifelong burden.

Psychoanalytic studies of adults who lost a parent through death in childhood show various serious effects on the adult's mental health (Deutsch 1937; Jacobson 1965). Some of our colleagues had treated such adults but noted different pathological resolutions and interferences in later functioning. In our contacts with parents of child patients we repeatedly encountered interferences in parental functioning, which appeared to stem from the parent's experience of bereavement in childhood.

EFFECTS OF THE PARENT'S DEATH ON DEVELOPING EGO FUNCTIONS

In patients who experienced the death of a parent as babies or toddlers the stress appeared to affect basic aspects of their personality development. Our observations of them at the time of the parent's death, and analytic work with them at a later point in their development, showed that, in some, the impact resulted predominantly in instinctual fixation points. In others it caused deficiencies in the narcissistic investment of the self-representation. Sometimes it appeared to affect especially the ego's ability to deal with anxiety as, at each level, they dreaded being overwhelmed. Our interest focused on several patients whose difficulties centered especially on interferences with developing ego functions.

Lisa was seen at eighteen months. She was a well-developed toddler with markedly good early speech development and comprehension and with even more advanced large- and small-muscle control. She used her motility safely and carefully with much pleasure and self-assurance and with justified trust and special enjoyment by her parents. During succeeding months her father's illness worsened rapidly. It was a period of turmoil and upset resulting in the parents' emotional withdrawal. They did not explain to Lisa anything about the father's illness or the reasons for their preoccupation. When Lisa was two years old her father died suddenly but Lisa was not told for several days. Already before the father's death Lisa's speech development had lost its impetus, apparently in response to the diminished parental investment and to the barrier in verbal communication about the parental illness and upset. Lisa's immediate reaction to the father's disappearance was that she abruptly stopped asking for him and about him but at once resumed this when her mother informed her that dad had died and would not come back. The mother subsequently maintained excellent verbal communication with Lisa in many areas, but a partial barrier persisted. The mother could not mourn and she discouraged Lisa's expression of sad and angry feelings about and memories of the father. Although she showed unmistakable interest, Lisa was never told the cause and circumstances of her father's death. Lisa's speech development began to lag and its infantile features were the more striking the older she got. By age five she spoke in an unclear babyish manner, often lisping and becoming almost inaudible. She evidently did not enjoy talking and tended to express herself in action rather than words. During her analysis her speech improved when its infantilisms and restriction could be linked to Lisa's fear of expressing her feelings, particularly anger, and to her need to hide her thoughts and fantasies, particularly in relation to her father.

With the father's death Lisa lost not only his admiration of her motor skills but her mother too changed her attitude to Lisa's motility. She became much more fearful for Lisa's safety and restrictive of her exploits, especially as Lisa age-appropriately ventured into outdoor play. Some of Lisa's activities in play suggested that she linked bodily harm to her vague knowledge of her father's illness. Increasingly, Lisa's motility became distorted. She remained very active bodily but derived little pleasure from it and became clumsy and often unaware of what her body was doing. In her analysis this difficulty too was related to inhibition of aggression and to aggression turned against the self. Aspects that appeared to be related to Lisa's ideas about her father's death could not be explored before the end of her analysis.

Some of Lisa's lack of motivation and difficulty in learning stemmed from her disinterest in perceiving what went on around her and from her not gaining gratification in making observations of her own. She had been an intensely aware toddler, ready to explore everything and to ask questions about it. It appeared that she had also observed more of her father's illness and death than she could understand or get answers to. Her mother welcomed Lisa's observations in some areas but not in others. Before the onset of the phallic-oedipal phase, Lisa's cathexis of perception appeared only somewhat diminished. Following her conflicts of that phase, her difficulty in this area increased greatly, although the mother had been able to answer Lisa's sexual questions. The function of perception now suffered secondary interference by defenses. The analyst supported Lisa's capacity to observe and explore her outer and inner reality and helped her to gain a partial analytic understanding of her defenses against conflicts about her father's death. This helped her to make the developmental step into latency and to regain her interest in learning sufficiently for adequate academic progress.

It seemed to us that the development of Lisa's functions of perception, motility, and speech had suffered interference through the father's illness and death as well as through their aftermath. Lisa lost her father's intense positive investment in these functions. The mother's earlier equally great pleasure and encouragement underwent a considerable change. In some respects she continued to support Lisa's skills, in others she discouraged and restricted them as a result of her own unresolved concerns about the father's death and its repercussions on her relationship with her daughter.

Danny's functions of perception, motility, and speech also regressed under the stress of the circumstances associated with the father's death. During his hospitalization he lost the father's and mother's libidinal investment and through the experience of medical procedures he apparently suffered damage to the narcissistic investment of his body image and early self-representation. These libidinal depletions were followed by a life in which his mother's affective attitude changed to some extent. Although her love for and devotion to Danny were undiminished, her preoccupation with practical demands caused a partial withdrawal. Her own mourning, with its restrained sadness and lack of joy, affected her emotional expression. Her relative difficulty in expressing and accepting anger influenced her interaction with Danny, as well as her tendency to take over her children's self-protective functions. The subject of the father's death however did not represent a direct interference. The mother could be helped to discuss the father's illness and death with her older children quite soon. She gauged sensitively Danny's ability to understand and integrate these facts, assisted him with his concerns and answered his questions. Perception, speech, and motility were always encouraged by her. No aspect of these functions was forbidden or linked to the father's death. In spite of these helpful factors, recovery of development was very slow with each of the affected ego functions. They showed some distortions and were subject to secondary interference by defenses.

Lucy was ten weeks old when her mother died suddenly. In contrast to Lisa and Danny, whose development could be observed through treatment-via-the-parent from the time of the parent's death and whose reactions could be studied later in analytic treatment during the phallic-oedipal phase, Lucy began her analysis in her eleventh year. The therapist had no previous knowledge of her development, and the family situation made it particularly difficult to obtain a consistent history. Lucy had attained a structured personality and was capable of establishing relationships in spite of many difficulties. Her entire personality, however, as well as her analytic work, was affected by her impaired synthetic function. Although many of Lucy's experiences throughout her childhood contributed to this problem, the analysis showed that the earliest damage to the developing integrative function was sustained during the first year of life. It affected the cohesion and stability of her body image and basic self-representation.

It appeared that the death of the mother when Lucy was ten weeks old constituted serious interference and ushered in a period of changes during the next few months which augmented the harmful effects, including damage to the developing synthetic function. The family's later handling of the topic of the mother and her death further interfered with the development and use of Lucy's capacity for integration. Subsequent secondary interference by the defenses of denial, isolation, and repression played an important part.

The maturation of certain ego functions proceeds autonomously. However, the apparatus must be activated by instinctual energy and only gradually comes under the control of the ego (Hartmann 1950). The effect of a positive object relationship on these processes was discussed by A. Freud (1952). A number of authors studied the influence of the parent-child relationship on ego functions and compared the relative importance of this factor for the development of specific functions. A. Freud and Burlingham (1944) found that toddlers raised in a group setting lagged in speech but excelled in motility compared with toddlers raised in families. Provence and Lipton (1962) also found that, in the institution children they studied, the development of motor activity was least affected by the absence of a mother-child relationship. They noted, however, that the motility of these children gained in grace, purposefulness, and pleasure after a period of foster home placement. The authors suggest that the close, consistent relationship with a parent figure helps to bring motility more under ego control. Pine and Furer (1963) studied the effects of varying maternal attitudes on some of the toddlers' developing ego functions. In regard to their observations of motility they stated (340), "In the normal toddlers, for example, the children not only worsen but also improve in certain kinds of functioning in the mother's absence, and also change in the quality of their functioning. In any of these cases there is a suggestion that the child's functioning is not yet autonomous but draws in some way upon the mother for its enhancement or impairment."

We compared our data from the study of bereaved youngsters with material gained in our clinical work with other young children (R. A. Furman and A. Katan 1969). Our experience suggests the following tentative formulation: each developing ego function requires a certain amount of instinctual investment, both from the child and from his main love object, in order to follow its maturational course and to establish itself as an autonomous function integrated in the service of the ego. A "good enough" emotional milieu is essential to these aspects of ego development. There is a critical period, from the beginning of the development of a function until it achieves autonomy and comes under ego control. During this period, withdrawal, imbalances, and changes in the instinctual investment may lead to interferences with the function. Although not altogether satisfied with the term, we called this a "primary emotional interference with an ego function." This enabled us to differentiate it from a primary organic interference due to physical defects in the apparatus, and from a secondary interference caused by defensive measures. A primary emotional interference can have a variety of outcomes. It may lead to total arrest of the development of the function, to regression, to impairment or distortion. When arrest occurs, the function does not progress beyond the achieved level, as happened with Lisa's speech. Regression results in loss of the function, as was observed in Danny's speech and motility. This phenomenon was described by A. Freud (1965) as ego regression under stress. We noted impaired or distorted development in Danny's motility and Lucy's synthetic function.

We discussed the possible relationship between primary emotional interference in a developing ego function and later forms of ego regression. A. Freud distinguishes several types of functional regression (1965). In developmental regression, due to fatigue or illness and regression under stress, it is always the last-acquired function which is first lost. "In contrast to drive regression, the retrograde moves on the ego scale do not lead back to previously established positions, since no fixation points exist" (104). As far as we know, Blos alone (1967) speaks of developmental ego regression harking back to specific points in early life. In his discussion of adolescent processes he writes, "Ego regression connotes the re-experiencing of abandoned or partly abandoned ego states which had been either citadels of safety and security, or which once had constituted special ways of coping with stress"; and, "Ego regression is, for example, to be found in the re-experiencing of traumatic states of which no childhood was ever wanting" (173).

Our case material showed that functions which had suffered a primary emotional interference were frequently subject to later interferences. This appeared to be in part due to the functions' delay in coming under ego control, in part due to secondary defensive interference. Could it be that a function which suffered primary emotional interference becomes the matrix in which later secondary interference take place? Does this function remain more vulnerable to defensive interference when there is an early interference of this nature and full ego control is not achieved or is labile? Our clinical findings are insufficient to provide answers to these questions.

We agreed on a hypothesis yet to be tested: While instinctual fixation points are caused by excessive amounts of energy remaining at earlier levels of development, ego functions may have "weak points" in their early development owing to a deficiency in instinctual investment. These weak points may cause delays or distortions of ego function development and may in some instances contribute to later secondary defensive interference with ego functions.

PARENTAL BEREAVEMENT RELATED TO EARLIER
AND LATER LOSSES

In initial discussions of bereavement we noticed how frequently an object loss in adulthood revived earlier, particularly infantile, losses and intensified the mourning. Many examples were given in which adult mourning was facilitated or handicapped by the manner in which object losses and developmental losses had been dealt with in childhood. In our child patients we also noted some instances where the child's reaction to his bereavement was affected by earlier experiences of loss. In others the bereavement in turn influenced the child's handling of subsequent losses. It seemed logical that such connections should exist, but their exact nature and extent were unclear. Does each bereavement revive all previous losses by association, so that mourning becomes a cumulative task, intensified with each additional loss? Are there only certain losses or forms of dealing with them that affect the later attitudes to bereavement? Does an appropriate mourning for a parent in childhood facilitate an individual's ability to cope with some or all later losses? In reviewing case material we focused on this topic and on finding some answers to our queries.

Does a Bereavement Revive All Previous Losses and Intensify the Current Mourning?

The following examples illustrate the complex nature of the clinical data.

Ken was thirteen years old when his father died suddenly. During the preceding three years Ken had experienced the deaths of a grandmother, uncle, and grandfather. Each of these deaths occurred after a prolonged illness which required his mother's involvement and resulted in her partial withdrawal from Ken. The relatives' deaths were handled realistically and with feelings by the parents as well as by Ken. His reaction was, however, affected by his difficulty in coping with the mother's partial withdrawal. Since the death of the father had been very sudden it was not preceded by a maternal withdrawal. This death did not revive Ken's mourning for his relatives nor his memories of earlier losses. In his mourning for his father Ken utilized those strengths which his family had helped him develop in connection with the previous deaths. He understood and accepted death in its concrete form. He could tolerate strong feelings of sadness. He could count on his mother's understanding of the need to mourn and on her support of his individual manner of mourning. Ken also drew on many other strengths derived from his advanced developmental position and from his particular personality makeup; for example, his aggression was sufficiently fused, his memory was intact.

Seth's mother died when he was three years old. She had been ill for a long time, increasingly unable to care for him. He had spent much of his time with an elderly aunt who lived with the family. The care she provided for him was also limited by her poor health. Internal and external factors combined to foil Seth's mourning. Following his mother's death he lived with his grandparents. He liked them and his widespread restrictions of affect and ego functioning enabled him to make a superficially adequate adaptation. During Seth's sixth year the father remarried and Seth joined the new family. In contrast to the defenses used after the mother's death, Seth reacted to the separation from the grandmother with instinctual and ego regression as well as symptom formation. The analysis showed that the loss of the grandmother reactivated the anal-sadistic conflicts which prevailed at the time of the mother's death and that the mother's death cast its shadow on the conflicts of the later phase: in the context of his recent phallic-oedipal relationships with father and stepmother, Seth reinterpreted his mother's death in phallic-sadistic terms and linked it to his ideas of sexual intercourse.

During this period Seth experienced another loss. His aunt, who had helped care for him during his mother's lifetime, died. He had continued to maintain his relationship with her through visits but had grown less close to her. Seth had no difficulty in understanding and accepting her death and in reacting to it appropriately. The aunt's death did not revive his memories of his mother's death, nor the separation from the grandmother, nor his experience of the parent's withdrawal in connection with their adult relationship.

These and similar clinical experiences suggested that a current object loss through death revives earlier losses in a selective manner. It is impossible to know all the losses a person has experienced if one thinks of losses in the wider sense, including partial and developmental ones. The revival of a specific past loss may, however, represent the telescoped experience of several losses.

We agreed that a current object loss and mourning does not necessarily revive previous experiences of loss. The circumstances and nature of the current loss and the framework of the individual's personality at the time appear to determine whether, which, and how many earlier losses are revived and how much they contribute to intensifying the present reaction.

Are There Certain Earlier Losses or Certain Earlier Forms of Handling Them That Adversely Affect the Individual's Capacity to Mourn a Later Object Loss?

Geraldine was almost eight years old when her mother died after years of illness and several hospitalizations (see chapter 24). She entered treatment in her twelfth year after she had developed a hysterical amnesia which extended back to just before her mother's death. Although Geraldine had a fully structured personality, it was noted during her analysis that she sometimes dealt with the conflictual feelings about her mother's death with primitive mechanisms of introjection and of merging. In some instances she employed the same mechanisms when her current love objects became ill and required hospitalization. Geraldine's use of these early forms of handling loss subsided when, through reconstruction, they could be traced to repeated short-term separations from her mother during her first two years of life. These early experiences with loss determined some, though not all, of her current reactions. Subsequent stressful factors appeared also to play an important part in reactivating these mechanisms.

From birth Sally had lived with a foster mother until, at twenty-two months of age, she was adopted into her present family. Sally was just over four years old when her adoptive father died suddenly. Sally could accept the father's death intellectually and realistically and, in contrast to her mother and siblings, could experience and contain her strong feelings about it. She talked about him and remembered him appropriately both in the family and with outsiders. In time the mother recognized Sally's mourning and began to share and support it. An important aspect of the work centered on helping the mother to understand Sally's feelings about the loss of her foster mother. Since her adoption Sally had played games with cosmetics and made requests for certain foods which led to some friction between mother and child. When the mother began to encourage her to express feelings in words, she learned of Sally's continued longing for the foster mother. It was now understood that Sally's special games and food requests represented memories of affectionate interactions with the foster mother.

Sally's appropriate reaction to her father's death appeared to stem in part from the personality strengths she had earlier developed in her relationship with her foster mother. Among these strengths were ability to tolerate feelings, inner and outer reality testing, and adequate drive fusion. Without help from her love objects, however, she could not come to terms with the loss of the foster mother. This resulted in some behavior difficulties and some interferences in her relationship with her adoptive mother. One does not know whether, without help, Sally's mourning for her father could have been completed. Her manner of mourning her father was, however, age-appropriate and did not repeat her earlier ways of coping with the loss of the foster mother.

In reviewing these and other clinical data it appeared to us that there are no specific previous losses or forms of handling them which directly impede the individual's capacity to mourn a later object loss. The effect of the experiences of earlier losses lies in the manner in which they contribute to the shaping of the total personality. The circumstances of the later object loss and the framework of the personality at that time are deciding factors in the individual's reaction. They determine which strengths can be utilized or which weaknesses are exposed.

Does the Appropriate Mourning of a Love Object Increase the Ability to Mourn Another Loss at a Later Time?

Billy's mother died in his sixth year. He was in analysis at the time and mourned her loss appropriately. In his prepuberty a young relative of Billy's died from an illness similar to the mother's. The relative's death reminded Billy of his mother's death. He mourned the relative appropriately.

Jim was seven years old at the time of his mother's sudden death. In his later treatment he worked on his bereavement for years, gradually allowing himself to experience the full extent of his feelings. During this period the death of an elderly relative affected him strongly. This loss appeared to revive the loss of the mother. His feelings intensified and extended from one death to the other. Some years later, at the time of finishing his analysis and coping with the impending separation from the analyst, Jim suffered another loss. A close friend died. Although this death revived memories of his mourning for his mother and relative, the losses did not become confused. There was no intensification of feelings and Jim dealt with the death of his friend appropriately.

These examples suggested that a completed mourning has a beneficial effect on the person's ability to mourn a subsequent death. It seemed inaccurate, however, to view the earlier and later loss reaction as directly connected. The death of a love object other than the parent cannot be compared to the death of a parent. Our patients' later experiences of deaths fortunately never concerned the only surviving parent. Even if that had been the case, the death of the second parent would place the child in a very different psychological situation. Moreover, the actual circumstances surrounding a death differ in each instance, as does the personality development and equilibrium of the bereaved.

In the cases studied we found many indications of indirect, rather than direct, favorable effects of a completed mourning on the reaction to later loses. We noticed that in the process of assisting a child in his mourning he was sometimes helped to mature in some areas. Among these were the ability to tolerate and verbalize affects, improvement in reality testing, fusion of ambivalence in relationships. With such gains a child stood a better chance of handling a number of later stressful experiences, including those of object loss.

All experiences, positive and negative, leave their mark on the personality and contribute to its individual makeup. At a time of severe stress, such as the death of a parent, developmental and individual strengths are helpful, and weaknesses tend to be exposed. If a child has developed adequately and learned to master stresses age-appropriately, he is better able to deal with a bereavement. If he has not been exposed to age-appropriate stresses or is burdened by unmastered ones, including earlier object losses, he tends to experience difficulty. The experience and handling of losses has a general effect on the personality rather than a specific effect on the ability to mourn. The extent to which earlier losses affect the reaction to later object losses in a specific manner depends mainly on the nature and circumstances of the later bereavement and on the framework of the bereaved individual's personality at the time. Appropriate mourning for a parent does not specifically strengthen a child's personality. At best it enables him to cope with the future without carrying a burden greater than it need be.

BIBLIOGRAPHY

Blos, P. (1967). The second individuation process of adolescence. *Psychoanal. Study Child* 22:162–87.

Bowlby, J. (1951). *Maternal Care and Mental Health*. Geneva: World Health Organization Monograph.

Deutsch, H. (1937). Absence of grief. *Psychoanal. Q.* 6:12–22.

Freud, A. (1952). The mutual influences in the development of the ego and the id. *Psychoanal. Study Child* 7:42–50.

———— (1965). *Normality and Pathology in Childhood*. New York: International Universities Press.

Freud, A. & Burlingham, D. (1944). *Infants Without Families*. New York: International Universities Press.

Furman, R. & Katan, A. (1969). (eds.) *The Therapeutic Nursery School.* New York: International Universities Press.

Gyomroi, E. L. (1963). The analysis of a young concentration camp victim. *Psychoanal. Study Child* 18:484–510.

Hartmann, H. (1950). Comments on the psychoanalytic theory of the ego. *Psychoanal. Study Child* 5:74–96.

Jacobson, E. (1965). The return of the lost parent. In M. Schur (ed.), *Drives, Affects, Behavior,* vol. 2. New York: International Universities Press.

Pine, F. & Furer, E. (1963). Studies of the Separation-Individuation phase: A methodological overview. *Psychoanal. Study Child* 18:325–43.

Provence, S. & Lipton, R. C. (1962). *Infants in Institutions: A Comparison of Their Development During the First Year of Life with Family-Reared Infants.* New York: International Universities Press.

Winnicott, D. (1949). *The Ordinary Devoted Mother and Her Baby.* London: Brock.

22. On the Concept of Mourning in Childhood: Reactions of a Two-and-One-Half-Year-Old Girl to the Death of Her Father

Christina Sekaer and Sheri Katz

Sue was twenty-eight months old when her father's death confronted her with a loss that her personality development and cognitive skills scarcely allowed her to comprehend. Sue's efforts to deal with her loss will be the focus of this paper and will be discussed with regard to the long-debated issue of whether or not children are capable of mourning (R. Furman 1964a, 1964b; Wolfenstein 1966; Nagera 1970; E. Furman 1974; Bowlby 1980). Sekaer (1986) suggested the term "childhood mourning" for the process by which children may work through a loss and proceed with normal development. The notion of childhood mourning emphasizes the differences from adult mourning, while at the same time stressing that decathexis, identification, reality testing, cognitive understanding of death, and other aspects of adult mourning may occur, but in a manner specific to children. Sue's reactions illustrate some of these similarities to and differences from adult mourning.

SELECTED LITERATURE REVIEW

For adults, Freud (1917) described the work of mourning as dealing with a conflict between the wish to maintain a libidinal tie to the internal representation of the lost object versus the demands of recognizing the reality of the loss. Memories of the lost one are hypercathected and then gradually decathected as the reality of the loss is accepted.

Arguing that children *cannot* mourn, Deutsch (1937) said that a young

Reprinted by permission of Yale University Press from *The Psychoanalytic Study of the Child*, vol. 42, 1986.

child's ego lacked the strength and development to tolerate intense pain, and that a child was unable to carry out the work of mourning. Nagera (1970) described the child's need for the parent to aid in his development as too strong to allow decathexis. Wolfenstein (1965, 1966, 1969) believed that decathexis of the internalized parental images as a normal part of adolescence must occur before a person can fully decathect a parent lost to death.

In contrast, Anna Freud (1960) argued that by the age of two or three a child who has achieved object constancy should be able to comprehend "the external fact" of the loss as well as to effect "the corresponding inner changes." For a child of two or older, she said, "the nearer to object constancy, the longer the duration of grief reactions with corresponding approximation to the adult internal process of mourning" (59). Bowlby (1960) stressed the similarity of adult and child reactions to loss, noting that even in the first year of life an infant may experience the "rupture of a key relationship and the consequent intense pain of yearning" (35). Bowlby (1980) discussed the development of the child's cognitive ability to maintain a representation of mother even in her absence, stressing object permanence rather than (libidinal) object constancy.

Robert Furman (1964a, 1964b) wrote that a child of three or four who has attained a postambivalent phallic phase of object relationships should be capable of "the painful internal decathexis of the lost object that is the essence of mourning" (322). Erna Furman (1974) said that children from the age of two years on could attain a sufficient understanding of death and "could apply this concept to the loss of a loved person when realistic and continuous help in understanding facts and feelings was available from surviving love objects" (125).

Lopez and Kliman (1979) describe Diane, bereaved at nineteen months, who, with the aid of analysis begun at age four, "experienced a process that did not in principle differ from what Freud (1917) called the 'work of mourning' " (265). In Diane's analysis fantasies, ideas, and affects stimulated by mother's death were revived and submitted to reality's verdict. Rather than a full decathexis followed by a hiatus before a new attachment was made, libido was withdrawn gradually and shifted to her stepmother, a process facilitated by the analyst.

When considering the prolonged and painful process of remembering and reality testing described by Freud (1917), one must keep in mind whose reality one is referring to. While it seems obvious that whatever mourning or adaptive processes children can carry out must occur within their own experience of the world, this realization is often overlooked. For example, Anna Freud (1960) refers to "the external fact," Erna Furman (1974) to "the concept of death," "the facts," "reality," "understanding," etc., and yet the meaning of these terms as perceived by the child is not made explicit. Thus Erna Furman (1974) discusses Sally, age four, "who clearly understood and accepted the meaning of death"; later in therapy, although "previously realistic about death, she now revealed a confusion . . . asking if [the dead] father was now too big for his clothes" (138). Clearly Sally had not "understood" on adult terms.

Piaget (1927) described a sequence of distinctions made by children about life: the term "life" is first applied to all activity or motion, then to self-initiated motion, then only to animals and plants. But things that cannot be directly experienced, such as the sun, moon, clouds, and wind, are still credited with life often until well into latency. Bemporad (1978) notes, "The child's concepts are in fact only preconcepts; they are sometimes too general and sometimes too specific . . . reasoning [sometimes] . . . is successful, but only when it does not go far beyond mere memory for past events" (82). A child's restating of adult teaching may not indicate understanding; Erna Furman (1974) reports Susy, a three-year-old, stating, "mommy is dead, and when you're dead you can't ever come back. That's right, daddy, isn't it?" (51). But how can she "know" that this is final if she is too young yet to conceptualize this fact? A child comprehends permanent loss without higher cognitive functioning to structure events in a context of time, space, and causality, and within a reality which is distorted by wishful fantasy and prelogical animistic thinking. His "mourning," if it occurs, must be done without comprehension of the implications of loss beyond his developmental level.

To compare the inner work following a loss requires consideration of what the concepts of decathexis and identification mean at different ages. Regarding decathexis, writers are generally agreed that when a child does *not* react with pain, it is due either to defenses against such painful work for pathological reasons or to defenses based on an inability to do the work because of age. But when painful reactions *do* occur, not all agree that decathexis is going on.

Wolfenstein (1966) criticizes the use of painful memories as evidence of decathexis, noting that the six-year-old boy who Robert Furman said "mourned" in fact "painfully missed his mother in many circumstances where formerly she was with him. . . . [But we] can miss and long for someone we still hope to see again'' (95). She felt children acknowledge, on the surface, the fact of the death, while on another level they expect the parent to return. Wolfenstein (1966) also described a ten-year-old boy who she said did not mourn but rather transferred his tie from his dead mother to his grandmother without a ''protracted sadness or withdrawal into painful preoccupation with memories of the lost object'' and without a hiatus before a new attachment was formed (121).

Very young children who are still internalizing parental functions that have not yet become autonomous may lose functions such as speech, walking, and perception (Anna Freud 1939–45; Erna Furman 1974). Decathexis, if one is to call it that, of a primary object may entail loss of part of himself. As Nagera (1970) states, ''Complete withdrawal of cathexis from the lost object will leave the child in a 'developmental vacuum' unless a suitable substitute object is readily found. . . . [Death] cannot lead to the type of decathexis that will be observed in the case of the adult'' (380).

As with ''decathexis,'' the term ''identification'' differs in meaning according to the age of the child. Jacobson (1954) describes the development from early primitive identifications to ''true ego identifications'' (43). She notes that primitive identifications ''disregard the realistic differences between the self and the object'' (46), whereas later identifications alter the child's ego realistically in selective ways. Diane, as described by Lopez and Kliman (1979), reacted to her mother's suicide by developing ''global identifications''; for example, she would fall and hurt herself in apparent copying of mother's suicidal leap. With an older child one would not expect such primitive identifications.

Identifications used by children in reaction to death may interfere with growth in that a child's normal development involves identifying with and differentiating himself from his parents. McDevitt (1980) describes identifications used in the resolution of the rapprochement crisis as important for building psychic structure. After the conclusion of rapprochement a bereaved child might be much less vulnerable to regression and loss of structure at least in part due to identifications formed by this age. Winnie, reported by Barnes (1964), might be such a case. Having lost her mother at 2½ years, Winnie was able to go through a ''mourning'' process at age three when assisted by her grandmother. She apparently did not become severely symptomatic after this (though a follow-up is not given).

Splitting of the ego is described as another defensive or pathological process that may occur when mourning is not completed. Wolfenstein (1966) considers it to be common in bereaved children. Freud (1927) describes such a split in the ego of an adult who maintained that his father (dead since he was two years old) was still alive and also knew that his father was dead. Nagera (1970) notes that secretly held fantasies of the continued existence of the dead parent are very common in bereaved latency-aged children who also are fully aware of the facts of the death. Splits in the ego prevent decathexis, leave the ego impoverished by the need to maintain such a split, and thus are considered pathological.

Unlike an adult, a bereaved child must deal not only with the immediate loss, but also with the impact of the loss at subsequent stages of his development. It may not be possible to separate reactions to a death from difficulties due to the "developmental vacuum" of a missing parent (Nagera 1970).

This is not to say that children cannot mourn. For each stage of development one may postulate an optimum degree to which mourning can be accomplished. If this is achieved, one may say that a normal childhood mourning is in progress; if this is *not* achieved, a pathological process may be occurring.

Childhood mourning delineates a process by which children may respond to bereavement and proceed with a relatively normal development. Based on a synthesis of the literature, Sekaer (1986) views this process not as a deficient version of adult mourning, but rather as one unique to the child's capacities. Thus a child needs adult help to understand death and still cannot do so beyond his own developmental level. A child also needs an adult, he cannot make use of a hiatus in attachment, by withdrawing into himself, in order to work through the loss. Identifications with a dead parent may interfere with identifications occurring as a normal part of a child's development. Full decathexis of the dead may not be possible or necessarily the best goal if a substitute attachment is not available.

In a further discussion of creative processes and transitional phenomena in bereaved children, Sekaer (1986) suggested the term "imaginary parent" to refer to fantasies of the dead parent as still alive; such imaginary parents may be gradually decathected as the child's need for the parent diminishes. Imaginary parents are an example, along with "mourning at a distance" through pets, toys, or fictional characters, of the bereaved child's heightened use of creative channels. Imaginary parents may serve a developmental purpose not unlike a transitional object or an imaginary companion; the fantasied person would "fade away" as no longer needed.

CASE REPORT

We shall discuss a 2½-year-old bereaved child whose reactions appear non-pathological and yet clearly limited by her level of development. Sue S., who had been attending full-time daycare from the age of three months, experienced the death of her father at twenty-eight months. The supportive structure of her experience at the daycare center and her therapeutic relationship with a teacher appeared to compensate for some of her mother's unavailability due to the loss. Thus the opportunity developed to observe the reactions of a 2½-year-old girl to the death of her father under circumstances which could facilitate rather than hinder their expression.

Developmental Data

Until her father's death Sue's development had proceeded in spite of recurrent tensions in the home. During Sue's early life her mother, while being generally warm and supportive, was occasionally unavailable due to personal preoccupations and physical health issues. Sue's father was also inconsistently available. Nevertheless he was strongly invested in her from the start, proud of her achievements, especially language, and pleased with her femininity. Sue lived with mother, father, and an older sister.

Sue's early development appeared normal in social, cognitive, motor, and emotional areas. At four months she sobered to strangers, at eight months she showed separation anxiety and formed specific attachments to her mother and daycare teacher. A normal recurrence of separation anxiety was noted at seventeen months at a time when tensions arose between her parents; for a while Sue avoided her mother when she came for her and turned to strangers. Although this appeared to resolve, at twenty-four months Sue again showed some signs of difficulty. Tension was again high at home, and Sue often shared her father's bed as her parents stayed apart. For a few weeks Sue showed isolation of affect, narrating anxiety-filled events without feeling; she developed a shallow seductive manner and sought out strangers while being provocative with her teachers. Sue was moved with her age group to the third year classroom, and individual play sessions with one of her new teachers were begun to assist Sue in developing a closer relationship with her.[1] These sessions had been in progress and a closer tie with this special teacher had begun to form when, at twenty-eight months, Sue's father became suddenly ill with a cardiovascular disorder. After a couple of days he was taken to the hospital in a police car. There, following a few days' illness with very poor prognosis, he died. Sue did not visit in the hospital, but did attend the open casket funeral.

Reactions to the Death

After Mr. S.'s death Sue's individual sessions with the special teacher were continued. These sessions did not constitute an analytic experience but rather an enriched extension of her daycare experience. Attempts to arrange for a more intensive analytic therapy were not made because of the lack of more severe or chronic symptom formation. The teacher's role was one of offering nurturance, verbalizing feelings, clarifying cognitive distortions, and encouraging Sue to express thoughts and feelings. Their relationship intensified after the death and became a focus for Sue's concerns about death. Sue used the sessions for fantasy play and expression of feelings often focused on her father. In the classroom she remained invested in the activities and play of the group; when issues about her father arose, she limited herself to more realistic comments and questions. Sue's teacher had a long-standing interest in childhood bereavement (Katz 1976). Such understanding is helpful to perceive the needs and to tolerate the stress of helping a bereaved child. Assisting a child with concerns and feelings about death can evoke deep feelings about an adult's own prior experiences of loss. For one student teacher, Sue's loss evoked intense memories of her own father's death when she was five, and led to her starting therapy. More frequently there is denial and inability to observe and sustain the painful responses of the young child (McDonald 1964).

Prior to the death, Sue's mother had made use of the daycare and her own weekly sessions with a staff social worker to plan for and then return to school and to discuss difficulties in her relationship with her husband. After the death, Mrs. S. did not hide her sad feelings from Sue, and they talked of the death. Mrs. S. tended not to be tolerant of regressive behavior and instead encouraged Sue's independence. Though empathic with Sue in general, her mother seemed not as available as the teacher to Sue regarding her father's death; for example, several months after the death Mrs. S. expressed surprise that Sue was still upset about it. As is true of bereaved parents in general, Mrs. S.'s struggle to cope with her own grief left her less able to be of help to Sue.

Sue was able to speak about her father's illness and death when they occurred and thereafter. In her sessions and in the class Sue began to show a variety of symptoms. She cried often. She became irritable, aggressive with peers, and clingy with adults. A sleep disturbance developed. Separation anxiety was renewed. These reactions diminished in intensity in the first months after the death. Following these initial reactions Sue continued to show preoccupation and concern with death, illness, and separation, while in other ways she resumed what appeared to be her normal development; she remained tied to her mother while social and cognitive development continued. As a very verbal child Sue received support, understanding, and clarification from her teachers and, to some extent, at home.

But what processes were going on as Sue continued with her life? How could her two- to three-year-old mentality deal with the fact of loss? The next part of the paper will deal with a closer examination of some of Sue's reactions between twenty-eight and thirty-six months as she struggled to comprehend and integrate events.

Cognition

Sue learned and remembered many facts about her father's death. Yet reality for Sue was subject to distortion according to her wishes, as is typical of primary process thinking. Thus the fact of death (if only as a label for her father's state) remained present in her mind along with its denial. Sue had known that her father was in the hospital and said that he went there to get better. After his death she often announced to familiar and unfamiliar people, "My daddy died." Once when her peers responded to this announcement by echoing in turn, "My daddy died," Sue angrily made the distinction: "My daddy's dead, not yours!" Although she knew this fact, she occasionally asserted the opposite without being disturbed by the contradiction, announced, "He at work" or "He coming to get me."

Sue's words reflected the irreversible nature of death as she said, "He's sleeping there," pointing to the sky, "He can't get out of the box" or on another occasion, "He can't come back." However, such comments were sometimes reversed as:

SUE: My daddy, he lay down on my mommy's bed and he sleeping on mommy's bed.
TEACHER: Does he sleep on mommy's bed now?
SUE: No, because he went up in the sky and that's why he died.

TEACHER: What does he do in the sky?

SUE: He dying.

TEACHER: Can he visit you?

SUE (pouting): Not anymore 'cause he died. He died up in the sky. Because he died in the sky. I miss my daddy. I know he comes to my house on Sunday.[2]

Her comment about missing daddy is followed by reassertion that he is alive and will visit. Typical of prelogical thought, she feels no need to integrate her wish with her contradictory knowledge of reality.

In a less affect-laden context Sue seemed to demonstrate more stable awareness of past-present-future, animate-inanimate, and of the irreversibility of death. A boy noticed a dead fish in the tank at the Center, asked why it was dead, and then said it was sick. Sue came in, asked, "The fish is dead? Let me see." She noticed its large open eyes. Her teacher clarified that it could not see anymore now that it was dead. Sue answered, "He can't see. He's dead. Like he dead. Like my daddy dead." They talked about things that the dead fish couldn't do (eat or swim or play with the other fish). Sue said, "He can't come back. Good-bye fish." As the teacher began to wrap it in a paper towel, Sue gently took over, wrapped the fish and put it in the garbage, saying, "There it goes. Away." When the teacher said this fish couldn't swim around anymore with the other fish, Sue went to the fish tank and announced, "Swimming! Look! These fish didn't die." When she saw her mother that afternoon, Sue said, "The fish died, like my daddy died." Sue did not continue to ask about the dead fish. It is possible that her "understanding" of the loss remained in her mind along with some ongoing notion of the fish's continued existence, as was the case for her father. It seems more likely that acceptance of the fish's death was due to a lack of emotional need for the fish to be alive and therefore a lack of continuing concern for it.

At one point, several months after the death, Mrs. S., following her own religious beliefs, spoke of her husband as though he were still present. Sue became quite confused and in class spoke of him as alive. Mrs. S. was advised not to share such ideas with Sue, and Sue's confusion subsided.

Sue's curiosity and need to understand her father's death were evident in her efforts to reason about it. These efforts incorporated ideas she had been told as well as her own experiences and remained limited to her developmental level of thinking. Such reasoning thus included application of memories of previous experiences to the present and transductive reasoning from particular to particular without true deductive or inductive reasoning (Ginsburg and Opper 1979). What follows are examples of Sue's thinking in several areas.

Sleeping was confused with death for several months. Sue had been told that her father was "sleeping in Heaven." She had seen him and kissed him good-bye in his coffin; she and her sister had played at being dead in a box after the funeral. In the weeks after this she fought sleep; she was fragile and whimpering at naptime and kept her eyes open despite fatigue. Her mother reported that Sue was waking up sobbing in the middle of the night. Sue said of her father, "He awake. No. He sleeping there" and pointed up to the sky. A few weeks later she said, "My daddy is sleeping. My daddy can't get out of the box!" Clarifications on a concrete level were helpful; thus after Sue was several times told of the difference between sleeping and being dead, her sleeping difficulty resolved.

Travel and "far away" are similar preconcepts that for Sue were associated with death. The fear was present that since one died in the sky, another might die in the sky. When her special teacher was leaving on vacation, Sue told her that she was flying away from her, that she wasn't coming back, that she would die like her daddy died; "He went far away." They discussed the difference between a trip on an airplane (a person can return, stays healthy) and dying. Sue said, "My daddy died. I didn't see him for a long, long time." She then asked about herself, "I'm not gonna die?" about the teacher, "You're not gonna die?" and then about each of her classmates in turn, "Doug's not gonna die?" etc.

Certain forms of travel such as taxis and planes were associated with dying. Sue talked about her father riding in cars, taxis, and school buses, and tied these memories closely to thoughts of his death. The memory of a taxi ride with her father maintained a special significance. Sue said, "My daddy went in the car, and me too. He told the taxi to stop." Several days later she told her friend Doug, "My daddy died. Did your daddy die?" Doug answered, "No," and Sue asked, "Did your daddy ride on a school bus?" She then asked her teacher if her daddy had died and whether he had gone in a school bus, adding that her daddy went in a taxi.

Sue's preconception of travel related to death is too general; thus since her father "went in a taxi," she appeared to associate taxis, buses, etc., with death. She reasoned with transductive logic that since he went in a taxi, others who did so might die too. Furthermore, Sue had no grasp of ideas of chance. As Piaget and Inhelder (1951) showed, children at her age (and older) have only a primitive notion of taking turns. She tried to reason within the small number of her peers whether death will occur to each of them. The concept of "chance," the idea that what happened to her father was very unlikely to happen to her mother or to her—that is, "statistically low odds"—could not be called upon as a reassurance. Instead Sue reassured herself concretely.

Sue was particularly confused about the difference between flying in airplanes and going to heaven. At one point without the teachers' knowledge Sue's mother had talked of taking a plane trip with Sue. In daycare Sue said, "I not sick. I not fly up in the sky. Mommy gonna fly up in the sky. Like daddy fly. You not fly up in the sky?" Her teacher talked of having flown in an airplane in the sky during her winter vacation. She explained that she wasn't sick or hurt and that she came back home on another airplane when she was ready, unlike Sue's father who was very sick and died and could not ever return. Sue then said, "I go fly with mommy and daddy. I go on horses with mommy and daddy." They talked about trips she used to take with her mother and father and further clarifications were made. When the teacher explained Sue's confusion to Mrs. S., they were able to continue these discussions at home and Sue's anxiety abated. One must also wonder what "in the sky" meant to Sue. Piaget (1927) quotes a boy of eight: "Is the sky alive?—Yes, because if it were dead, why then it would fall down" (289).

Sue associated medical things with dying and avoided medical play for several weeks after her father's death. She averted her eyes from a stethoscope saying, "It's not here. Forgot in room. Lost it"; or she tossed it aside. After a few weeks this shifted to a strong interest in playing doctor, as she gave shots and Band-Aids and talked about her father.

One day while reading *Nicki Goes to the Doctor,* she called the instrument a "deathoscope" and then denied feeling afraid of shots "because people don't need shots and daddy didn't need a shot." On another occasion death was associated with a Band-Aid as Sue, her teacher, and a classmate conversed:

CLASSMATE: My mommy died.
SUE: Your mommy not die. My mo—my daddy died.
TEACHER: What happened to your daddy?
SUE: He died.
TEACHER: How did that happen?

SUE: My daddy had a Band-Aid. My daddy died. My mommy didn't die.
CLASSMATE: My daddy didn't die. He go to work.

That afternoon when the classmate's father came for him, Sue said to him, "See, your daddy not dead."

In part because of her inability to specify causes, Sue seemed to wonder about her ability to precipitate death. On a walk Sue started to pull some ivy vines that another child had just been told not to pull up. A volunteer teacher told her to stop because she was making the plants die. Sue pulled back, looked very frightened, gazed around her at the trees and plants, and asked, "Everything gonna die?" She was then reassured and agreed she had been very scared. The volunteer's comment became quickly generalized, as it touched on a source of anxiety in Sue.

Separation Anxiety

Sue's heightened separation anxiety immediately after the death, and through the ensuing months with her special teacher, indicated fear of further loss. "Because" there was one loss there may be another. Brief separations from her teacher evoked a variety of behaviors from Sue that seemed to be efforts to master this fear. These behaviors did not occur in isolation. Experiences involving separation were linked together by association either with events recognized as similar and/or with the affects involved in these past events. The following incidents illustrate how Sue, when threatened by separation from her teacher, referred either through action or words to specific, past, related experiences.

When her teacher told Sue about a brief trip she was taking, Sue immediately grabbed a child's pacifier and answered in a stream of infantile syllables. She then asked to read a book, *Hop on Pop,* which she had read daily with a temporary summer worker who had left three months earlier (when Sue was twenty-five months.) Sue sang, "Daddy, daddy, happy birthday" and suddenly broke into sobs, asked to join the teacher on her trip, and shook her head "no" in disbelief about reassurances that the teacher would return and that she would be taken care of safely. That afternoon Sue had a difficult time separating from the teacher, throwing herself on the floor, demanding a bottle, and then threatening to "tell daddy." The turning to the remembered book appeared to be an attempt to control her reaction to the threatened separation.

Bemporad (1978) makes the point that for a young child affective experiences are "of the moment" and that moods are not held over time due to the child's lack of inner mental continuity unless the outer circumstances continually provoke certain feelings. Sue did not become depressed in the adult sense. She did not go into a continued, lasting depressive mood. She did, however, remain sensitized to separation experiences and associated memories over time.

In the following example, an incident is remembered and referred to four months later. On a walk with her group Sue announced to some porcelain figures in a store window, "My daddy died." Soon after, Sue saw her sister, walking by with her school class. The sister hugged Sue and then left. Sue cried and called for her sister and her daddy. Her temporary caregiver, Anny, picked her up and Sue clung to her neck whimpering. Sue's special teacher, who was busy with the others, left Sue to calm down with Anny and went on with the rest of the group to the park. As soon as Sue arrived in the park, she stumbled, fell, and ran to her special teacher crying in her arms for a long time. Sue had been upset at being left with Anny.

Sue referred to this incident four months later when her teacher was again unavailable. The teacher had just returned from a four-day illness during which Sue was cared for by her group's second regular teacher, Mary. Sue arrived, saw her special teacher, and asked for Mary. She slapped her special teacher who tried to help her with her coat and let Mary help instead. Her teacher initiated a conversation, saying "You haven't seen me in a long time." Sue then rushed to her and pulled herself onto her lap. The teacher told her that she must have been angry at her for having been gone for so long, and that Sue must have been worried because she was sick even though she had been told she was getting better. Sue asked if the teacher lay in bed and watched television, if she took medicine, and if she "drank lots of soda to get better." Then Sue said, "I was very mad." The teacher asked at whom, and she said at Anny for picking her up when she saw her sister.

Sue was clearly angry with her teacher for being out sick as she slapped her and turned from her. She talked of a time when she had wanted her teacher and had instead been left with Anny. As she again felt close to her teacher, she shifted the anger to Anny and to the past incident. One may presume that Sue was also angry at her father, but this was not expressed directly.

Object Constancy, Separation-Individuation

Sue showed clear evidence of having achieved some degree of (libidinal) object constancy. She often sang or recited to herself the phrases "I want mommy" or "daddy" to comfort herself. She remembered specific incidents with painful longing. When Mary was describing her sadness at the death of an uncle to Sue's special teacher, Sue called the two teachers by name and said, "Remember my daddy in the picture? My daddy went far away. My daddy got me an umbrella." Her face fell sadly, and she added, "I saw my daddy in the picture."

The ability to see the other as separate from oneself assists one in modulating the fear that what happened to another person may happen to oneself or mother or specific others. This ability was not fully developed in Sue. Thus when mother returned from visiting father in the hospital, Sue asked, "Are you feeling better mommy?" as though it were mother who was sick. Sue frequently reassured herself, "My daddy died. My mommy didn't die." She also used her peers to compare whose fathers had died and whose hadn't.

Illness in her mother increased Sue's fears, and with this stress her sense of self merged with her mother as she feared they both would die. Once when mother was ill with a bad cold and her attention was inconsistent to Sue, Sue was very distressed and fearful that her mother's illness would cause them all to die. She showed her teacher scrapes on her face where she had fallen and told her of getting a shot at the doctor's the day before. She then said, "I went in an airplane in the sky with my mommy and daddy. No, I didn't. My daddy died."

Because Sue could not reason in a generalized causal way, she could not clearly comprehend what made people die and therefore could not use even concrete operational logical thought to comprehend as an adult can and to reassure herself that she too would not die or that others would not. Adults with helpful explanations cannot "correct" this logic or raise it to a higher level, which must wait for later development.

Thus Sue did not let this unresolved issue rest. In a follow-up visit[3] Sue still feared her mother too would die. She used the toilet; when she flushed it, she asked her teacher, "Do it bother you?" and reassured herself, "People don't go down." After a few minutes she began to sing, "Where's my mommy? She died? No, she didn't," and continued, "My mommy didn't die. Only my daddy. Doug's daddy didn't die. He said his mommy died. She didn't. I miss my daddy."

Affective Reactions

Sue's reactions to her father's death included varied expressions of affect. To integrate affective experiences one must tolerate affect and also limit it so as not to be overwhelmed. Sue did not become overwhelmed and disorganized by her father's death. She did not constrict or omit affect but instead experienced a wide affective range.

A storybook in which a hunter shoots and kills the mother of Babar, the elephant, became a focus for a variety of feelings and primitive fantasies as Sue would open the book to the page of the shooting on different occasions. Sue usually expressed anger at the hunter, shouting and hitting his picture. But she also slapped the dead mother or slapped at the crying Babar. Sue feared Babar would die: "Babar [was shot], not his mommy." Another time the gun going off was associated with her daddy dying.

Although Sue played out murderous and angry impulses, she did not acknowledge directly anger at her father for dying. For example, Sue excitedly called a policeman the daddy. Then she put down the policeman and picked up the lion and the horse.

SUE: Lion angry at horse. Biting him.
TEACHER: Why is the lion so angry with the horse?
SUE: Because she died.
TEACHER: The lion is mad that the horse died. Your daddy died too. Are you angry at daddy?
SUE: He awake. No. He sleeping there [pointing to the sky]. Sue picked up the elephant and threw it, saying, "He died." She then threw the horse, "He died," Then two mothers, "She died."
TEACHER: They're all dying.
SUE: They awake.

Sue put them away and asked to end the session.

Here the suggestion of anger at her father interrupted the play; Sue had the dolls "die," denied this, and then ended the session. Such direct interpretations were rarely made. Playing out various emotions, especially anger, was encouraged to help her accept and express her own feelings on the level she presented them. It is possible that unspoken feelings, such as anger at her father, could become a focus for later conflict and symptom formation or for resolution at a later age. For example, Sue's lack of anger directed at her father may represent splitting and idealization of him with the anger displaced to others.

Although Sue often gave in to the impulse to cry, she stressed that she did not cry; e.g., hearing another child cry, she said, "Somebody's crying. I'm not crying. I don't cry." In another example, Sue climbed into the teacher's lap, began to stroke her hair, and said, "You look pretty like a queen. I hold you. You won't cry." She soon asked if the teacher would always stay her teacher when she grew older. The teacher explained that, after Sue left, Sue would have new teachers who would help her and that she could visit the Center. Sue responded, "My daddy can't come for me yet. He at work. I didn't cry home sick. Mommy cried home sick. Daddy at work." Her face fell suddenly and she said, "I never see my daddy."

Sue stressed she didn't cry, mommy cried. Crying must be controlled and is also unpleasant as she reassured her teacher, "You won't cry." Anticipation of separation from the teacher seemed to stir feelings for her father, which she tried to ward off. As Wolfenstein (1966) suggests, children fear that pain or anger "may continue without letup and increase to intolerable intensity" (103). Sue also needed to feel independent and not to regress.

Although Sue stressed not crying and maintaining control, she often cried. In a follow-up session she showed her teacher a bruise on her elbow and said that she fell running but that she didn't cry because she was a big girl. In her play she put lady bugs "in the oven so they got burned up. They not gonna cry." She made a play-doh roller coaster that went fast and said it was not scary. She said that if the teacher thought a roller coaster was scary, she should have held on. She asked, "Did you let go? Was you crying?" That same session she told of pinching her finger in the door and that she didn't cry. The school director noted that in fact Sue had screamed very loudly when she pinched her finger.

In the following example Sue shows her continued need to deny crying while at the same time she is able to label sadness and to articulate a cause. On the sixth follow-up visit Sue was interested in a story about a boy's pet dog who became ill and died in a book entitled *Grownups Cry Too*. Sue renamed the book *Grownups Don't Cry*, asking to see the dog, and saying, "That boy misses the dog. That dog gonna be fine." On the next and final session Sue asked to see "the boy who missed the dog," adding, "Not my dog died." The teacher answered that someone else special to her had died and she said, "My daddy died. That's why I get sad."

Psychosexual Development

Psychosexually, Sue appeared to be between an anal and an early phallic phase. She had achieved toilet training and did not regress. She struggled to control her impulses and for the most part succeeded. This process of increasing control continued after her father's death along with increased verbalization of affect. For example, Sue used play to express and master ambivalent feelings after an aggressive act. Although biting was not a frequent occurrence for Sue, one day she bit a peer without provocation and announced, "I talk to daddy." She sang lustily, "I bit Larry, da da da da da da," then regressed into a stream of babytalk. She then noted the alligator emblem on her teacher's shirt, put her finger on it, cried, "ouch," shook her finger, and told the teacher, "I take your alligator off." She covered it with her palms, "It went away," and then played peekaboo with it under her hand. Sue bit, attributed the urge to bite to the alligator, was herself bitten, and made the alligator come and go.

Sue's play often expressed ambivalence, particularly in association with issues of illness and death, as the following examples from play sessions illustrate:

Sue threw a doll, Ernie, then nursed him with a Band-Aid and threw him again. She said, "Ernie, a Band-Aid. My finger hurts," and showed the teacher her finger. She found Ernie, threw him again, and expressed concern that he felt sad. Later she refused to bid Ernie good-bye, saying, "I don't want to kiss him good-bye."

Sue gently put a large doll, Betsy, to sleep saying, "Don't bother my Betsy. She needs a Band-Aid. For everything. You bothering my baby!" (to her teacher). She lifted the phone to say that her teacher was "bothering my Betsy sleep. I asked her not to bother Betsy. Betsy." Then she stomped angrily on Betsy. She pointed a finger at the teacher and said loudly, "You step on her. You did it." Sue then smiled and said, "I'm gonna be a monster."

Precursors of Guilt

As one would expect at her age, Sue did not express guilt or self-reproach. She did show, however, a transient tendency to fall and hurt herself. This was marked particularly just after her father's death and again just after her move to the new school. That getting hurt had significance is suggested in the following example. Sue picked up the book about Babar, flipped to the page where the hunter shots Babar's mommy, and said, "The boy had to shoot the hunter." She then turned and scrambled up the back of the couch to a precarious position, leaning out over the back of the couch above the floor. The teacher told her that she had to get down, that she might hurt herself. She answered, "I want to go hurt myself," but came down. The teacher told her she wouldn't let her do things where she could get hurt as she helped her down. Sue then commanded, "Finish that book!" in a stern voice. "Who's shot?" Sue asked, and answered, "Babar, not his mommy." Then Sue closed the book again.

Sue seemed to want the child to be hurt rather than the adult. Self-hurting did not lead to real danger, nor did it become a chronic symptom for Sue. That such behavior was noted occasionally seemed consistent with the view that Sue had many unintegrated feelings, reactions, and unelaborated primitive fantasies.

Other examples reflecting precursors of guilt might include an incident wherein she noted her big teeth in a mirror and commanded to herself, "No biting!" and also her fear "Everything gonna die?" in response to her pulling up a plant.

Identification

Adults and children are often noted to identify with the lost object in a global or partial way, more global reactions occurring when less differentiation from the object has been achieved before the loss. Although Sue feared she would die, she did not seem to identify in a global way with her dead father. That is, she did not act as though she were her father. Instead Sue showed some interest in, or selective identifications with, aspects of her father, consistent with having achieved a more differentiated view of him. Thus she liked beaded necklaces. She commented that she had big eyes like her daddy, and she sang particular songs noting that they were songs he had sung. She also referred to daddy as a "monster daddy" as a time when she was playing "monster," scaring her peers. But none of these were persistent or intense interests.

DISCUSSION

Sue's reactions to her father's death appear consistent with the concept of childhood mourning (Sekaer 1986) in that Sue reacted to bereavement without developing serious fixations or conflicts, at least at the time, and appeared able to proceed with her development. Sue did not "mourn" like an adult, according to Freud's definition, since reality was tested only on a primitive level. Sue appeared to fit Anna Freud's criteria, but with the following limitations: she "understood" the "external fact" while at the same time maintaining contradictory facts in mind. Death was viewed as a departure: "He went far away . . . in the sky"; although Sue stated, "he can't come back," she did not accept the finality as she complained at thirty-six months, "I never see my daddy," and said, "He at work. . . . He can't come for me yet." The "fact" that she knew he "died" and "can't get out of the box" did not conflict with her other ideas. She appeared at least transiently to comprehend irreversibility with regard to a fish, but with her father she continued to view death as reversible. The dead cannot "do things," as she agreed the fish could not swim, and yet her daddy (as she said under stress) was "at work" and "can't get out of the box."

Causality was not understood by Sue, and instead, with her primitive logic she associated by juxtaposition medical phenomena, forms of transportation, etc. She reacted fearfully to sleep as death. She also could not understand the low statistical likelihood of death at a young age. She had primitive notions of her own power, pulling up a plant and fearing "everything gonna die." Reality testing occurred with adult prompting: "Can he visit you now?" "No because he died." But the reasons for the death continued to be not understood and its irreversibility to be contradicted. Within these cognitive limits, clarifications of some of Sue's concrete confusions were definitely helpful. Thus explaining that sleep did not mean death alleviated her sleep difficulty, and explanations that flying in a plane was not "dying in the sky" resolved her fears about a trip. These explanations did *not* become generalized, nor did they lead to a higher cognitive level of thought.

Nagera (1970) says that the latency child's lack of acceptance of death is due to the child's *need* to keep the tie. The cognitive *inability to comprehend* the finality of death can also account for the split in the acceptance of "facts" of death and the continued belief in life of the lost one. Sue, typical for her prological level of thought, maintained many contradictory "facts" and ideas in her mind; this could not truly be called a split in her ego until she reached the level where more integrated thought is present. It is possible that Sue's mother conveyed to Sue some lack of acceptance of the finality of her husband's death and *her* wishes for his return, thereby undermining Sue's reality testing, but this appeared to play a minor role compared to Sue's cognitive limitations. Lopez and Kliman (1979) and Erna Furman (1974) argue that with adult help the "reality" can be understood and accepted. Yet, without follow-up one cannot rule out the existence or development of splits in the ego wherein the expectation of return of the parent is maintained even after such apparent childhood acceptance of "the facts."

The timing of bereavement in childhood is particularly important. Sue's personality development at the time of the death was at a plateau, perhaps more stable than it would have been a few months earlier or later. Sue had apparently achieved resolution of rapprochement. She gave evidence of libidinal object constancy as she talked of both her mother and father in their absence to reassure herself and continued to long for and talk of her father eight months after his death. Sue had not yet shown evidence of oedipal conflicts at the time of the death. The stability of her personality is evidenced by the fact that she did not regress cognitively nor develop evident fixations on oral or anal levels. Similarly she did not regress along lines of separation-individuation nor deviate toward a less than optimal rapprochement outcome as described by McDevitt. Winnie (Barnes 1964) appears to have been at a similar stage, whereas Diane (Lopez and Kliman 1979) at nineteen months was much more disrupted by her loss.

Sue did not appear to use identification with her father as a way of maintaining his presence. Though she played at being dead in a box after the funeral, she did not go on to reenact the death as did Lopez and Kliman's patient, who imitated, in jumping and falling, her mother's suicidal leap. Sue did not become confused about sexual identity nor act out being her father in other ways. Instead there were minimal selective imitations and identifications, such as singing songs he had sung or playing monster at a time she spoke of him as a monster. Perhaps there was less need to identify with him because her cognitive abilities did not exclude her maintaining a conscious belief in his existence. Or perhaps Sue as a preoedipal child did not need her father as strongly, being still more tied in with her mother. Sue's identifications with her mother were evident in her internalized controls, in her feminine manner and appearance, and in her play with mothering activities. She seemed to have had less of her personality dependent on identifications with her father. Or it is possible that Sue will identify more with her father in the future, for example, when she goes through the oedipal stage.

According to the Furmans, Anna Freud, and others, Sue should have been capable of decathecting her father. She did not appear to do this in the adult sense of detaching libido from the mental representation of the dead one, at least not fully detaching libido. But she did react affectively and cognitively in a prolonged struggle to deal with the death. One might infer decathexis from her observed sadness and longing for her father and from specific painful memories she described, e.g., "My daddy got me an umbrella." But the pain did not derive from knowledge that he would never return so much as from an awareness of his current absence, "I never see my daddy. . . . My daddy died. I didn't see him for a long, long time." Since she still talked of him as returning, "He at work. He can't come for me yet," she had clearly not gotten rid of the libidinal tie to him and held on to a belief in his continued existence.

Sue did not omit affect as did Deutsch's patients. But a great deal of her affect about the death emerged only in the private play sessions in her relationship to her special teacher. Sue's use of this tie, which intensified after her father's death, does not fit Wolfenstein's description of an "adaptation reaction" because it was not used *instead of* expressing pain over her loss. Sue could not turn inward alone to a preoccupation with thoughts about father as adults do, but was able to express feelings about the loss in the context of this relationship. Left alone, Sue may well have covered up her feelings and "omitted affect." Unlike an adult in grief, Sue needed an adult to share her feelings. It is doubtful that Sue would have worked through her loss with her mother. Her mother was herself bereaved, and thus less available to Sue, and also was inclined to minimize Sue's reactions to the death. Barnes's case omitted affect at two and a half after her mother's death until her grandmother was able to share the affective experience with her; one wonders if Winnie would have gone on to become symptomatic if grandmother had not become available to her. Diane used her transference tie to Lopez as a focus around which to organize her feelings, wishes, and memories about her mother.

If one follows the adult model, one might focus on assisting the child to accept the finality of death and to decathect the dead. If one, like Wolfenstein, views mourning as decathexis of the dead followed by a hiatus and then a recathexis of a new person, one may decide that a transfer of cathexis to another person is not mourning, but only an "adaptation." But if a child is better off avoiding a developmental vacuum, the optimal response for the child may be to transfer the tie to someone else or to maintain the cathexis of the dead one until it can be more slowly withdrawn. Sue did not have a substitute for her father at home onto whom she could transfer cathexis. Maintaining the fantasy of the dead's continued existence may allow the child to go on with crucial steps in development without interfering with reality testing in other areas.

Adults develop conscious and unconscious fantasies that embody and express the meaning of death to them. In normal mourning, realistic causes of death are accepted and irrational or pathological beliefs (e.g., that one's bad wishes caused a death) are given up. In a case cited by Neubauer (1967), "Mommy has killed Daddy . . . by giving him 'doody' to eat" was apparently a precocious formulation by a 2½-year-old. In Sue's play a single clear-cut theme representing the meaning of the death did not emerge. The death was viewed as a separation loss for which no single clear cause was articulated. Instead several possible themes were touched on: her ambivalent play, e.g., with the doll, Betsy, may have been a displacement of her mixed feelings of concern for and anger at her father. Her wish to have "Babar shot, not the mommy" and to hurt herself may have represented some early primitive guilt reactions. Her lack of expression of anger directed at her father may have meant such feelings were being denied or split off and could become a focus for later conflict. Or it may be that the death did not need to take on a pathological meaning based on inner or external conflicts on Sue's part. The fact that she did not become seriously symptomatic in the eight months following his loss may mean she was reacting to the death in a nonpathological way within the limits for her age. In fact, it is this lack of development of serious or chronic symptoms that seems most comparable to *normal* mourning in an adult. Clearly Sue did react to and struggle to integrate her loss, facilitated by her therapeutic experience with her teacher, and yet without overt signs of pathology.

Children often find their own creative solutions to developmental or traumatic stresses. Infants create transitional objects to assist with separation from mother. Older children create imaginary companions to cope with a variety of stresses. Bereaved children sometimes maintain their dead parent as though still living in fantasy, as an imaginary parent (Sekaer 1986). Sue readily expressed thoughts about her father as living ("He at work" . . . "My daddy can't come for me yet"). Her talk of father as returning at times and as not coming back at other times can be explained as typical inconsistencies of prelogical thought rather than a fantasy. However, her use of her father in remembered and fantasied roles took several forms. He assuaged loneliness and undid the loss ("I know he comes to my house on Sunday"). She invokes him as a punisher when angry at her teacher ("I'll tell daddy''); here he is also her rescuer helping her deal with the teacher. She spoke of her father as a scary monster who got shot, and seemed to identify with him as she played monster and scared other children. She thought of him as at a distance, unable to reach her (''He at work. . . . My daddy can't come for me yet''). While these fragments hardly constitute an integrated fantasy of an imaginary parent, nevertheless they may represent the roots of such a fantasy which could become more integrated as her relationship to this imaginary father develops over time. The fact that she is motivated to think of him in these ways may represent the beginnings of a specifically cathected use of creativity. If Sue is able to use other substitutes along the lines of her special teacher (or a stepfather), she may feel less need for her father and may elaborate fewer fantasies about him, investing instead the substitute.

Children may also mourn at a distance (Wolfenstein 1966), expressing affect for the dead one displaced onto toys, fictional characters, or pets. Sue appeared to do this in a primitive way through her use of the book about Babar, the elephant, and with the dolls, Betsy and Ernie, insofar as she played out themes of loss and death with them. Though she certainly was able to express sadness and longing for her father, she seemed able to express more anger and ambivalence with Babar, Betsy, and Ernie, than with her father.

One may argue that the impact of the trauma, for Sue, may still have pathological effects in the future, that the loss may take on other meanings, e.g., as Sue goes through the oedipal stage, and that symptoms may form later. This is a problem inherent in discussion of any childhood trauma (Nagera 1966). Since the child is growing and developing, any trauma may be reactivated if it resonates with later developmental conflicts even without further traumatic events. If one would call this a delayed pathological response, then one cannot speak of any childhood trauma as resolved until the child is grown. It is possible that analysis would have accomplished more by way of integrating Sue's feelings and fantasies. But perhaps not.

We may consider that Sue went through a childhood mourning with the help of her therapeutic relationship with her teacher to the extent that she resolved her reactions to the death as much as possible for her developmental level. Not all children who lose a parent react in a pathological manner; further studies are needed of bereaved children who do well, with or without therapeutic intervention, and of how they accomplish this.

NOTES

1. The special teacher was Sheri Katz. The daycare supervisor was Virginia Flynn.
2. Excerpts are taken from a daily record kept by Sue's special teacher. This record was rewritten in narrative form and parts have been published (Katz and Flynn 1982).
3. The daycare center enrolled children only up to the age of three years. Sue's special teacher continued to meet with Sue after her move to the new school for a series of weekly follow-up sessions.

BIBLIOGRAPHY

Barnes, M. J. (1964). Reactions to the death of a mother. *Psychoanal. Study Child,* 19:334–357.

Bemporad, J. R. (1978). A developmental approach to depression in childhood and adolescence. *J. Amer. Acad. Psychoanal.,* 6:325–352.

Bowlby, J. (1960). Grief and mourning in infancy and early childhood. *Psychoanal. Study Child,* 15:9–52.

——— (1980). *Attachment and Loss.* New York: Basic Books.

Deutsch, H. (1937). Absence of grief. *Psychoanal. Q.,* 6:12–22.

Freud, A. (1939–45). Infants without families. *W.,* 3.

——— (1960). Discussion of Dr. John Bowlby's paper. *Psychoanal. Study Child,* 15:53–62.

Freud, S. (1917). Mourning and melancholia. *S.E.,* 14:243–258.

——— (1927). Fetishism. *S.E.,* 21:149–57.

Furman, E. (1974). *A Child's Parent Dies.* New Haven: Yale Univ. Press.

Furman, R. A. (1964a). Death and the young child. *Psychoanal. Study Child,* 19:321–333.

——— (1964b). Death of a six-year-old's mother during his analysis. *Psychoanal. Study Child,* 19:377–397.

Ginsburg, H. & Opper, S. (1979). *Piaget's Theory of Intellectual Development.* Englewood Cliffs, N.J.: Prentice-Hall.

Jacobson, E. (1954). The self and the object world. *Psychoanal. Study Child,* 9:75–127.

Katz, S. (1976). The development of a child's concept of death. Unpublished thesis, New College.

Katz, S. & Flynn, V. (1982). A young child's response to death. *Daycare & Early Education,* fall, pp. 22–25.

Lopez, T. & Kliman, G. W. (1979). Mourning in the analysis of a four-year-old. *Psychoanal. Study Child,* 34:235–271.

McDevitt, J. (1980). The role of internalization in the development of object relations during the separation-individuation phase. In *Rapprochement,* ed. R. Lax, S. Bach & J. A. Burland, pp. 135–150. New York: Aronson.

McDonald, M. (1964). A study of the reaction of nursery school children to the death of a child's mother. *Psychoanal. Study Child,* 19:358–376.

Nagera, H. (1966). *Early Childhood Disturbances, the Infantile Neurosis, and the Adulthood Disturbances.* New York: Int. Univ. Press.

——— (1970). Children's reactions to the death of important objects. *Psychoanal. Study Child,* 25:360–400.

Neubauer, P. B. (1967). Trauma and psychopathology. In *Psychic Trauma,* ed. S. Furst, pp. 85–107. New York: Basic Books.

Piaget, J. (1927). *The Child's Conception of the World.* New York: Littlefield, Adams, 1979.

Piaget, J. & Inhelder, B. (1951). *The Origin of the Idea of Chance in Children.* New York: Norton, 1975.

Sekaer, C. (1986). Toward a definition of childhood mourning. *Amer. J. Psychother.* 41:201–19.

Winnicott, D. W. (1953). Transitional objects and transitional phenomena. *Int. J. Psychoanal.,* 34:89–97.

Wolfenstein, M. (1965). Death of a parent and death of a president. In *Children and the Death of a President,* ed. M. Wolfenstein & G. W. Kliman, pp. 62–79. New York: Doubleday.

———— (1966). How is mourning possible? *Psychoanal. Study Child,* 21:93–123.

———— (1969). Loss, rage, and repetition. *Psychoanal. Study Child,* 24:432–460.

PART VI

CASE REPORTS ILLUSTRATING ASPECTS OF MOURNING IN CHILDREN, ADOLESCENTS, AND ADULTS

Introductory Notes to Chapter 23

Rita V. Frankiel

Erna Furman describes her work with a mother on behalf of her bereaved three-year-old son after the suicide of her husband. In the case report provided here, Furman shares how she decided whether to use analysis of the child or treatment-via-the-parent. First, she carefully evaluated the child's symptoms, his development, and his defenses, using an implied continuum of flexibility-rigidity. She also evaluated their adequacy in binding anxiety, the mother's capacity to understand her child, her competence as a parent, and their mutual empathy. Over and above these considerations, it was felt that the introduction of an outsider should be delayed and used only if really necessary. In this regard, this technique is a most interesting option in helping a family recover from a traumatic and sudden loss without introducing yet further fragmentation. One important factor in this situation that is not available in the usual private practice or clinic situation is that this treatment took place in the context of a therapeutic nursery school and kindergarten; data were available to the therapist from teacher's observations, and her own classroom observations of the child in his group.

Erna Furman's treatment of a young child via his mother after the suicide of his father is an excellent example of one form of work with bereaved young children. This is a form of treatment that Furman and her group have been identified with in this country, and it is but one of the forms offered in their program.

This technique has not been universally accepted. There are some (e.g., Glenn 1980) who feel that the technique promotes regressive attachment and fosters the child's feeling invaded by parental omniscience. Such critics usually hold out for separate analysis or psychotherapy for the child and counseling or psychotherapy for the parent. Despite this, there may be a developing trend among child therapists and even some child analysts to work much more actively with parents and families in connection with child patients than had been favored in traditional child treatment. For example, at the spring meeting of the Division of Psychoanalysis of the American Psychological Association in April 1992, about 75 percent of the papers involving treatment of children under five and children with severe difficulties older than five involved substantial involvement of the therapist or analyst with the mother or both parents. It was a widely accepted observation at that meeting that this seems to be a current trend in work with children in the United States.

23. Treatment-via-the-Parent: A Case of Bereavement

Erna Furman

INTRODUCTION

In this report I shall portray three crucial years of Steven's development, from the time of his father's death—just prior to Steven's third birthday—till the beginnings of latency at age six. I shall focus on tracing how aspects of the father's illness, death and the subsequent fatherless years affected Steven's development. He was helped by his mother, with whom I worked throughout this period in a weekly treatment-via-the-parent and by the teaching staff of the Hanna Perkins Therapeutic Nursery School and Kindergarten where Steven had attended since he was three and a half years old (R. A. Furman and A. Katan 1969). The therapeutic work was based on the mother's and teachers' observations, augmented by my own weekly visits at the school.

Although we kept open the option of individual analysis for Steven, during this period of work we considered treatment-via-the-parent to be the treatment of choice for several reasons; in spite of phase-appropriate difficulties, some neurotic manifestations, and a tendency to instinctual regression under stress, Steven maintained a progressive development. His defences had not calcified to the point of rigidity, nor had they been inadequate to binding his anxieties. Thus no serious inner obstacles interfered with access to his psychic life. The mother-child relationship was characterised by age-appropriate closeness and empathic mutual understanding as well as a shared knowledge of the past. Even at the height of distress at the beginning of our work, the mother functioned well in her parental role, was familiar with emotional development and its handling and keen on actively helping

Reprinted by permission of the author and the Association of Child Psychotherapists from *Journal of Child Psychotherapy* 7 (1981):89–101.

her boy. Aware of some of her weaknesses, she struggled valiantly to overcome them and largely succeeded. Apart from these more usual indications for treatment-via-the-parent, it seemed particularly important that, following the loss of the father, the mother-child relationship should not be interfered with by the introduction of an outsider—which the analyst inevitably is—unless it proved absolutely necessary.

INITIAL PICTURE

Steven's mother contacted me about two weeks after the father's death, on her return with Steven from a brief stay with her family out of state and just before Steven's third birthday. Her main concern was prophylactic although Steven was showing some behavioural difficulties: he had recently become very afraid of aggressive people, especially a girl he sometimes played with, but, at other times he also provoked "potential" aggressors, e.g. his older teasing cousin and their own gentle but huge dog. Steven had periods of getting "high," i.e. excited, loud and somewhat hyperactive, especially when visitors came to the home. This difficulty had preceded father's death and the mother had linked it then with times when she and her husband had tense arguments. Judging by their content, however, Steven's most recent "high" episodes appeared also linked to experiences with a neighbour-policeman who often had his police car with blaring radio parked near their house and liked to regale the children on the street with excited accounts of his cop-and-robber activities. Further, Steven had started to withhold bowel movements and occasionally urine, a difficulty that had been much less in evidence during his toilet training a year earlier. There was occasional night wetting. Steven was also quite concerned about any separation from mother. We learned later that, occasionally and since about eighteen months of age, Steven had suffered from *pavor nocturnus* during which he could be neither woken nor comforted. It usually started with his crying in distress and walking toward the door that led to the bathroom but sometimes he ended up rocking on his rocking horse. He always wet himself at these times either before, during, or after leaving his bed. He had no memories of these episodes and neither original onset nor current occurrences could be linked to known events.

In general, however, Steven appeared age-appropriately developed in the early phallic phase, bright and very verbal.

HISTORY

Steven is his young parents' first and only child and the mother eagerly looked forward to his arrival. The father, in spite of a successful professional career and loving relationship with his wife and son, struggled with a self-destructive depressive illness. The mother learned that he had been quite depressed before she had known him, but she became aware of his difficulty only during Steven's first year and, increasingly, in the latter part of Steven's second year. Periodic bouts of withdrawal coupled with misuse of alcohol and drugs showed at times of stress. To Steven the father's illness manifested itself at first in sleeping, not being available when Steven wanted him, not responding to him, and, occasionally, in teasing. By the time Steven was two, the mother realised the seriousness of father's illness. At that time she also had to undergo a breast operation for removal of what turned out to be a benign tumor. It was a period of great anxiety plus several days of physical separation from Steven, the only one he experienced. The grandmother cared for Steven and noted his overt sadness and listlessness in spite of many phone and gift contacts with the mother. But he felt immediate relief when mother returned. Steven's third year was chaos as father's health deteriorated, unalleviated by psychiatric treatment which he reluctantly accepted but never utilized. Mother never knew when or in what state father would return home, whether she might be called to pick him up at work, or whether they would have to cancel and change all plans if he was not well. Although the parents tried strenuously to protect Steven from the impact of the father's illness and from their quarrels about it, the tension mounted. Mother, who tended to be loud, angry and controlling when very anxious, felt that Steven often bore some of the brunt of her mood. She tried to discuss her trouble with him but could not alter her behavior. She finally decided to get a divorce.

The mother told Steven only that he and she would, the next day, go for a short vacation to his aunt's family. When she informed the father of her wish for a divorce and plans to leave town, he reacted with an irrational fit of fury in which he bodily threw her against the wall. Steven watched the scene and pleaded with father to leave mummy alone. At that point the mother decided to leave with Steven at once "to go to grandma to be safe." While they were getting ready the father, demented, threw furniture and houseware into the street as if to get rid of wife and child, while Steven anxiously yelled at him to spare his and mummy's things. The paternal grandmother came to stay with the father and his doctor was informed, but Steven did not know that.

The next day, when the mother returned alone for some of her belongings she found the father dead, called the police and, since she had to stay on for official business, she called Steven to say that she would be late. On returning to Steven she told him that daddy had died. Steven asked, "Did the police come?" which mother affirmed. Steven stayed with a family friend during the funeral and burial and was told of all the details except for the cause of death. Later autopsy proved it to have been caused by an injection of cyanide. The suicide took place after both the paternal grandmother and doctor assumed the father had calmed down and left him according to his wish. After the funeral mother and Steven visited the aunt as had originally been planned and then returned to their house which has remained their home.

It has been our experience that the exact circumstances of the parent's death play an important part in the child's understanding of the event (Furman 1974). This was confirmed in the case of Steven where each detail proved to be significant.

COPING WITH THE DEATH AND MOURNING

The initial months of work focused on clarifying with Steven the concept of death, the circumstances and cause of the father's death, and on helping him to differentiate himself from the father's fate.

Steven knew from his earlier experiences with small dead animals that dead meant the absence of the functions of living, such as motility, eating, feeling pain, and he even knew about burial and bodily decay. His many questions showed how he applied this knowledge to his father's body: "Do the worms eat him?" "Can one dig him up and see?" "Does it hurt him?" He wondered, "Did every part of him die?" and asked specifically whether father's penis was dead too, which the mother confirmed. He worried whether all this would happen to his mother and to him, either now or when he would become a daddy. His fear intensified on later visits to the grave when he noted how many graves there were, but he also used these occasions to master his concerns.

Steven asked reproachfully why someone had not stayed with daddy and was relieved to learn that the paternal grandmother and the doctor had indeed been called in. Steven became very aware of what made other people or animals die but did not question the cause of his father's death. However, he repeatedly turned to gun and police play. When the mother wondered with

Steven about this play he brought out that he thought the police had come because daddy was out of control and had killed him—hence his initial question, "Did the police come?" which the mother had affirmed because she had misinterpreted its meaning. Over a period of time Steven absorbed the information that daddy had suffered from a mind sickness which had muddled up his thinking and had made him want to die—so different from healthy people—and that it had made him give himself a shot of stuff that made the body die. He learned that the father had been calm when he was left alone on the fatal night and that the police were called the next morning by mother to take daddy to the hospital so that the doctors could either help him or officially pronounce him dead and that this was a doctor's special job. Later, in connection with many remembered episodes, the earlier signs of father's illness were discussed as well as related issues—the proper and improper use of medicine, the unusual and noninfectious nature of father's illness, and how father's aggressive behaviour differed from the anger of healthy people.

Steven's withholding of bowel movements and urine yielded to interpretations of a mixup between bowel movements and "daddy feelings," and his wish to control things inside him because he had not been able to control what happened outside. Nightwetting, although it persisted longer, was related to "big feelings" which Steven could gradually verbalise—helplessness, sadness, and especially anger. Steven's excited teasing behaviour was linked primarily to an identification with the aggressors—the anxious mother who had been defensively angry and the fearsome uncontrolled father. There were many recountings of the scene of the attack which had overwhelmed Steven and his mother with fear for their bodily safety.

During this period Steven's *pavor nocturnus* recurred. The mother was able to help Steven become aware of this symptom and when the first content reached consciousness it was seen to relate to Steven's recent observation of his little girl friend's nudity during a beach outing. This led to clarification of sexual differences and conception but also increased Steven's phallic sadistic behavior with big sticks and pretend guns with which he attempted to poke holes into objects. He felt very badly about this and feared that big men would be angry with him. In pursuing this concern with Steven he reminded his mother that, already as a little toddler, he used to be in the bathroom with daddy when the latter shaved and urinated. He described father's genitals in detail, confessed that he had always wanted to take daddy's big penis, and after his death, had hoped that now he would be able to have it for himself—

hence his earlier question, "Are all parts of daddy dead, even his penis?" which had not struck the mother as so meaningful at the time.

Steven's *pavor nocturnus* subsided after these discussions and did not recur, although the underlying experiences and feelings were to reemerge in later years, attached to new developmental concerns.

As Steven came to grips with the realities concerning the father's death, mourning proper began with great intensity and lasted unremittingly for well over a year and, episodically, throughout the second year, comparable to but not imitative of his mother's mourning. In words, actions and activities Steven remembered and longed for all the gratifying aspects of the father-child relationship. He tolerated deep prolonged sadness and even considerable anger. Over and over he bemoaned the fact that nothing could be done to help daddy. When he saw children play a particular game he began to cry as it reminded him of daddy playing it with him. He could not join in because it would be no fun without daddy. Several months later he did join in, saying he liked to play this game because it reminded him of how nice it was when he played it with daddy. Strikingly, both longing and identification repeatedly took the form of performing previously shared activities and keeping joint interests, with very little need for concrete reminders and hardly any magical identifications of the more primitive preoedipal kind. He utilized well his relationships with an older neighbour and with his grandfather without substituting them for the father. For Steven, as for other under-fives with an immature sense of time, anniversaries were not of great significance. Rather, he missed his father during daily routines (mealtimes, going-to-bed stories), when visiting places where father had been with him (the park, picnics), and with new developmental steps (starting nursery school). Steven was acutely sad when other fathers visited the school. When he was told that his daddy knew the Hanna Perkins School and would have been glad for Steven to attend there he sighed, "Now I can like my school."

Steven also experienced the loss of the father as a narcissistic depletion. In comparing himself with other children he felt he was inadequate because he had no daddy at home, no big power to bolster his boyish self-esteem. He felt insignificant in having no daddy to talk about or to show to his peers, although he referred proudly to his father's profession and to memories of times with him.

As we were to learn, Steven's cathexis of the father remained strong throughout the oedipal period and affected his superego formation although by that time the acute mourning of the real father had subsided and he had sought and enjoyed relationships with potential fathers.

SOME EFFECTS OF THE FATHER'S DEATH ON
STEVEN'S PHALLIC PHASE

When Steven was three and a half years old, about seven months after his father's death, the mother began to prepare him for entry to Hanna Perkins Nursery School. With this news, and with mother occasionally going out in the evenings, Steven developed severe tempers around separations, even in the home, especially at bedtime. He provoked his mother with his disobedience and several times ran away from her just after she returned. When she interpreted this as a passive into active defence, Steven began to express his anger at her verbally and complained that he felt very "left out" when she was not with him. We learned that his anger was also a defence against his feeling of utter helplessness in the face of loss of object and against a deep narcissistic hurt at the imagined rejection that loss implied for him. Steven's separation difficulty subsided with this work and never recurred, but the feelings of being alone, helpless and rejected continued to manifest themselves in other areas.

In the initial weeks of nursery school, during a very gradual separation from the mother, Steven achieved a good intellectual mastery of the new environment but he kept himself aloof emotionally from the teachers, preferring independence to relying on their help whenever possible and using the school rocking chair rather than the relationship with the teacher to comfort himself when he missed his mother. Although eventually he formed a close relationship with his teachers, Steven remained aloof with people to the point of rejecting their friendly overtures and rarely initiating contacts. The mother brought this to his attention and once when he ignored a family friend's gracious greeting she pointed out to him how much he had hurt the man's feelings. Steven was surprised and chagrined. He empathised acutely with the man saying, "Oh, he felt all alone," and added wistfully, "I have known that feeling for a long time." A next step in understanding came when it was observed how much even minor rebuffs hurt Steven's feelings. One time he felt deeply and permanently rejected when his little friend refused to play with him just then because he was busy. Steven could appreciate that his reaction to the friend's "no" was unrealistic and perhaps belonged to another situation. He could also be shown in many instances that he warded off his painful "all alone" feeling by rejecting others. This brought memories of times when his father had, in his illness, withdrawn from Steven and rejected his overtures. With much work on this topic Steven's identification with the father lessened but it was not till Steven's fifth birthday that he was able to integrate fully his "all alone" feelings with his experience with his father. Many friends and relatives over-celebrated Steven's fifth birthday in an attempt to make up for the missing father, but when the nice party was over Steven wept inconsolably for his daddy and at feeling rejected by him through the latter's death. The mother and he could then discuss the "all alone" feelings Steven had so often experienced due to father's illness and which had culminated in the father killing himself and thus seemingly rejecting his child. This helped Steven considerably. As we were to learn, however, his propensity to feel rejected coloured Steven's attitudes to some men mother dated and made the mother's oedipal rejection of him especially difficult to tolerate.

I have already mentioned the narcissistic depletion Steven experienced with loss of the father. Steven's feeling of phallic adequacy was no doubt threatened much earlier when he enviously viewed the father's penis but a number of events during the phallic phase further enhanced his concerns. Just prior to the start of nursery school Steven had a swollen testicle which led to a traumatic hospital visit where a surgeon physically overwhelmed him. The swelling later subsided without treatment. He also had a dead tooth which caused intermittent pain and interfered with eating. In addition, there were repeated colds and ear infections during the first year of school. This resulted in considerable hearing loss with anxiety about the possible need for an operation like his little girl friend had to undergo. Actually, conservative but tiresome medical measures corrected the condition. All these factors affected Steven's feeling of competence in the nursery. Whereas at home he was quite skillful and interested in a variety of activities, at school he avoided them or expended minimal effort. Sometimes he scribbled up or destroyed his work and, instead of using his own creative ideas, he imitated others. At times he turned to "high" teasing fantasy play to ward off his fear of not measuring up to tasks. When the mother paid a morning's visit at school, however, Steven's self-esteem was enhanced and he took greater interest and pride in his achievements.

Likewise, Steven used the mother initially as a protector against his fears of the "bigger boys." This prolonged his need for her at the time of entry.

Actually only a few other boys were physically bigger and more capable but Steven viewed all of them as superior, displacing on to them his feelings about the father. Steven's conflicts manifested themselves in provocative teasing behaviour. It was observed that he generally teased potentially aggressive or teasing men and boys. When his defence of identification with the aggressor was interpreted Steven could express his fear of these people and could be shown that he overreacted to them because they reminded him of the times when his father's disturbed teasing frightened him. Steven vividly recalled many such occasions. Likewise, Steven often became silly and teasingly excited when something unusual happened, for example when their car was almost mired in a muddy parking place. At other times Steven annoyed adults by "copying" the naughty behavior of others, e.g. when a peer turned off the lights, Steven immediately followed suit. When the mother discussed these and similar incidents with Steven it gradually emerged that he became acutely anxious when people or events surprised him or appeared out of control. The mother helped Steven by linking this to his earlier fear of his father's outbursts and unpredictable moods. To some extent Steven's defences also represented an identification with his mother who reacted in a somewhat loud, excited and controlling fashion when helpless—both with the sick father of the past and with Steven in the present when his teasing behaviour reduced her to helplessness and made her anxious. The mother struggled hard to exercise conscious control over this difficulty within herself, discussed it with Steven and told him she hoped he would be able to cope differently.

In his second year of nursery school Steven mastered his phallic narcissistic difficulties to a considerable extent. He invested his activities and achievements independently and could utilize and enjoy his good potential. His aloofness and provocativeness subsided and his relationships improved and deepened. With other boys he was able to compete and show off his skills appropriately. The positive aspects of his earlier experiences with his father found their way into friendship with peers and ever more satisfying times with his grandfather and adult men friends with whom he engaged in a comfortable working-together relationship. These hard-won masteries were shortlived as oedipal conflicts intensified and revived earlier experiences in a new context.

STEVEN'S OEDIPAL PHASE

When Steven was almost five years old, the intense period of mourning came to an end for mother and him. Steven began to wish for a new daddy. The mother dated a man, Mr. A., who loved Steven as the son he had always wanted and Steven soon reciprocated with genuine fondness. Increasingly, however, Steven's teasing and provoking of old returned. With the teachers he defied requests, ignored admonitions and indulged in excited doll corner play and misuse of toy materials. We learned that at home Steven's similar baiting of his mother usually ended up with her giving him a couple of smacks on the bottom. In this way she provided regressive gratification of an oedipal nature which further stimulated his excitement. The mother came to recognise how unhelpful this was. She explained to Steven that she would no longer smack him because she did not love people in a toddler way and wanted to help him to grow up so that one day he would be able to love a lady his own age in a grown up way too. Steven reacted to the mother's oedipal rejection first with fury and increased determination, then with a desperate feeling of depletion and helplessness, a return of the "all alone" feelings. He began to have a problem with wriggling and inability to sit still. When the mother wondered with him about this he confessed very guiltily that he was withholding faeces and urine because "it feels nice." Steven had used this autoerotic gratification at earlier stressful times during the height of the father's illness and again immediately following his death. For Steven as for other fatherless boys it was especially painful to recognize that whereas he wooed his mother as the ideal loved partner, she sought out a newcomer, apparently spurning what her boy offered her. When Steven, his mother and her friend planned a joint spring vacation trip, the following incident took place on the day before they left:

> Steven was hunched down sitting in the sandbox in the park adjacent to their home. He was joined by a man who hunched down next to him. The mother observed the two from her kitchen window, eventually went out, found the man to be a stranger who at once tried to "pick her up" and she quickly left with Steven. When she asked him what he and the man had been doing, Steven had told her that the man rubbed Steven's penis and asked him to show it, which Steven did not do. Steven hugged his mother, said how glad he was she had come and taken him away because he had

been so scared. The mother sympathized, told him that the man had a trouble and that Steven should always call for her to help him.

During the subsequent trip there was no reference to the incident or behavioural reaction. Steven acted very grown up, tried to identify with manly behaviour in many ways but, toward the end, complained bitterly at not being allowed to share mother's single hotel room. On their return, when the boyfriend gave the mother a goodbye kiss, Steven kicked her. During the following weeks Steven was exceedingly angry, excited and defiant. Some of this was clearly related to his oedipal disappointment in his mother and anger at her, some of it related to the seduction. Mother overheard Steven tell his friend, the policeman's son, about it. The boy suggested they go to "look for the man to see if he is still in the park" and Steven was ready to join in. The mother stopped them and later told Steven that he must have got very excited by the man's touching of him and perhaps felt badly that his excitement had kept him from running away and calling mummy at once. She related Steven's recent persistent excited behaviour at home and school to this, "I can't stop myself and I don't want you to stop me."

Steven's reactions to the trip and seduction were overshadowed and confused by the fact that mother's relationship with her boyfriend changed to a mere friendship and she began to go out with a new man, Mr. B., a widower with two prepubertal sons. Mother and Steven spent a great deal of time in activities with this family. Mr. B. was fond of Steven and enabled him to share in many of his and his boys' interests, but he was more reserved than Mr. A. (the previous boyfriend) and less in need of a son. Steven felt keenly how little he was compared to these three tall males and considered himself rejected and left out. He endowed Mr. B. with his own father's negative attitudes just as he had attributed his father's positive aspects to Mr. A. Although Steven again tried to be very grown up and manly on the joint family outings, his anger and excitement manifested themselves at school and in seeking renewed regressive gratification from his mother. Steven also became quite curious about sexual matters but refused verbal explanations; "Don't give me that talk, I want to see," he insisted. One day he revealed a "secret" to another boy while both were using separate closed stalls in the nursery school bathroom. Steven said he had been using the dressing room at Mr. B.'s club and seen adult men urinate. He was greatly relieved when the teachers reported this secret to his mother and he then confided to her that he tried to use the urinal but could not reach. In discussing the incident with Steven it could be linked to his recent excitement and anger, to how little and "teased" he felt when he compared himself to men. His wish to see was related back to the seduction in the park when the man wanted to see Steven's penis and Steven perhaps wished to see the man's. Steven himself brought up his memories of seeing his father nude when he was a toddler. He added that when he saw his father's penis he took it. The mother questioned this and Steven surprised himself when he explained, "I think I was so little that seeing and taking was like the same thing. I just didn't know then that they are different."

Steven's oedipal feelings reached their crest during the summer when, on a brief joint vacation, Mr. B. and Steven's mother shared a room. Steven had always reacted strongly to mother's private times with her men friends— delaying going to bed, coming down from his room with needless requests, checking used ashtrays and glasses in the morning, and being outspokenly angry at mother before and after she would go out for an evening, but he had never had to face proof of mother's adult intimacy with her friend. Now he was both furious and deeply hurt and behaved accordingly. However, he managed quite well during a later vacation week without Mr. B. which they spent with Steven's aunt's family.

On their return, a week prior to the start of school, Steven had a severe anxiety dream: "A big bird flew down from the sky." He later added vaguely that maybe the bird tried to pick up or hurt a little boy who lived nearby. Steven was anxious for several nights after that, feared going to his room to sleep and wakened a few times. With the start of school Steven's anxiety subsided markedly except for wanting his light on "because monsters are on the walls when it's dark." Almost from the first day Steven misbehaved in the Hanna Perkins Kindergarten. He was disinterested in learning activities, could not settle down or play or work and spent his time either imitating a couple of uncontrolled boys' outbursts or provoking them to lose control. When isolated he always asked whether the other boy was back in control and only when the answer was affirmative did Steven calm down. He was impervious to and defiant of the teachers' admonitions and requests and acted as though he had forgotten all school rules and means of self-control.

In talking with mother Steven was only aware of his fear of the uncontrolled "bigger boys" and complained that "nobody can stop them." The mother suggested to Steven that the turmoil he saw in others might really be his own and that, when the others were not around, this very turmoil appeared on the walls of his room at night. As Steven began to enlist himself in working on his trouble many aspects could be understood. He displaced his anger at mother's nights with the boyfriend to the teachers and, with his omnipotent defiance, made them feel helpless in order to ward off his own helplessness in the face of mother's rejection and of his imagined inadequacy at school tasks. He did not try to learn for fear of not being able to compete with other boys successfully. Steven managed to be nice and obedient with adult men by displacing his oedipal competition to the classroom situation, projecting his own anger to his peers and controlling, through provocation, their feared retaliatory outbursts. When Steven faced his underlying anger at men sufficiently to voice it to his mother she suggested he tell his feelings to Mr. B. Steven whispered in terror, "But I could never tell a big man that I'm mad at him. The bigger the man, the less you can be mad at him." Why? Apparently the consequences were unspeakable. Nevertheless, the mother arranged a meeting between Steven, Mr. B., and herself to give Steven a chance to discuss specific complaints of being left out. Steven plucked up all his courage and stated his feelings. Mr. B. assured him that he was not angry back and said he well remembered when his own boys and even he as a child had felt that way. Steven was greatly relieved.

Other layers of his difficulty now became accessible. Steven recognised from his descriptions of the out-of-control schoolmates' behaviour that they reminded him of his father's outbursts which had preceded his death. In his own anger Steven also identified with the father—he was unstoppable and devastating. He was finally able to associate to his earlier anxiety dream, recalling some events which had precipitated it: he had attended a museum talk about birds of prey with live specimens; during their visit to the aunt he had learned that her dog had been killed by a car; and on a visit to the village cemetery there he had read the inscription of a child's tombstone, "and the angel of the Lord came down from heaven and touched him." The bird who flew down from the sky in Steven's dream represented the killer-avenger father. Steven again went over the father's outburst and asked if daddy had been mad at him because he, Steven, called to him to leave mother alone. In retrospect he interpreted events differently: mother had chosen him, Steven, to go away with, and when daddy found out about that he felt so left out and angry that he lost his temper and wanted to kill them and killed himself. This helped to clarify Steven's fear of his own left-out feelings and of expressing anger at men. It was also his masturbation fantasy as we learned that one aspect of Steven's explosive behaviour at school related to his renewed withholding of urine and increased touching of his genital.

Steven's negative oedipal conflict and its passive antecedents had manifested themselves periodically. Although Steven's withholding of faeces and urine had many active and masculine aspects, there were also passive ones. Steven knew that his passing a large motion probably precipitated the swelling of his testicle which in turn led to his being overpowered by the surgeon who examined him. Minor swellings occurred a couple of times since without requiring medical attention. Steven felt discomfort along the canal to the testes at these times and it was unclear whether his withholding was designed to anticipate or control these feelings. Steven had the earlier experience of being teased by his father and later provoked and teased men and boys who appeared unpredictable to him. He provoked his mother to smack his behind. He had his penis rubbed by the stranger in the park. Steven often "appropriated" Mr. A., mother's boyfriend. His feelings came to the fore most clearly at a later point when the mother informed him that she had decided against marrying either Mr. A. or Mr. B., although she liked both of them. Steven was very upset but only with much help could finally express his great anger at the mother for depriving him of these potential fathers as well as of his own father, as though she had been responsible for his death.

THE BEGINNINGS OF LATENCY

Steven's anxiety dream and subsequent school problem represented not only the latter phase of his oedipus complex but also the first superego internalisations. When Steven's school behaviour improved his anxieties at going to bed increased and he still dared not sleep without the lights on. Focusing on this problem, Steven described his fear that the monsters of the dark would come and do bad things to him. Why? Steven answered by drawing the teachers' attention to his excited waterplay with the faucets in the school bathroom and the mother became aware of how long it took Steven to bathe in the evening as he splashed around in the tub. It was now possible to show Steven that he felt very guilty over his play with his own body-faucet and over the genital excitement he felt from holding back urine—so guilty that it seemed safer to pass on to the grownups the job of knowing the rules and of controlling him than to listen to his own conscience. But when he was alone at night, the guilty feelings caught up with him as though they were monsters and threatened to punish him. Steven's newly harsh introject was evidently modelled on the killing angry father.

The concomitant working through of Steven's memories of the father's aggression in the context of his current oedipal anger at men seemed to help Steven modify his superego sufficiently to tolerate and utilize its injunctions more comfortably. He gradually involved himself more in his schoolwork, took pride in learning and achieving and especially enjoyed his gift in mathematics. Peers became friends and partners in play and work. He could structure his free time better with more available neutral energy and heeded the adults' reminders to check with himself whether this or that really seemed the right thing to do when Steven appeared to be on the verge of wrong-doing or loss of control. The withholding of urine stopped and he bathed more quickly. Steven thought ahead much to first grade in primary school where he wanted to do well and be a regular schoolboy. At home he managed nicely, pursued new interests and no longer needed his night light.

FOLLOW-UP

Steven has progressed well during his latency years. When he was about eight years old, his mother shared with me this conversation which he had happened to overhear between Steven and his new friend while the boys looked at toys and momentoes in his room: "You don't have a Dad, do you?" "That's right. My Dad died." "I know he died but how did he die?" "He had a mindsickness." "You mean he died of that mindsickness?" "No, his mindsickness made him so mixed up that he made himself die. The doctors tried to help his mindsickness but they couldn't." "Your Dad was a great swimmer, wasn't he?" "Yes, this is one of the trophies he won. He was a great swimmer."

It is too early to gauge whether Steven resolved his conflicts in such a way that they will not encroach upon his development or encumber his adolescence. His mother knows he may experience difficulties and may need an analysis at a later point.

REFERENCES

Furman, E. (1974), *A Child's Parent Dies*. New Haven: Yale University Press.

Furman, R. A. and Katan, A. (1969), *The Therapeutic Nursery School*. New York: International Universities Press.

Introductory Notes to Chapter 24

Rita V. Frankiel

This case report is an exceptional contribution to the literature on object loss because it provides a detailed narrative of the unfolding of transference in the treatment of a young girl quite seriously disturbed after the death of her mother. Not only is transference used effectively and reported in detail by the analyst, but the analyst also includes more information about her interventions and reactions than was typical at the time she was writing up this case, or even today, for that matter. This paper is therefore an exceptionally useful tool for teaching and learning about the analytic treatment of object loss.

Geraldine, eight at the time her mother died, was eleven years and eight months old when she began analysis with McCann. Her symptoms included amnesia and severe repression. The treatment, which began in prepuberty, continued until she was eighteen. The case report focuses on the analysis of the defenses that prevented her mourning and the use of the transference in illuminating the relationship with the mother, the circumstances of the mother's death, and the pathological mourning state that developed. Suitable replacement objects were not available and the girl was cared for for a time by a neighbor and later by maternal relatives. Treatment began when she was placed in a residential treatment center for emotionally disturbed children.

24. Mourning Accomplished by Way of the Transference

Marie E. McCann

In *Mourning and Melancholia* (1917), Freud asks the question, "In what, now, does the work which mourning performs consist?" and then proceeds with his answer:

I do not think there is anything far fetched in presenting it in the following way. Reality testing has shown that the loved object no longer exists and it proceeds to demand that all libido shall be withdrawn from its attachments to that object. This demand arouses understandable opposition—it is a matter of general observation that people never willingly abandon a libidinal position, not even, indeed, when a substitute is already beckoning to them. This opposition can be so intense that a turning away from reality takes place and a clinging to the object through the medium of hallucinatory wishful psychosis. Normally, respect for reality gains the day. Nevertheless its orders cannot be obeyed at once. They are carried out bit by bit, at great expense of time and cathectic energy, and in the meantime the existence of the lost object is psychically prolonged. Each single one of the memories and expectations in which the libido is bound to the object is brought up and hypercathected and detachment of the libido is accomplished in respect to it (244–45).

I shall attempt to show in the analysis of Geraldine how mourning the death of her mother was made possible via the transference. Geraldine was eleven years eight months of age when I first met her, and it had been three years and eight months since the death of her mother. She was a child who had not been capable of mourning her mother's death, which had occurred just one week before her eighth birthday. Geraldine had had the developmental readiness for mourning in that she had entered latency at the time of her loss of her mother but she had lacked several other factors essential to the accomplishment of mourning (R. Furman 1964). That is, she had not been prepared for her mother's death in that she had never been helped to under-

Reprinted by permission of the author and Quadrangle Books from *The Analyst and the Adolescent at Work*, edited by M. Harley, 1974.

stand the realities of the terminal illness; she had lacked the assurance that her needs would be met after her mother's death; and her environment had failed to offer her any of the support necessary to enable a child to mourn.

During her mother's terminal illness and following her death, Geraldine had utilized the defense of denial of all affects and in action, by being good instead of bad. Eleven months before Geraldine had begun treatment, she had developed amnesia, and repression had blotted out not only the associated affects but also the actual reality of her mother's terminal illness and death, and her own life in the two years and nine months subsequent to the loss of her mother. Geraldine began analysis with no real memory of her mother's death, thus eliminating reality testing by which memories are assigned to the past. Her analysis continued for six and one-half years and ended when she was a little over eighteen years of age, a week after her graduation from high school.

From the analytic work which extended from pre-puberty into late adolescence, I have selected the work related to the analysis of defenses which had prevented her mourning; the shifting and lifting of mechanisms; and the working through of the relationship with her mother, with facilitation of her mourning, via the transference. This thread is the focal aspect of her analysis and weaves throughout the entire period of her treatment.

PERTINENT HISTORY

Geraldine was an only child. She had a half-brother, seventeen years older than herself, and a half-sister, fourteen years her senior. The half-siblings were the children of the mother's first marriage. The mother married a second time and separated but had not yet obtained a divorce from her second husband when she began her relationship with Geraldine's father and when Geraldine was conceived. Actually, owing to further delays in obtaining the divorce, Geraldine was approximately three years old when her parents married.

Geraldine's father, now in his late sixties, worked as an independent waiter in a rather sporadic manner, earned minimal wages, and was constantly in debt. His history of chronic alcoholism and severe pathology (on occasion involving hallucinations and paranoid ideations) interfered with his functioning as a father, as a husband, and as a contributing member of society.

Geraldine's mother died of cancer at the age of forty-eight, one week before Geraldine's eighth birthday. Verified history revealed the mother's pregnancy with Geraldine as very difficult because of the presence of many uterine tumors. She was hospitalized six days prior to Geraldine's birth, which was by Caesarian section. She also had a hysterectomy at that time, with a history of multiple fibroid tumors for several years. The mother had excision of papilloma, left breast, when Geraldine was almost four and a half. Cancer was first diagnosed when Geraldine was almost seven years of age, and the mother had a mastectomy of the right breast, at which time there was a marked involvement of axillary glands. She was again hospitalized for X-ray therapy, was home briefly, then was hospitalized for a left breast mastectomy. She had a rapid metastasizing type of growth, with weight loss (her top weight had been 275 pounds), anorexia, vomiting, weakness, shortness of breath, and severe chest pain. She went to the emergency ward four months after her last surgery, was admitted, and died one day later.

The mother was described as having been extremely bright, a "whiz" at math, and employed in the accounting departments of several government offices. In personality, she was portrayed as a difficult, demanding, domineering, and stubborn woman. She was volatile and at times had an uncontrollable temper.

Early history was almost totally lacking because of the father's hazy and unreliable memory. Geraldine's mother stayed at home to care for Geraldine and tried to alleviate dire financial problems by caring for other babies and by sewing. She returned to full-time employment when Geraldine entered nursery school. The parents had violent fights, with many separations. The fights also involved Geraldine's half-brother, who left when she was quite young, and her half-sister who remained in the home. The wild fights were always very upsetting to Geraldine who was described as having clapped her hands over her ears and having run out of the house.

Following her mother's death, Geraldine stayed with her half-sister for one week, went to an aunt's for another week, and then moved to the home of a neighbor who had often cared for her when the mother was either working or ill. She remained at the neighbor's for a little over a year. The following summer she spent with maternal relatives on a farm and then, at the age of nine and a half, went to live with her maternal aunt and uncle. She remained there until her treatment began, which was when she was placed at the Children's Aid Society, a residential treatment center for emotionally disturbed children. Residential placement during her analysis was considered essential to insure continuation of her treatment by offering her controls and stability which her relatives could not provide because, against Geraldine's wishes, her father would occasionally take her for visits with him. Neither Geraldine nor the father described what occurred on the visits, but they became increasingly upsetting to Geraldine and she eventually asked her aunt not to allow the father to take her away from the aunt's home. She also needed protection in the event that there was further exacerbation of the amnesia.

The causative factors in the onset of the amnesia are still only partially understood. The initial knowledge was that the amnesia had followed her deceptively having changed D grades in music to B's (she was an excellent student); and she had responded to a reprimand for the deception by running away for several hours; that she had received threats by her father of being sent away to a "bad girls' " school; that she had gone to school the following day and had failed to return home at the close of school that day. Only during the subsequent years were other factors learned which doubtlessly related to the grossly overdetermined causes of the amnesia. These precipitants included a weakening of her denial of sexuality and of her femininity upon seeing a school film on menses (she had forged her aunt's signature on the permission slip, too guilty to mention it); and a pelvic examination subsequent to the trouble at school because she had described a man following her on that runaway day. Other important events, revealed much later in her treatment, included her aunt's angina attack; her father's proposal that the two of them move to another state; his telling her at that time of her illegitimate birth; and a false report of the sudden death of her father which had been given to her by one of the father's friends.

When Geraldine had been found wandering in a dazed state, she had known neither who she was nor where she lived. She had said that she had a severe headache; she had realized that she was on the wrong bus; she had known that her mother was not with her; and she had asked a strange man to take her to a hospital. She had been returned to her aunt with the aid of the police. The father had had Geraldine hospitalized for complete neurological studies, and no organic basis had been found. She had then been referred to a child psychiatry clinic. At the onset of the amnesia, Geraldine had recognized only her father, then later her half-sister. She had had no memory of her mother's terminal illness and death. The eleven-month delay until her placement at the Children's Aid Society and the beginning of treatment had been due to the fact that no analytic opening was yet available.

The aunt gave a full description of Geraldine as she had known her. She referred to her as strong-willed and determined, with "lots of grit." She felt the closeness in their relationship had developed after the onset of the amnesia when she had remained out of school for the semester. Prior to the amnesia, Geraldine had been withdrawn and distant. She had never cried and had controlled her anger, although she had expressed it in looks of cold fury and in devious ways. She was of very superior intelligence and had artistic and musical talent (her mother had played the piano and had sung well, often participating in church services). Geraldine had been transferred to Major Work classes (for children of superior intelligence) when she was ten and a half. Her amnesia had not affected her reading, but she had forgotten all of her math except simple addition. Geraldine had no close friends and chose only children whom she could dominate and rule. She was competitive and jealous. After the amnesia, she withdrew from peers completely.

REVIEW OF THE TREATMENT

Geraldine at eleven was of average height and of slightly stocky build, with beginning breast development and mild acne. Her complexion was light brown; her large eyes were intense and in no way shadowed by her dark-rimmed glasses. Her shoulder-length hair was worn in two braids. She had an air of quaintness about her—in her dress but even more in her overall appearance. In conversation, she spoke voluminously with a vocabulary far advanced for her age, avoiding slang and with stress on propriety and impressing others. She often used literary references quite aptly and as proof of how well read she was. She presented herself as calm, self-assured, and in command of the situation. Her posture had a stiffness and rigidity. Most striking was her lack of true affect, and her deceptiveness at times through her effort to portray the affect which she felt was appropriate and expected of her.

Geraldine approached me and treatment with wariness, caution, and a manifest attitude of cooperation: she came promptly and talked incessantly. She set out to impress and to please me. Early in her treatment, she offered factual statements about her amnesia, describing its onset or saying, "I know my mother is dead, but I cannot remember it." Such statements disappeared as she tried to keep the amnesia hidden from all others: it was a defect, to be hidden and ashamed of. The most notable aspect in those early months was Geraldine's lack of any genuine affects, the frozen quality of her personality and the shallowness of her relationships.

The character of her relationship with me initially was clearly a need for my presence, which was most evident in her reaction to my three absences during that first year. While I was there, all was fine; when I was away, everything seemed very different and her self-control seemed to vanish to an alarming degree. Her need for my presence was gradually understood as her need to have me there to support her "proper girl" self. The origin of this was her tendency to adopt the behavior which various parent substitutes had expected of her and which, to a great extent, coincided with the ideal of a good daughter which her mother had held up for her (although she had failed to serve her as a model).

My first absence resulted in Geraldine's acting out an identification with her mother in her verbal attack on her father for his neglect, thus displacing her anger toward me to him. This outburst stunned the father. Geraldine had never spoken to him like that and "it was just as if his wife had returned from the grave." A few months later, I was away for one week and she repressed the approaching separation. But while I was gone, she was depressed, cried frequently, and had serious fights with the other girls in the cottage. Although these reactions frightened her, the most terrifying aspect was the extent of the emotional impact of my absence. When I returned, all was fine; she described affectlessly what had occurred and added reproachfully, "I don't understand it at all, and I don't know why I'm so certain, but I'm positive that none of this would have happened if you had been here."

I agreed that such strength of feelings did not make much sense unless we understood that they were not just of the here and now but were feeling memories from older times in her life. She had felt then that things got out of control when that very important person—her Mama—was not with her. Although she scoffed at such an explanation, there ensued the first meaningful discussion of her mother, a partial lifting of her amnesia. She told of the week following her mother's death when her sister had carried out the plans for Geraldine's eighth birthday party, plans that had been initiated by her mother. She said, "I know my sister Joanne was trying to cheer me up, make me happy"; and we could now talk of this reversal of affect, the "happy good mood" which was the affective counterpart of denial, a defense which, as I have already mentioned, was often employed by Geraldine. Her further talk of her mother was bland and affectless as she described how unavailable her mother always had been: "She did little for me as she was always either working or ill." However, in her poems and plays Geraldine presented repeated themes of loneliness and having to fend for herself. When we could view the clear loyalty conflict in one of her plays, true affect began to enter the sessions.

The fourth anniversary of her mother's death was now near and Geraldine told of her envy of her mother who had gotten chocolates Geraldine longed for but never could get and who could play the piano beautifully by ear while Geraldine had to learn to read notes laboriously. She had been unable to compete with her mother and had demonstrated this by dropping piano lessons. She became openly depressed and self-injury was evident in a fall and a painfully injured knee on the actual anniversary date of the mother's death.

As my summer vacation approached, Geraldine could never remember it, the dates and details, but negated my reference to her tendency to forget unpleasant things. This repression was accompanied by an intensification of all of her other defenses: denial, isolation, denial of affect, and rationalization. During my vacation, she became very upset, feared she would "crack up," and accused a male staff member of trying to kiss her. She wrote me an unmailed letter of reproach. Geraldine was experiencing added internal pressure at this time in that her menses had started shortly before I left for vacation. She could not even mention this to me and when I brought it up, her reply, "It's a perfectly normal, natural thing that happens to every girl sometimes between the ages of twelve and twenty-one" was bereft of any feeling. I asked if she had read this in a book somewhere and her shy reply was, "Sure, that's how I have learned most things." We could then speak of her turning to books, rather than to people, for answers and we could also identify this as her "learning through her head and not through her heart" (with feelings via a human relationship).

When I returned from vacation, she told me of the events which had transpired, but she had no feeling whatsoever. We could then see how, during my absence, she had become terribly anxious and out of control. When I came back, the crisis was over, she had lived through it, and the anxiety was gone. This pattern she repeated many times. And thus she often repeated her tremendous anxiety of being overwhelmed, of being annihilated, engendered by a fear that her needs would go unfulfilled.

A new quality of a positive mother-child relationship emerged in the treatment as she read fairy tales and sang lullabies to me. When I said that her Mama must have done such things with her, she disagreed with annoyance: her mother had been too busy.

President Kennedy's assassination brought forth her initial denial and incredulity of death news, then an appropriate but most intellectual description of her reaction. Her only affective response was to seeing the casket lowered into the ground. When I spoke of an earlier funeral—her Mama's—she vehemently denied that this was relevant. "I was too young, I knew nothing of Mama's funeral, I wasn't even there." The following week, she fell in the gym and broke her left leg, requiring a toe-to-thigh cast for ten weeks.

However, she missed only one treatment session, the day of the fracture. She described her trip to the emergency ward, her pains and fears. She expressed an unrecognized loneliness as she described the miserable day. Very soon afterward, she began asking me personal questions: where did I live, what was my home like? She reminisced about how her mother used to take her up "that hill" to the suburb where I live. She recalled how it used to seem to her "like going into a different world."

At Christmas, Geraldine spoke of having, for the first time in her life, a feeling of Christmas—of love—inside herself. Within a few days, she openly professed her deep love for me but could not bring into analysis her subsequent frustration and anger engendered by my lack of reciprocation. It was at this point that a cottage parent's mother died of cancer and Geraldine was hospitalized overnight for severe abdominal pains, with no positive physical findings. She told me of her desolate loneliness in the hospital, negating that her longing was for me, and proceeding to displace her feelings for me to the resident at the hospital. She developed an open crush on him, wrote him notes, and at times chastized him for his double talk to her. My attempts to bring this into the treatment were met with vehement disagreement, criticism of me and the conclusion that I was "a nut."

Through the month of January she showed no anxiety about leaving elementary school. However, she fell twice the first week of February, her first week in the overwhelming junior high school. That was also the week in which her cast was removed. I reminded her of this pattern of not permitting anxiety ahead of time, her fear of being overwhelmed, having to get through the crisis and then letting her feelings out in some way. I went on to say that it must have been this way at the time of her mother's death, when she had had real needs and no idea of how they would be met. She furiously disagreed on the basis that her loss was minor since her mother had never been able to do that much for her anyway. (This feeling was omnipresent in the transference.) However, that night she sobbed unconsolably for hours, slipped and twice fell in the hall.

Geraldine was steadily becoming more upset; her old defenses were no longer effective. She regressed (was infantile in her play), isolated herself to her room, and withdrew from peers; her school work deteriorated; she was furtive and suspicious, and talked of seeing a man in a brown suit lurking around. I knew all of these things about her but not from her; with me she was angry, short, and sarcastic, refusing to discuss anything. She had a wild, out-of-control episode one stormy night when she crawled out the music room window, ran around the campus, and crawled into the senior boys' cottage, where she was found sleeping on the floor. Her diary explanation, which she sent to my office, was that she thought she was going crazy, that an adolescent boy, Carl had made her go out, that she felt as if she were standing aside watching herself, and later realized that Carl was really part of herself.

I can only speculate on precipitates for this acting out of Geraldine's bisexual conflict, and the data for my speculations came only years later. A few days preceding this episode, she had seen a sex-education film at school, and the science teacher had asked for a volunteer in an experiment. Geraldine had volunteered and was asked to lift something from a can. The object proved to be the heart of a cow. She had been filled with horror, repulsion, and had felt ill. It seems clear that Geraldine denied affects and facts regarding sexuality just as she did regarding illness, surgery, and death. To her, growing up and becoming a woman meant being attacked sexually, being attacked surgically and dying.

It was quite soon after this incident, on the fifth anniversay of her mother's death, that Geraldine truanted, spent the day in a church, and reported taking forty aspirins over a three-day period. She would not discuss any of this with me (the aspirin taking, the trip to the emergency ward, the day spent in church, the truancy, and so on) but soon began to treat me openly like a mother, asking me what her dress size was and instructing her father to leave her birthday gifts with me. Within a few days, she had reversed her positive feelings for me to hate and had then projected them onto the other girls— they hated her, were out to hurt her, to kill her.

This behavior reached a height one day when she refused to leave school to return to the residential treatment center: she was not safe, was subject to attack, was mistreated, and she feared her amnesia would return. She was brought home from school by a cottage parent and came to her session looking horrible: drawn, tense, masklike. Walking in like a robot, she said, "I have taken all I can. I can stand no more." When I replied that this must be exactly as she had felt much earlier in her life, she began sobbing, "Yes, but it's five years now since Mama died. I should be over it, but I'm not. I want more than anything for someone to hold me tight and really mean it." She told, in detail and with tremendous affect, of her mother's final trip to the hospital, of having been told by Joanne of Mama's death. Joanne had told her that Mama had gone to join Jesus and that Geraldine would join her there one day. Geraldine had sat staring and Joanne had asked if she had heard and Geraldine had replied, "Yes, Mama is dead." She had not cried until that night at a neighbor's home; she had been afraid to cry lest she might not be able to stop. She recalled having cried for twelve hours, alone, without comfort or support.

Geraldine told of the funeral, the hymns sung, the trip to the cemetery, the adults discussing whether she should go to the graveside, and their decision that she was too young. Thus she had sat alone in the car. She explained she had not seen Mama lowered into the ground; the first time she had seen that was with President Kennedy. We talked of her longing for reunion with Mama (a merged relationship), of her taking the aspirin as a gesture which reflected this longing; yet this was not what Mama would have wanted for her. She was now thirteen, her needs for Mama were less than at age eight, she had capabilities, could do more for herself. After this, she was better able to deal with her positive feelings toward me—once offering herself to me in her wish to be my cat, to be loyal and loved.

A new resistance now emerged in the treatment: Geraldine refused to take in my words and was repulsed by anything I said. On the one hand, she showed an oral inhibition by missing meals, and, on the other hand, out-of-control orality by eating paper in the sessions. I spoke of her inability to eat what she should, yet her reaction to my words was as if she were saying, "Don't feed me that line." She responded by narrating an early experience when she had foolishly made a hot dog, and, using her finger and a piece of paper, she bit herself. She looked repulsed as she added, "How can cannibals do it—eat humans?" I equated her affect with her response to my words, as if taking them in were devouring me as well, being cannibalistic. It was following this work that Geraldine for the first time seemed truly allied with me in the treatment. She progressed in many ways: showed increased self-esteem, evidenced a Negro identity which she had consistently denied, looked and dressed more like an adolescent, and was, in general, more attractive. Her domination of peers shifted to more genuine leadership, with an exchange of affection in her relationships.

Geraldine now also manifested a difference in her reaction to my summer vacation. She showed no repression. She was angry with me and equated my trip with her mother's "trips" to the hospital. Her mother, she said, had always deceived her. She had never spoken of cancer, had told her she was going to the hospital for an examination, yet had always returned having had surgery. Geraldine voiced these complaints with annoyance and irritation, a preamble to a later expression of stronger aggression toward her mother. Yet these complaints were memorable as the first nuances of direct angry feelings toward her mother. Her own guilt and defense of undoing were discernible as she told how her father had drunk and worried her mother, as if worry caused cancer. In contrast, she had avoided worrying her mother by helping at home and by getting very good grades.

There was also a gradual change in Geraldine's relationship with her father. She became openly glad to see him and was eager to meet some of his relatives who were visiting from a nearby state. She made her father a birthday card, then quickly and guiltily made one for me. Thus there appeared, in the transference, the first oedipal jealousy with concomitant guilt and the need to atone. Geraldine's guilt still prevented her from identifying with her mother, but she began to identify with her aunt by an interest in cooking and by working with younger children at church.

Geraldine's progress was interrupted by the very serious and for some time undiagnosed illness of her aunt, the one who was so meaningful for her and with whom she had lived. She repeated her earlier denial of illness by asking friends into the home on one of her regular Sunday visits and thus acting as if her aunt were feeling fine. I pointed out this repetition to her and she acknowledged that she was terrified; her aunt "looked like a ghost." She had thought "Here it is again. Where will I go, where will they send me?" She felt like running away, but where? This acknowledgement led to her recall of events preceding the amnesia: her conviction that her aunt would die when she had had an angina attack; her memory of her father's proposal to take her away to live with him in another state, and his disclosure then of the fact that the parents had not been married until she was three years old. She described how she had suddenly felt that she did not care about anything and as though her head were held on by strings. It was after this partial lifting of the repression that, for the first time, Geraldine recalled the woman with whom she had lived during the year following her mother's death. Her conclusion about this return of the repressed was "I am getting help."

Her aunt's physical condition improved, but she then had a relapse at the end of December and told Geraldine she expected to enter the hospital for tests during that week. That same day she also reprimanded Geraldine for secretly wearing lipstick at church and expressed strong disapproval of Geraldine's forwardness at church with an adolescent boy with whom she was infatuated. Simultaneously, Geraldine experienced two other very upsetting events. She visited her father's apartment for the first time in two years and saw evidence of the fact that his lady friend had recently moved in with him. This was a repetition of earlier experiences of having been rebuffed by her father. Now he had a lady friend living with him and Geraldine was again "out."

Earlier, the father had seductively encouraged her ideas of living with him and keeping house for him after her mother's death but in reality had clearly offered nothing. Then again, prior to the onset of the amnesia, he had proposed that the two of them move together to another state. It seems clear that Geraldine's oedipal guilt was intensified at the time of her father's rebuffs. In the treatment, she was extremely upset by my news that I would be leaving the residential treatment center, even though she knew intellectually that her treatment would not be interrupted. Again, she could voice no anxiety about any of these events, yet acted out the anxiety by running away, taking Sominex, and appearing late that night at the hospital emergency ward, asking for a reevaluation. She told of her worry about her aunt's health, her fear of cancer, and her feeling that her birth had been responsible for her mother's illness and eventual death.

Subsequently, Geraldine refused to talk with or visit her aunt, declaring that her aunt's heart could stand no more, that she had already caused her aunt enough trouble. I interpreted her identification with her aunt, explaining that she had heard of her expectation that she would go into the hospital and that she had then brought about her own trip to the hospital, as if what happened to her aunt also happened to her. Now in the sessions, Geraldine excluded me and tried to hurt my feelings—employing again her defense of reversing passive to active. She feared she would contract epilepsy, saying good people did not get epilepsy, and equated illness with loss of control to a murderous degree. In her sessions she acted like Jesse James, but refuted her own murderous thoughts and subsequent guilt in relation to me. While negating all interpretations, she tentatively acknowledged the existence of the unconscious (referred to by her as "things in the back part of my mind") in her discussion of her slips of the tongue, described by her as "skid talk"—a topic which was being currently discussed in her English class.

As Geraldine again became friendlier toward me, both positive and negative oedipal elements appeared in the transference. She was jealous of me in reference to her father: he always seemed so eager to see me, so hurried to end their visits so that he could spend time with me. Then she displaced her excitement with me onto the girls at school and described how embarrassed she had been when they had hugged and kissed her after her original song had been played in a school program. She said she wished that she could avoid the girls and "all that excitement." When she missed her next session with me, I pointed out her displacement and her concomitant avoidance of excitement with me. To this she replied, "You're a nut—a real nut."

Geraldine reacted strongly to the fact that she was the only Children's Aid Society child whom I would continue to see after my job change. She was excited and elated at being my "chosen child" yet filled with guilt. We could relate her concept of "chosen child" to its popular equivalent in that an adopted child is often referred to as a "chosen child." This stirred her guilt about eliminating her competitors, that is, the other children, and also stirred her loyalty conflict. Her wish to be my chosen child meant being disloyal to her mother, to her aunt, and ultimately to her own race. In her fantasy, it also represented being male in that she thought she would literally come with me and that I would be working with boys in the adolescent residence which was housed in the same building where I would have my office. She felt she would live there and would have to cut her hair and wear boys' clothing to be acceptable to me.

With the approach of the sixth anniversary of her mother's death, I mentioned Geraldine's failure to say anything about this. Her angry retort was: "What do you expect me to do, celebrate?" But once more she brought nursing books and renewed her interest in becoming a nurse, this always having occurred as an undoing when her aggression toward her mother became strengthened. Her father then requested a birthday visit to his home and, on the day following his request, Geraldine fainted in school. She confirmed my suggestion of a connection between these two occurrences by telling of many early trips with her father to various churches, where wild orgies took place and "women were fainting all over the place." That was a time when she was terrified of her father but this no longer was true. She wanted a visit but felt that attending church with him was not a good idea. The visit went well.

With me, Geraldine became increasingly disappointed and frustrated by my not doing enough for her. These feelings were now displaced onto her young, male French teacher. In one session, she performed for me the interpretive dance that she had choreographed to the song "Somewhere." She took the part of "Len," treating me as her partner, and the dance represented a search for love, love of a mother. The next day in school she had a panic reaction, fell, backed into a corner, and felt as if she were being stabbed. I interpreted her reaching toward me in the dance as reaching toward a mother, as well as her disappointment, deep frustration, and killing (stabbing) wishes. Her guilt ultimately resulted in her feeling that it was she who was being stabbed. This led to her musing about the incident a few months previously, when she had taken the Sominex and had gone to the hospital. She said she was "truly glad" that had happened because it had brought about a change in her: prior to that she had felt like "half a person" and that whatever happened to someone dear to her was happening to her. Suddenly she had realized that she was Geraldine, a separate person, and that the Sominex would have hurt her.

Subsequent analytic unfolding included many references to the superiority of males. Geraldine wrote a poem as if depicting herself as a tall, lanky farm lad; she identified herself with the soldiers in Vietnam. Her original songs were songs of love—search, unworthiness, declaration, rebuff, reunion—in which a strong male identity was apparent. And we could now discuss her belief that being male meant being first and crowding out all competitors, including her father, for her mother.

Geraldine's anger about being female was basically directed toward her mother but appeared in relation to her sister. Joanne's advanced pregnancy was the impetus for revealing her fantasies in respect to conception. She said she knew that the father determined the sex of the baby. She knew that with her brain. Yet she still harked back to her earlier belief that the mother had the baby and controlled the baby's body formation: sex, coloring, and so on. We could then look at her conviction that it was her mother who denied her the "number one status," that is, to be male. She often referred to herself through her parody of a national car rental advertisement: "I'm number two, but I try harder."

Geraldine's anger at her mother as the source of her femininity emerged in the transference several months later. We were discussing Joanne's uterine hemorrhaging, or, more accurately, I was verbalizing this, while Geraldine sat in icy silence which reflected her controlled rage. She then reproached me for giving her "nothing good, only the bad." She wanted nothing from me: no news, no explanations. "Female troubles" were repulsive to her and she wanted to know nothing of Joanne's physical condition. At the end of this session, as she scooped up her books and papers, she took my ballpoint pen. She was embarrassed the next day when I inquired about this and apologized for forgetting to bring the pen back. She continued to forget it, finally lost it, and later replaced it with a pen she begged from her father. We could see her strong need for something from me, who gave her nothing. And I suggested that she had earlier felt this way about her mother.

Geraldine's aggression to women increased in many directions. She was angry with her aunt for not extending an immediate invitation to her upon the resumption of her (Geraldine's) relationship with her. She was hurt and furious because Joanne did not tell her directly of her son's birth. She was jealous of her eighteen-year-old girl cousin when the latter visited her aunt for the summer and used her old room. She became angry at her father's lady friend when she saw the robe this woman had given him for his birthday; such an intimate gift seemed to shatter her denial that their relationship was a platonic one. She proceeded with her requests for visits with her father and her aunt two weeks before my vacation. She was angry with me about the vacation and wished "much wrath on my head."

Geraldine had these two visits and became very upset. She saw her nephew for the first time and was most offended because her sister had subtly prevented her from holding him. The next day she swallowed three safety pins (my unspoken thoughts were of diaper pins), one of which had to be removed surgically from her esophagus. When she returned to treatment, after her two days in the hospital, I interpreted to her her aggression toward the introject. I spoke of how earlier it had seemed that when something happened to someone else, it seemed to be happening to her. This seemed to be the other side of the coin. Her anger toward others was taken out on herself, as if it were not happening to her at all but to someone else instead.

Geraldine was definite about not wanting any visits while I was away. She felt discouraged about her treatment but was buoyed up by my speaking of how she had gotten through difficult times before and could again. The last day before my vacation, she brought her guitar, sang the Beatles' song "Help," and smiled when I said I felt I had gotten the message. She added,

"Sometimes I can sing what I cannot say." She managed well as a model citizen while I was away.

I have given some fairly detailed accounts of the first two and three-quarters years of Geraldine's analysis to illustrate the quality of her object relationship and how its development via the transference made mourning possible. The ensuing three and three-quarters years followed more typical analytic unfolding. She engaged in relatively little acting out, showed increasing tolerance for anxiety and an ego capacity to involve and ally herself in the treatment. She now became my sole source of information; and she brought material, albeit at times with much resistance. External reality events (illness of her sister and of her father) ushered in regressions for brief periods, but these regressions never reached the point of a merging with the object.

Sequentially, the analysis unfolded with many ups and downs. There was a period of resistance, this time anal in form. For a time, Joanne then became a focus for her ambivalence. As her aggression toward women became more conscious and more tolerable, she had less need to deny it in action, that is, in being good instead of bad. Originally, this need to be good had taken the form of being a good student so as not to worry her mother. During this period of our work on her aggression toward her mother, her grades declined markedly. Later they rose but this time not as a defensive maneuver.

After more work on her bisexual conflict and on her oedipal rivalry, Geraldine no longer denied her sexuality. She began asking for sexual information, stating that for one who was sixteen, she was grossly naive. She produced many of her sexual fantasies, the majority of which emerged more readily after I had given her a bit of factual information.

Primal scene material entered the treatment via dreams, screen memories and, later, through transference manifestations. Only after this work was Geraldine truly able to learn the details of her mother's illness. She had condensed the two mastectomies into one, yet was puzzled because her recollection involved two separate apartments at the time of surgery. She asked for clarification by way of doctor's reports and hospital records. This clarification of the reality was indeed helpful to her as she was then able to recall more details of the timing of surgery and the places where they had lived. Thus memory of the two separate mastectomies returned.

Typically adolescent, she worked at arriving at her standards and choices regarding many things, including the choice of a church; which was preceded by a period in which she was an agnostic. As for the type of radical identity which was "right" for her, she "knew she was no Uncle Tom," and finally concluded that she was aggressive for blacks' rights but not revolutionary.

During the process of adolescent object removal (A. Katan 1937) as she moved into dating, she spoke of the conflicting standards in her background. Her mother had married twice, had lived with her father, had had her, then had married him only much later. Her identification with this aspect of her mother became apparent in her strong identification with a friend who thought she was pregnant. Geraldine told of having morning nausea, adding, "Who ever heard of a pregnant virgin?" and it was she, Geraldine, who fainted when the friend found that she was not pregnant. When Geraldine had first heard of the friend's suspicions of being pregnant, she had been shocked, had disapproved, and had spent several days crying uncontrollably in her sessions.

She could see that her degree of affective reaction was out of proportion to the current reality and agreed to a connection with her first knowledge of her mother having been unmarried when she had become pregnant and of her illegitimate birth. Her tears could then be understood as a piece of her mourning—her mourning the death of her idealized mother when she had learned from her father the circumstance of her conception and birth. This information had followed the actual death of the mother by two and one-half years and had preceded the onset of her amnesia. We could also gain some insight into a major determinant in her symptom of falling as an identification with the "fallen woman," her mother.

Geraldine also talked of her father's double standard: he lectured her to be a "good girl" yet he still failed to marry the woman he had been living with for years, "just like with Mama." Her aunt represented severe morality: she was extremely rigid and considered card playing, dancing, dating before age eighteen as all evil. Geraldine decided, "I have to look at these standards of others and come up with my own."

Her reactions to separation and loss occurred several times with favorite teachers as well as with those staff members of the residential treatment center when she moved, at age sixteen and a half, to a group home for twelve adolescent girls. Of course, the end of her analysis loomed steadily during the final fifteen months of treatment, even through she would be in touch with me in the future (which she has been). She was able to deal with these losses with most appropriate affects. When the termination date was about four months away, she had three brief periods of amnesia (called "lapses" by her), two of them occurring as she left my office. In our discussion of these "lapses," we could see how the old pain of loss (the fear that the feeling was too great) was intolerable since she not only felt nothing, but she knew nothing—the blank of amnesia. These three incidents took place within a two-week period and did not reoccur.

I might conclude with some of Geraldine's reflective comments during the final months of her analysis. As to her many struggles with her aggressive feelings and how she dealt with them: "With Mama, I was scared to death to step out of line. I saw with my own eyes how she attacked, in words and actions, my Dad and sister and after all I was just a little kid—very power-less." And, "Mama didn't treat Dad too well at times. I remember once when I was about five, he was hospitalized with pneumonia. We moved and Mama didn't even tell him because she was mad at him." Another description of her dilemma was: 'How could I ever be mad at Mama; she was really the only security I had. You really have to side with the parent who looks after you."

Geraldine had always known that her mother was regarded as the black sheep by all of her relatives and that she, Geraldine, was never thought of as a person, only as "Helen's daughter." In her early years, relatives were never around or interested in her, and her aunt had taken her in, after her year with the family friend, more from a sense of family duty than because of any genuine love for her. She recalled that her aunt could never tolerate "back talk" and she was convinced that her aunt could know if she had even an angry thought. But Geraldine was equally in touch with the positive factors in these relationships. She spoke of her gratitude to her mother for imbuing her with a love for music, and reading, both of which were great pleasures in her life. She was realistic about her aunt, "We will always disagree on many things; my aunt is old and won't change and, after all, she has a right to her own opinions too." Her aunt's husband she had always regarded with fondness and admiration; she admired his sensitivity, patience, and industriousness.

As to her earlier denial of all affect, again Geraldine's own statements are more descriptive than any I might make. "You know, I think my treatment, or really my life, has been sort of in three phases. At first, I blotted out all feelings—things happened that were more than I could endure—I had to keep going. If I had really let things hit me, I wouldn't be here. I'd be dead or in a mental hospital. I let myself feel nothing and my thoughts were all involved with fantasies, fairy tales, science fiction. Then, in the second phase, my feelings took over and ruled me. I did things that were way out.

And in the third phase, now, my feelings are here, I feel them and I have control over them. One of my big assets is that I can experience things, with genuine feelings. At times it hurts, but the advantages, the happiness, far outweigh the pain.''

Her reflection on her relationship with me she expressed when she brought her boy friend to meet me, several months after ending her analysis. She explained that she had told her husband-to-be all about herself, her life, her treatment. She referred to me as her friend, then turning to her boy friend, she said, "She never lectured me, blamed me, chastized me, praised me—she let me be me, she helped me know and to sort of like myself.''

Her gains were notable in this period of adolescence, when she had to try to accomplish the developmental tasks as well as the major task of mourning a loss which had had to be blotted temporarily from her memory and which took along with it the capacity to feel herself worthy of living. Life events will help determine her future since her tendencies toward somatization and action under great anxiety remain, although they are under relatively good control. Many aspects of this lengthy analysis I have, of course, excluded in my attempts to focus on the task of mourning which was accomplished via the transference.

BIBLIOGRAPHY

Freud, A. 1960. Discussion of Dr. John Bowlby's "Grief and mourning in infancy and early childhood." *Psychoanalytic Study of the Child* 15:53–63.

Freud, S. 1917. Mourning and melancholia. *Standard Edition*, vol. 14. London: Hogarth Press, 1955.

Furman, R. 1964. Death and the young child: Some preliminary considerations. *Psychoanalytic Study of the Child* 19:321–34.

Katan, A. 1937. The role of "displacement" in agoraphobia. *International Journal of Psycho-Analysis* 32:41–50.

Introductory Notes to Chapter 25

Rita V. Frankiel

Lerner describes the need to search for, find, and symbolically reclaim in the external world a version of a love object lost in early childhood. In the course of treating patients trying to recover from the sequelae of early losses, Lerner observes that this recapture of the lost object serves essential functions in restoring their sense of narcissistic intactness. It is Lerner's impression that what is accomplished is a more complete and acknowledged internal representation of the lost object that can then be more fully mourned. Jacobson's contribution on this subject (chapter 14), while not cited by Lerner, is a significant contribution to understanding these phenomena.

25. The Treatment of Early Object Loss: The Need to Search

Paul M. Lerner

With his publication in 1917 of *Mourning and Melacholia,* Freud laid the conceptual groundwork from which most subsequent psychoanalytic theories of loss have arisen. In that work Freud described the mental features of mourning (i.e., feelings of painful dejection, a loss of interest in the outside world, an inability to love, a massive inhibition of all activity), outlined the mourning process (i.e., a gradual relinquishment of and severing of emotional ties to the lost object and a corresponding displacement of the libidinal cathexis onto other objects), and distinguished mourning from melancholia. He noted that melancholia, like mourning, may be a reaction to the loss of a loved object; at the same time it differs from mourning in that the individual "cannot see clearly what it is that has been lost. . . . He knows whom he has lost but not *what* he has lost in him" (245). Freud went on to observe that "in mourning it is the world which has become poor and empty; in melancholia it is the ego itself" (246).

Anna Freud (1960), in a deceptively simple way, described mourning as "the individual's effort to accept a fact in the external world and to effect corresponding changes in the inner world" (54).

Debate abounds in psychoanalysis over whether children are capable of mourning in a comparable way to adults (A. Freud 1960). Authors point to the complex ego functions involved in mourning, including a concept of reality, an ability to take cognitive distance, a capacity to bear pain, and a capacity to summon an inner image of the object in its absence. They question whether children have these capacities.

Other questions are raised with respect to at what age children reach sufficient levels of ego development to comprehend the concept of death and

Reprinted by permission of Lawrence Erlbaum Associates, Inc., from *Psychoanalytic Psychology* 7(1) (1990):79-90.

the idea of its finality (Furman 1974; Schur 1960; Shambaugh 1961; Spitz 1960; Wolf 1958; Wolfenstein 1966). Developmental achievements including self-other differentiation, grasping the distinction between animate and inanimate objects, understanding time (especially a future perspective), and reality testing appear essential in order for the child to conceive of death as involving the cessation of certain functions.

In contrast with far-ranging disagreement as to when the child is capable of comprehending death and experiencing mourning, there is a consensus that early parent loss is traumatic and that the younger the child, the more devastating the effects. Authors have drawn attention to the impact of early object loss on the child's drive development (Meis 1953), formation of intrapsychic structures (Jacobson 1964; Loewald 1978; Mahler, Pine and Bergman 1975), and emerging sense of self and concept of the other (Atwood 1974; Tahka 1984; Tyson 1983; Wolfenstein 1966). Collectively, these writers have noted that although the impact is dramatic and pervasive, it is also complex and depends on a multitude of internal and external factors including the mitigating aspects of defense, the availability of substitute objects, and the degree to which inner psychic structures have become autonomous from the supporting objects (Lerner and Lerner 1987).

Although several clinical reports (Meis 1953; Shambaugh 1961; Wolfenstein 1966) have described the treatment of children who have experienced a significant loss, there is sparingly little in the literature regarding the treatment of adults who, as children, experienced a major loss.

In treating several such adult patients I have repeatedly observed a particular phenomenon that seems coincident with a good treatment outcome. Specifically, it has been my experience that the treatment process itself sets in motion within the patient a compelling need to seek out, rediscover, and then symbolically reclaim the lost object in the real world. These patients are not satisfied with simply experiencing the object anew transferentially in the person of the therapist. Rather, they seem bent on capturing something more concrete and more directly related to the object, and their quest invariably takes them beyond the bounds of the treatment setting. I present excerpts from two cases to illustrate the importance for the patient of setting out on such a search and then discuss the phenomenon in terms of our understanding of the mourning process. The cases also serve to illustrate the delicate interplay that occurs between the treatment process and the external search.

CASE EXAMPLE 1

The patient, a 36-year-old, twice-divorced, interior designer, sought treatment soon after the painful termination of a nine-month relationship with a married man five years her junior. With the realization that her brief, highly romantic involvements with married or otherwise unavailable men were becoming a distinct pattern, she became obsessed with the thought that she was destined to spend the remainder of her life unmarried and essentially alone. This coincided with a palm reading in which the reader pointed out that she had been fated by her father's death.

The youngest of three girls, she experienced the first of several losses at age five when her father died of a brain tumor. Four years later, when the patient was nine, her mother had a severe stroke resulting in paralysis of one side of her body and the loss of speech. Following her mother's stroke, a distant, uninvited uncle intruded on and split up the family. The two older sisters were sent to boarding school while the patient and her mother were taken to the uncle's farm in a small, rural community. During the next several years a maternal grandmother died, her oldest and favorite sister married and moved to a distant city, and she and her mother were frequently and thoughtlessly shifted from relative to relative. When the patient was sixteen, her mother suffered another stroke and died. Thus, by mid-adolescence, the patient had lost both parents and a grandmother through death and a sister through marriage, and had essentially raised herself.

The patient began her analysis by providing, in a highly controlled and typically affectless manner, a comprehensive, exhaustively detailed chronicle of her life beginning with her father's death and extending through other deaths and losses, her two marriages and subsequent divorces, the birth of her daughter, her cervical cancer confirmed and operated on soon after her daughter's birth, and her many and varied affairs. As she spent each analytic hour meticulously recalling and detailing each of these events in their entirety, I gradually became aware of her inordinate need for control, defensive use of compliance, excessive investment in self-sufficiency, yearning for but intense fear of belonging, longstanding search for the ideal man who would love her, and overriding desire to feel genuine. Throughout this period, I, paradoxically, felt like an ignored bystander watching her, in her characteristically self-reliant manner, conduct her own analysis. I also felt like a captive audience constantly being monitored to ensure that my attention did not wander off. As well, I experienced the sensation that I was a protective container into which she was pouring the hardships and suffering life had visited on her. Mindful of the dangerous, unwanted, intrusive uncle of childhood, the infrequent remarks I did make involved attempts to empathize with her and recognize the immense pain and sadness that had accompanied her much of her life. She responded to these comments with genuine but controlled and muted gratitude—as if they were unexpected, unsolicited, mildly intrusive, but nonetheless, precious gifts.

In the eleventh month of treatment, the first extended separation from analysis occurred. During the three-week break, the patient's efforts to be in control and entirely self-sufficient failed to quiet and contain intense feelings of emptiness, loneliness, and isolation. She also suffered the unbearable but persistent thought that her analyst would never return to her. As we explored these more spontaneous and genuinely painful thoughts and feelings, with their accompanying defenses, the patient became able to openly grieve the father's death thirty years earlier. She began to recapture a veritable flood of early memories: painful ones, such as the recollection of having to direct both of them home when her father got lost one day at the onset of his illness, but also fond, pleasurable ones, including her recollection that, before his illness, he had infected her with his joyful, devil-may-care attitude toward life.

As she filled her analytic hours with these forgotten experiences, she spent time away from treatment in a singularly determined, unwavering, sometimes desperate attempt to totally reclaim her lost father. For the first time since his funeral she began to visit his gravesite, not once, but on a weekly basis. In her search for more information about him, she contacted neglected relatives, secured hospital records, and hungrily explored stashed-away photo albums. One photo, which she brought to treatment to share with her analyst, had particular importance. It was a picture of her and her father. She was sitting on his lap reading a book, and he was affectionately gazing at her with deep tenderness and admiration. Amid a flood of tears while looking at the picture, she could recapture and fully experience the feeling at age four of having been totally loved by her father.

Soon after sharing the photo she reported the following dream:

I went to the hospital to visit my father. Two people were in the room and my father was furthest away. It was the first time in a very long time I had seen him. I walked into the room and he recognized me. He had only one eye. Covering one eye was a layer of skin. I felt that he felt self-conscious. I hugged and held him for a long time with my hand behind his head and kissed the right side of his face, the side with the missing eye. I sensed that he knew I was not repulsed by him. Later, I moved to the other side of the bed. I had vague sexual feelings toward him which I can't explain.

Two associations to this dream, one involving her view of her father from the right side and the other view from the left side, were especially meaningful for the patient. Seeing him in the dream with the right side of his face covered over by a layer of skin evoked a highly painful, previously lost memory. She recalled that during his illness he was sent to a world-renowned hospital in another city for brain surgery. Meeting him on his return at the local railroad station, she remembered being stunned, mortified, and horrified by his appearance. He looked like a broken, damaged, deformed shadow of the father she had once known. Clad in pajamas and a bathrobe with a large bandage covering one side of his head, he had lost considerable weight, was ashen, and was helplessly confined to a wheelchair. His fly lay open exposing his genitals. This sight she found profoundly humiliating, both for him and for herself. Her other association, to the view from the left side, involved dramatically different feelings. She felt elated, almost ecstatic, and rather disbelieving that for the first time since his death, her mind could conjure up a full, total, undisguised inner image of him.

CASE EXAMPLE 2

The patient was referred for intensive psychotherapy by her family physician amid a depressive episode precipitated by a psychiatric resident who had confronted her with his belief that she was psychosomatic. She took his comment as a severe moral condemnation and soon thereafter became highly self-punitive and self-reproachful, felt inordinately guilty, and was convinced, more than ever, that she was basically "bad."

The patient, a White, 38-year-old divorcée, is the mother of three children, two natural daughters and a Black adopted son. Following her divorce some eight years earlier, she worked as an office manager for two years, and then took a leave of absence because of a host of disabling symptoms including vertigo, headaches, nausea, intense pain throughout her body, and continuous feelings of tiredness and depletion. At times her symptoms reached the point that she would be confined in bed for up to a week. Although positive findings have been reported on various lab tests (i.e., abnormally high temperature, abnormal EEG, etc.), because of the inconsistency of results, various specialists have been unable to establish a definitive diagnosis or provide long-lasting symptomatic relief. Lupus and encephalitis have been repeatedly mentioned, but again, not conclusively substantiated.

Born and raised in a large, northwestern city, she was the older of two children with a brother two years her junior. Most vivid in her early memories was her sense of the family home. She recalled the house as grey, dingy, constantly in need of repair, and a place she felt embarrassed to bring friends. Her father, an insurance agent, suffered from a severe alcoholic problem. Although he was able to work without interruption, on weekends she recalled his repeatedly drinking himself into a stupor. Her mother worked full time, as a secretary-typist. With shame and disgust, she reported how each morning her mother would awake for work, eat breakfast, and then become nauseous and vomit until it was time to leave for work. Because both parents worked, the patient was expected to perform numerous family chores including cleaning the house, looking after her brother, and preparing most of the family meals. She felt her parents robbed her of her childhood and that from an early age she was expected to mother her mother and ask for little caretaking in return. The relationship between her parents was characterized by intense strife and turmoil.

In contrast with her desolate home life, the patient experienced school as a haven and excelled academically. Upon graduation she accepted a scholarship from the state university, and in spite of her parents' protests, she left home to attend college. In her second year she met and, after a brief courtship, married her husband, and then set about putting him and herself through school. Upon graduation he accepted a sales position which entailed frequent and numerous moves. Within the next three years they had two daughters. Despite the many moves and the accompanying disruptions, and her husband's increasing drinking, the patient invested much of herself in her children and obtained immense pleasure from mothering. When her children were four and five respectively the patient desired another child. Unable to become pregnant, she convinced her husband to adopt, and soon thereafter they adopted a three-month-old abandoned Black boy. This infant quickly became the focus of the patient's life and up until she entered treatment, one senses, her very worth and being were intimately connected with restoring this youngster to wholeness. As the patient became increasingly preoccupied with this child, her husband's drinking reciprocally increased and their relationship became more strife torn. Amid mounting dissatisfaction they decided to separate, and six months later, divorced.

Within a year and while attending a party the patient met a man who was in the city on a business trip. After spending the evening together, he decided to extend his stay so that they could be together over the weekend. They quickly became quite intimate and close, shared with each other the loneliness in their private lives, and found they had mutual interests. A nuclear engineer, he was especially unhappy in his marriage and felt little sense of relatedness with his two children. They spent several weekends together, and in less than a year, he left his family, arranged with his company for a transfer, and moved in with the patient and her children.

The relationship has endured and deepened over the past several years. In many respects he has been the loving mother she felt she never had. He has been and continues to be responsible, reliable, attentive, cherishing, and singularly concerned with her welfare and well-being. Paradoxically, however, as their relationship has grown her physical symptoms have worsened.

I discuss aspects and vicissitudes of the patient's treatment beginning when I had been seeing her for about two years. Over the two-year-period, the patient had improved considerably and we were beginning to identify and explore certain patterns which seemed related to exacerbations of her physical symptoms. For example, times in which she functioned relatively independently and with competence were quickly followed by bouts of intense pain and disabling feelings of fatigue and depletion.

During a comparatively symptom-free period, the patient announced to me that she was to begin volunteer work at a local social service agency and that she was charged with routinely transporting a small group of infirm elderly patients to their doctor's appointments. Because of her own illnesses and her affinity for the elderly, she felt especially suited for the task. Within a week she found herself enmeshed with several of the patients to the point of spending extra time filling their prescriptions, volunteering her children to help clean their apartments, and even offering to prepare meals. It was clear to both of us that her frantic activity would result in a return of symptoms and I pointed out her driven need to prove her "goodness." The patient responded by re-acknowledging her inexplicable feelings of guilt, but soon thereafter provided, for the first time, highly important material.

While reflecting upon the guilt, she related that throughout her childhood her paternal grandmother had played a major role in her life. In contrast with her grey home and her unsatisfactory relationship with her mother, she recalled her grandmother's house as bright and cheery and their relationship as one of excitement and pleasure. She recaptured and related experiences with her grandmother including shopping when her grandmother bought her books, preparing meals together, and participating in her grandmother's hobby of collecting dolls. Then in a rather thoughtful way she mentioned that perhaps her grandmother had viewed her as a replacement for a lost daughter. The patient went on to note that her grandmother had had a daughter who had died in her first year of life from burns suffered after falling into a pot of scalding water. Preoccupied with her lost daughter and her own feelings of negligence and responsibility, the grandmother recounted this story often to my patient and would add that the patient resembled her baby daughter. My patient, then, regarded herself as the benefactor of the infant's death and the "good" experiences she had with her grandmother were drenched with guilt. I reminded the patient of past times when she had reported to me images of a little baby inside of her whom she had described as needy, pained, vulnerable, unattended, and "raw." Although we had both assumed that this image represented a sense of herself as an infant, perhaps the image also represented her sense of (and identification with) the grandmother's lost child.

Several months later and after much discussion the patient decided to return to her city of birth. She felt compelled to learn more about the dead child. Toward the end of the stay she visited her grandmother's gravesite. Mindful that she had never seen a stone for the infant, she arranged for a marker to be place next to her grandmother's grave. Upon returning to treatment the patient described this incident and wondered aloud if perhaps she had been able, concretely and symbolically, to finally bury her grandmother's daughter.

DISCUSSION

In both cases, treatment provided a context within which the mourning process could be completed. That neither patient had fully mourned her significant losses was not surprising or uncommon. Nagera (1970) noted that in children legitimate developmental needs oppose the normal mourning process. He pointed out:

It is not sufficiently taken into account that if the relevant objects are absent, especially during certain stages, it is in the nature of many of these developmental phases to recreate the object anew: to make them come to life in fantasies or to ascribe such roles as the developmental stage requires to any suitable figure in the environment. Thus, relevant objects are brought to life again and again in order to satisfy the requirements of psychological development (367).

The fact that children defend against loss and the accompanying pain for the adaptive purposes of negotiating developmental tasks that lie ahead is understandable. I am still perplexed over the compelling need in these patients to take action in the real world and to recover something concrete and directly related to the lost object.

It was noted previously that mourning is a complex process that involves various ego functions including a concept of reality, an ability to take cognitive distance, a capacity to tolerate pain, and an inner representation of the object. Based on case material, it was my understanding that neither patient had developed a full inner representation of the lost object.

With the first patient, her dream was both telling and foretelling. One association to the dream, as noted, involved feelings of elation and disbelief that for the first time since her father's death she could summon a complete and clear image of him. Also in the dream the patient reported "vague sexual feelings toward him which I can't explain." Following the dream, oedipal issues readily emerged, both in the content of her sessions and in the transference. The patient filled her treatment hours with material related to her current and past heterosexual relationships including her tendency for involvement with unavailable men. As we explored these relationships in depth it became apparent that her oedipal struggles were compounded and influenced by the earlier failure to completely internalize and represent her father. As in Freud's description of melancholia, she was strikingly vague and uncertain as to what she desired in and from men. In addition, she seemed invested in being rejected and disappointed by them. The repeated rejections related to oedipal defect; also involved, however, was the need to repeat the loss of her father.

In the second case, the patient became enmeshed in the loss suffered by a significant other. Having felt used by an exploitive mother she had turned to her grandmother for positive maternal supplies. Because of feelings of guilt associated with being the beneficiary of the tragic death of a baby, her acceptance of her grandmother's offerings was painfully conflicted. The split in maternal objects together with guilt associated with positive offerings continued into adult life. With her first husband and her adopted son she felt exploited. By contrast, with positive nourishment from her common-law husband and the guilt it evoked, she regressed and experienced a multitude of physical symptoms.

In time, we came to understand her somatic symptoms as a defense against the guilt through identification with the lost object (i.e., the burned infant). However, this must be qualified. Following the search the patient spent considerable time discussing the infant. From these sessions it became clear that previous to the search the patient had known little about the infant other than that it had died tragically by falling into a pot of scalding water. Thus, her representation of the infant was confined to and determined solely by its death. Her identification, therefore, was not with the infant per se but with the dying infant. As her sense of the infant developed, this brought into sharp relief the specific nature of the identification. Once we worked through the identification, she could fully mourn the infant's death.

Through their respective searches, then, each patient was able to symbolically reclaim a lost object. Paradoxically, this also created the conditions whereby they could lose the object as part of completing the mourning process. With the evolving of the inner representations, however the mourning involved a more completely internalized representation of the lost object.

When a child loses a significant object he or she does not lose only the object. In addition, he or she loses a part of the self that had been complementary to the object. Tyson (1983), for example, noted that the impact of the loss will vary depending on the child's degree of self-other differentiation and developmental level of mental representations. He emphasized that psychic structure formation is dependent on objects for growth and maintenance, and that the impact of loss on these structures will co-vary with the degree to which the structures are internalized and thereby autonomous from the object's actual presence.

Tahka (1984) drew a useful distinction between loss of a poststructural object and loss of a prestructural object. Whereas loss of the poststructural object involves loss of the object proper, loss of the prestructural object also entails loss of parts of the self. That is, with prestructural loss the subject experiences the loss not as the loss of a whole person but, rather, as the loss of a self-function.

For Joffe and Sandler (1965), what is lost in object loss is ultimately a state of the self for which the object is a vehicle. Accordingly, even if a level of object love has been achieved, the object is, in the end, the means whereby a desired state of self may be attained, in fact or in fantasy. For the child, the state of self relates to feelings of well-being, safety, and security. Thus, when a child loses its mother he or she loses not only the mother but also the sense of well-being that occurs as a result of that relationship.

In both cases, treatment and the external search it promoted served to restore aspects of the self which were lost with the loss of the object. For the first patient, in first reclaiming her father and then losing him and fully mourning his loss, she was also able to recapture an important part of herself related to him, namely, a previously held but lost sense of having been preoedipally loved and cherished by him.

With the second patient, intimately connected with her grandmother were feelings of well-being and safety, strikingly similar to those feelings described by Joffe and Sandler (1965). Symbolically finding and then losing and mourning the infant enabled this patient to fully integrate the feelings of well-being associated with her grandmother, without the previously accompanying guilt.

The loss of a human love object initiates processes which attempt to resolve the situation created by the loss. The defensive processes employed by children have been identified and described by several investigators. Both Meis (1953) and Wolfenstein (1966) indicated that object loss in children and adolescents leads to a heightened defensive identification with the lost object that differs in significant ways from the normal process of identification and the commonly accepted definition of mourning. Specifically, the identification does not involve a gradual decathexis or "letting go" of the lost object but an intensification of the loss. In combination with idealization of the object and denial of the loss, a study by Wolfenstein (1966) found that children and adolescents harbor a fantasy that the dead parent will return. For Wolfenstein the denial and fantasy serve the adaptive purpose of maintaining ego integrity.

The massive defensive response to childhood loss is described by Shambaugh (1961) in his account of the analysis of a seven-year-old boy who began treatment because of the impending death of his mother. The child's mourning reaction was not visible to the adults around him. Following the death he did not appear to have suffered a loss but, rather, became energetic, hyperactive and restless, distractible, and almost euphoric; there was a global suppression of actual events and associated feelings. Mention of the loss evoked anger and denial, play was laden with aggression, and there was an increase in oral and dependent needs. There was also a marked increase in magical thinking and enhanced narcissism manifested in fantasies of omnipotence, independence, and invulnerability.

In keeping with Shambaugh's (1961) observation, several authors have reported a defensive flight into narcissism occasioned by object loss, taking the form of enhanced omnipotence and grandeur. Atwood (1974) described a child who had had a nonambivalent relationship with a lost parent and then developed salvation fantasies in which he assumed the role that the lost parent had played for him. The child's feelings of despair and helplessness were projected onto others, thus allowing him to indirectly satisfy his own needs for comfort and security by administering to others.

Another defense I have observed which also constitutes a major resistance typically encountered in the early phases of treatment involves a flight into and intensification of self-sufficiency. Modell (1975) suggested that severe and accumulative trauma can induce the formation of a false self-organization including the illusion of omnipotent self-reliance. Because the sharing and communication of affects is object seeking, the illusion that nothing is needed from others and that one can be the source of one's own emotional sustenance removes the individual from the fear of closeness to objects. For example, in the first case presented, associated with closeness and defended against by the illusion of self-sufficiency were the patient's profound fears of loss and abandonment as well as fear of losing her autonomous sense of self.

CONCLUSION

In this article I have attempted to demonstrate that when a therapist or analyst is dealing with issues of early object loss in which mourning has been incomplete and specific psychic structures have not achieved total autonomy from the presence of the actual object, discussing, re-enacting, and reexperiencing the loss in the transference is not enough. In such instances treatment mobilizes in the individual a need to take action in external reality to rediscover and symbolically reclaim the lost object. Such action in certain cases permits the patient to complete the internal representation of the lost object. For these patients this step is necessary before they can fully mourn the object's loss and restore to the self functions that were lost with the object. It is important to note that the external search arises from the evolving treatment and is not prompted by extratherapeutic activities on the part of the therapist.

REFERENCES

Atwood, G. (1974). The loss of a loved parent and the origin of salvation fantasies. *Psychotherapy: Theory, Research, and Practice, 11,* 256.

Freud, A. (1960). Discussion of John Bowlby's paper. *Psychoanalytic Study of the Child, 15,* 53–62.

Freud, S. (1917). Mourning and melancholia. *S.E., 14,* 243–258.

Furman, E. (1974). *A child's parent dies: Studies in childhood and bereavement.* New Haven, CT: Yale University Press.

Jacobson, E. (1964). *The self and the object world.* New York: International Universities Press.

Joffe, W. & Sandler, J. (1965). Notes on pain, depression, and individuation. *Psychoanalytic Study of the Child, 20,* 394–424.

Lerner, H. & Lerner, P. (1987). Separation, depression, and object loss: Implications for narcissism and object relations. In J. Bloom-Feshbach & S. Bloom-Feshbach (Eds.), *The psychology of separation and loss* (pp. 375–395). San Francisco: Jossey-Bass.

Loewald, H. (1978). Instinct theory, object relations, and psychic structure. *Journal of the American Psychoanalytic Association, 26,* 493–506.

Mahler, M., Pine, F. & Bergman, A. (1975). *The psychological birth of the human infant.* New York: Basic Books.

Meis, M. (1953). The oedipal problem of a fatherless child. *Psychoanalytic Study of the Child, 7,* 216–219.

Modell, A. (1975). A narcissistic defense against affects and the illusion of self-sufficiency. *International Journal of Psychoanalysis, 56,* 275–282.

Nagera, H. (1970). Children's reactions to the death of important objects: A developmental approach. *Psychoanalytic Study of the Child, 25,* 360–400.

Schur, M. (1960). Discussion of John Bowlby's paper. *Psychoanalytic Study of the Child, 15,* 63–84.

Shambaugh, B. (1961). A study of loss reactions in a seven-year-old. *Psychoanalytic Study of the Child, 16,* 510–522.

Spitz, R. (1960). Discussion of John Bowlby's paper. *Psychoanalytic Study of the Child, 15,* 85–94.

Tahka, V. (1984). Dealing with object loss. *Scandinavian Psychoanalytic Review, 7,* 13–33.

Tyson, R. (1983). Some narcissistic consequences of object loss: A developmental view. *Psychoanalytic Quarterly, 52,* 205–224.

Wolf, A. (1958). *Helping your child understand death.* New York: Child Study Association.

Wolfenstein, M. (1966). How is mourning possible? *Psychoanalytic Study of the Child, 21,* 93–123.

PART VII

OBJECT LOSS AND CREATIVITY: MOURNING AND REPARATION

Introductory Notes to Chapter 26

Rita V. Frankiel

In this extraordinary paper, Hanna Segal writes about the creative process and its rootedness in the acceptance of death and loss. She undertakes to connect acts of creation with aspects of the depressive position, and the creative impulse with the need to reestablish an inner harmony after the internal chaos and violence that follow in the inner world after a loss or profound disappointment. The paper includes case material from the treatment of individuals with inhibitions of work and creativity. It is an indispensable supplement to Freud's "Creative Writers and Daydreaming" (1908). It builds a bridge between the experience of bereavement so often noted in the history of creative persons and the resolution such people seek through art. In a postscript to this paper (Segal 1981, 204), Segal mentions that she would also like to connect aspects of creation with idealization and the phenomena of the paranoid-schizoid position. She cites her agreement with the art historian Adrian Stokes (1965) on this point. She also wishes to forge a link with the work of Jaques (1965) on the midlife crisis; like him, she argues that before the midlife crisis the artist seeks a more ideal object in his art whereas after the midlife crisis he searches to recreate the object seen in the more resolved depressive position.

26. A Psycho-Analytical Approach to Aesthetics

Hanna Segal

Denn das Schöne ist nichts
als das Schrecklichen Anfang, den wir noch gerade ertragen,
und wir bewundern es so, weil es gelassen verschmäht
uns zu zerstören.

In 1908 Freud wrote: "We laymen have always wondered greatly—like the cardinal who put the question to Ariosto—how that strange being, the poet, comes by his material. What makes him able to carry us with him in such a way and to arouse emotions in us of which we thought ourselves perhaps not even capable?"[1] And as the science of psychoanalysis developed, repeated attempts were made to answer that question. Freud's discovery of unconscious phantasy life and of symbolism made it possible to attempt a psychological interpretation of works of art. Many papers have been written since, dealing with the problem of the individual artist and reconstructing his early history from an analysis of his work. The foremost of these is Freud's book on Leonardo da Vinci. Other papers have dealt with general psychological problems expressed in works of art showing, for instance, how the latent content of universal infantile anxieties is symbolically expressed in them. Such was Freud's paper "The Theme of the Three Caskets,"[2] Ernest Jones's "The Conception of the Madonna through the Ear,"[3] or Melanie Klein's "Infantile Anxiety Situations Reflected in a Work of Art and the Creative Impulse."[4]

Until recently such papers were not mainly concerned with aesthetics. They dealt with points of psychological interest but not with the central problem of aesthetics, which is: what constitutes good art, in what essential

Reprinted by permission of the author and *The International Journal of Psycho-Analysis* 33 (1952):196–207. Copyright © Institute of Psycho-Analysis.

respect is it different from other human works, more particularly from bad art? Psychological writers attempted to answer questions like: "How does the poet work?" "What is he like?" "What does he express?" In the paper "The Relation of the Poet to Day-dreaming," Freud has shown how the work of the artist is a product of phantasy and has its roots, like the children's play and dreams, in unconscious phantasy life. But he did not attempt to explain "why we should derive such pleasure from listening to the day-dreams of a poet." How he achieves his effects is to Freud the poet's "innermost secret."[5] Indeed, Freud was not especially interested in aesthetic problems. In "The Moses of Michelangelo"[6] he says: "I have often observed that the subject-matter of works of art has a stronger attraction for me than their formal and technical qualities, though to the artist their value lies first and foremost in this latter. I am unable rightly to appreciate many of the methods used and the effects obtained in art." He was also aware of the limitations of analytical theory in approaching aesthetics. In the preface to the book on Leonardo da Vinci[7] he says that he has no intention of discussing why Leonardo was a great painter, since to do that, he would have to know more about the ultimate sources of the creative impulse and of sublimation. This was written in 1910. Since that time the work of Melanie Klein has thrown more light on the problem of the creative impulse and sublimation, and has provided a new stimulus to analytical writers on art. In the last fifteen years a number of papers have appeared dealing with problems of creation, beauty and ugliness. I would mention in particular, those by Ella Sharpe, Paula Heimann, John Rickman and Fairbairn in this country, and H. B. Lee in the U.S.A.

Maybe it is possible now, in the light of new analytical discoveries, to ask new questions. Can we isolate in the psychology of the artist the specific factors which enable him to produce a satisfactory work of art? And if we can, will that further our understanding of the aesthetic value of the work of art, and of the aesthetic experience of the audience?

It seems to me that Melanie Klein's concept of the depressive position makes it possible at least to attempt an answer to these questions.

The "depressive position," as described by Melanie Klein, is reached by the infant when he recognizes his mother and other people, and amongst them his father, as real persons. His object relations then undergo a fundamental change.[8] Where earlier he was aware of "part objects" he now perceives complete persons; instead of "split" objects—ideally good or overwhelmingly persecuting—he sees a whole object both good and bad.

The whole object is loved and introjected and forms the core of an integrated ego. But this new constellation ushers in a new anxiety situation: where earlier the infant feared an attack on the ego by persecutory objects, now the predominant fear is that of the loss of the loved object in the external world and in his own inside. The infant at that stage is still under the sway of uncontrollable greedy and sadistic impulses. In phantasy his loved object is continually attacked in greed and hatred, is destroyed, torn into pieces and fragments; and not only is the external object so attacked but also the internal one, and then the whole internal world feels destroyed and shattered as well. Bits of the destroyed object may turn into persecutors, and there is a fear of internal persecution as well as a pining for the lost loved object and guilt for the attack. The memory of the good situation, where the infant's ego contained the whole loved object, and the realization that it has been lost through his own attacks, give rise to an intense feeling of loss and guilt, and to the wish to restore and re-create the lost loved object outside and within the ego. This wish to restore and re-create is the basis of later sublimation and creativity.

It is also at this point that a sense of inner reality is developed. If the object is remembered as a whole object, then the ego is faced with the recognition of its own ambivalence towards the object; it holds itself responsible for its impulses and for the damage done to the external and to the internal object. Where, earlier, impulses and parts of the infant's self were projected into the object with the result that a false picture of it was formed, that his own impulses were denied, and that there was often a lack of differentiation between the self and the external object; in the depressive phase, a sense of inner reality is developed and in its wake a sense of outer reality as well.

Depressive phantasies give rise to the wish to repair and restore, and become a stimulus to further development only so far as the depressive anxiety can be tolerated by the ego and the sense of psychic reality retained. If there is little belief in the capacity to restore, the good object outside and inside is felt to be irretrievably lost and destroyed, the destroyed fragments turn into persecutors, and the internal situation is felt to be hopeless. The infant's ego is at the mercy of intolerable feelings of guilt, loss and internal persecution. To protect itself from total despair the ego must have recourse to violent defence mechanisms. Those defence mechanisms which protect it from the feelings arising out of the loss of the good object form a system of manic defences. The essential features of manic defences are denial of psychic reality, omnipotent control and a partial regression to the paranoid position and its defences: splitting, idealization, denial, projective identification, etc. This regression strengthens the fear of persecution and that in turn leads to the strengthening of omnipotent control.

But in successful development the experience of love from the environment slowly reassures the infant about his objects. His growing love, strength and skill give him increasing confidence in his own capacities to restore. And as his confidence increases he can gradually relinquish the manic defences and experience more and more fully the underlying feelings of loss, guilt and love, and he can make renewed and increasingly successful attempts at reparation.

By repeated experiences of loss and restoration of the internal objects they become more firmly established and more fully assimilated in the ego.

A successful working through of the depressive anxieties has far-reaching consequences; the ego becomes integrated and enriched through the assimilation of loved objects; the dependence on the external objects is lessened and deprivation can be better dealt with. Aggression and love can be tolerated and guilt gives rise to the need to restore and re-create.

Feelings of guilt probably play a rôle before the depressive position is fully established; they already exist in relation to the part object, and they contribute to later sublimation; but they are then simpler impulses acting in a predominantly paranoid setting, isolated and unintegrated. With the establishment of the depressive position the object becomes more personal and unique and the ego more integrated, and an awareness of an integrated, internal world is gradually achieved. Only when this happens does the attack on the object lead to real despair at the destruction of an existing complex and organized internal world, and with it, to the wish to recover such a complete world again.

The task of the artist lies in the creation of a world of his own.

In his introduction to the second Post-Impressionist Exhibition, Roger Fry writes: "Now these artists do not seek to give what can, after all, be but a pale reflex of actual appearance, but to arouse a conviction of a new and different reality. They do not seek to imitate life but to find an equivalent for life." What Roger Fry says of post-impressionists undoubtedly applies to all genuine art. One of the great differences between art and imitation or a superficial "pretty" achievement is that neither the imitation nor the "pretty" production ever achieves this creation of an entirely new reality.

Every creative artist produces a world of his own. Even when he believes himself to be a complete realist and sets himself the task of faithfully reproducing the external world, he, in fact, only uses elements of the existing external world to create with them a reality of his own. When, for instance, two realistic writers like Zola and Flaubert try to portray life in the same country, and very nearly at the same time, the two worlds they show us differ from each other as widely as if they were the most phantastic creations of surrealist poets. If two great painters paint the same landscape we have two different worlds.

> . . . and dream
> Of waves, flowers,clouds, woods,
> Rocks, and all that we
> Read in their smiles
> And call reality.

How does this creation come about? Of all artists the one who gives us the fullest description of the creative process is Marcel Proust: a description based on years of self-observation and the fruit of an amazing insight. According to Proust, an artist is compelled to create by his need to recover his lost past. But a purely intellectual memory of the past, even when it is available, is emotionally valueless and dead. A real remembrance sometimes comes about unexpectedly by chance association. The flavour of a cake brings back to his mind a fragment of his childhood with full emotional vividness. Stumbling over a stone revives a recollection of a holiday in Venice which before he had vainly tried to recapture. For years he tries in vain to remember and re-create in his mind a living picture of his beloved grandmother. But only a chance association revives her picture and at last enables him to remember her, and to experience his loss and mourn her. He calls these fleeting associations "intermittences du coeur," but he says that such memories come and then disappear again, so that the past remains elusive. To capture them, to give them permanent life, to integrate them with the rest of his life, he must create a work of art. "Il fallait . . . faire sortir de la pénombre ce que j'avais senti, de le reconvertir en un équivalent spirituel. Or ce moyen qui me paraissait le seul qu'était-ce autre chose que de créer une œuvre d'art?" ("I had to recapture from the shade that which I had felt, to reconvert it into its psychic equivalent. But the way to do it, the only one I could see, what was it—but to create a work of art?")

Through the many volumes of his work the past is being recaptured; all his lost, destroyed and loved objects are being brought back to life: his parents, his grandmother, his beloved Albertine. "Et certes il n'y aurait pas qu'Albertine, que ma grandmère, mais bien d'autres encore dont j'aurais pu assimiler une parole, un regard, mais en tant que créatures individuelles je ne m'en rappellais plus; un livre est un grand cimetière où sur la plupart des tombes on ne peut plus lire les noms effacés." ("And indeed it was not only Albertine, not only my grandmother, but many others still from whom I might well have assimilated a gesture or a word, but whom I could not even remember as distinct persons. A book is a vast graveyard where on most of the tombstones one can read no more the faded names.")

And, according to Proust, it is only the lost past and the lost or dead object that can be made into a work of art. He makes the painter, Elstir, say: "On ne peut recréer ce qu'on aime qu'en le renonçant." ("It is only by renouncing that one can re-create what one loves.") It is only when the loss has been acknowledged and the mourning experienced that re-creation can take place.

In the last volume of his work Proust describes how at last he decided to sacrifice the rest of his life to writing. He came back after a long absence to seek his old friends at a party, and all of them appeared to him as ruins of the real people he knew—useless, ridiculous, ill, on the threshold of death. Others, he found, had died long ago. And on realizing the destruction of a whole world that had been his, he decides to write, to sacrifice himself to the re-creation of the dying and the dead. By virtue of his art he can give his objects an eternal life in his work. And since they represent his internal world too, if he can do that, he himself will no longer be afraid of death.

What Proust describes corresponds to a situation of mourning: he sees that his loved objects are dying or dead. Writing a book is for him like the work of mourning in that gradually the external objects are given up, they are re-instated in the ego, and re-created in the book. In her paper "Mourning and Its Relation to Manic-Depressive States,"[9] Melanie Klein has shown how mourning in grown-up life is a reliving of the early depressive anxieties; not only is the present object in the external world felt to be lost, but also the early objects, the parents; and they are lost as internal objects as well as in the external world. In the process of mourning it is these earliest objects which are lost again, and then re-created. Proust describes how this mourning leads to a wish to re-create the lost world.

I have quoted Proust at length because he reveals such an acute awareness of what I believe is present in the unconscious of all artists: namely, that all creation is really a re-creation of a once loved and once whole, but now lost and ruined object, a ruined internal world and self. It is when the world within us is destroyed, when it is dead and loveless, when our loved ones are in fragments, and we ourselves in helpless despair—it is then that we must re-create our world anew, re-assemble the pieces, infuse life into dead fragments, re-create life.

If the wish to create is rooted in the depressive position and the capacity to create depends on a successful working through it, it would follow that the inability to acknowledge and overcome depressive anxiety must lead to inhibitions in artistic expression.

I should now like to give a few clinical examples from artists who have been inhibited in their creative activities by neurosis, and I shall try to show that in them it was the inability to work through their depressive anxieties which led to inhibitions of artistic activity, or to the production of an unsuccessful artistic product.

Case A is a young girl with a definite gift for painting. An acute rivalry with her mother made her give up painting in her early teens. After some analysis she started to paint again and was working as a decorative artist. She did decorative handicraft work in preference to what she sometimes called "real painting," and this was because she knew that, though correct, neat and pretty, her work failed to be moving and aesthetically significant. In her manic way she usually denied that this caused her any concern. At the time when I was trying to interpret her unconscious sadistic attacks on her father, the internalization of her mutilated and destroyed father and the resulting depression, she told me the following dream: "She saw a picture in a shop which represented a wounded man lying alone and desolate in a dark forest. She felt quite overwhelmed with emotion and admiration for this picture; she thought it represented the actual essence of life; if she could only paint like that she would be a really great painter."

It soon appeared that the meaning of the dream was that if she could only acknowledge her depression about the wounding and destruction of her father, she would then be able to express it in her painting and would achieve real art. In fact, however, it was impossible for her to do this, since the unusual strength of her sadism and her resulting despair, and her small capacity to tolerate depression, led to its manic denial and to a constant make-believe that all was well with the world. In her dream she confirmed my interpretation about the attack on her father, but she did more than this. Her dream showed something that had not been in any way interpreted or indicated by me: namely, the effect on her painting of her persistent denial of depression. In relation to her painting the denial of the depth and seriousness of her depressive feelings produced the effect of superficiality and prettiness in whatever she chose to do—the dead father is completely denied and no ugliness or conflict is ever allowed to disturb the neat and correct form of her work.

Case B is that of a journalist aged a little over thirty, whose ambition was to be a writer, and who suffered, among other symptoms, from an ever increasing inhibition in creative writing. An important feature of his character was a tendency to regress from the depressive to the paranoid position. The following dream illustrates his problem: "He found himself in a room with Goebbels, Goering and some other Nazis. He was aware that these men were completely amoral. He knew that they were going to poison him and therefore he tried to make a bargain with them: he suggested that it would be a good thing for them to let him live, since he was a journalist and could write about them and make them live for a time after their death. But this stratagem failed and he knew that he would finally be poisoned."

An important factor in this patient's psychology was his introjection of an extremely bad father-figure who was then blamed for all that the patient did. And one of the results was an unbearable feeling of being internally persecuted by this bad internal father-figure, which was sometimes expressed in hypochondriacal symptoms. He tried to defend himself against it by placating and serving this bad internal figure. He was often driven to do things that he disapproved of and disliked. In the dream he showed how it interfered with his writing: to avoid death at the hands of internal persecutors he has to write for them to keep them immortal; but there is, of course, no real wish to keep such bad figures alive, and consequently he was inhibited in his capacity for writing. He often complained, too, that he had no style of his own; in his associations to the dream it became clear that he had to write not only for the benefit of the poisoners, and to serve their purposes, but also at their command. Thus the style of his writing belonged to the internal parental figure. The case, I think, resembles one described by Paula Heimann.[10] A patient of hers drew a sketch with which she was very displeased; the style was not her own, it was Victorian. It appeared clearly during the session that it was the result of a quarrel with another woman who stood for her mother. After the quarrel the painter had introjected her as a bad and revengeful mother, and, through guilt and fear, she had to submit to this bad internal figure; it was really the Victorian mother who had dictated the painting.

Paula Heimann described this example of an acute impairment of an already established sublimation. In my patient his submission to a very bad internal figure was a chronic situation preventing him from achieving any internal freedom to create. Moreover, although he was trying to appease his persecutors, as a secondary defence against them, he was basically fixed in the paranoid position and returned to it whenever depressive feelings were aroused, so that his love and reparative impulses could not become fully active.

All the patients mentioned suffered from sexual maladjustments as well as creative inhibitions. There is clearly a genital aspect of artistic creation which is of paramount importance. Creating a work of art is a psychic equivalent of pro-creation. It is a genital bisexual activity necessitating a good identification with the father who gives, and the mother who receives and bears, the child. The ability to deal with the depressive position, however, is the pre-condition of both genital and artistic maturity. If the parents are felt to be so completely destroyed that there is no hope of ever re-creating them, a successful identification is not possible, and neither can the genital position be maintained nor the sublimation in art develop.

This relation between feelings of depression and genital and artistic problems is clearly shown by another patient of mine. C, a man of thirty-five, was a really gifted artist, but at the same time a very ill person. Since the age of eighteen he had suffered from depression, from a variety of conversion symptoms of great intensity, and from what he described as "a complete lack of freedom and spontaneity." This lack of spontaneity interfered considerably with his work, and, though he was physically potent, it also deprived him of all the enjoyment of sexual intercourse. A feeling of impending failure, worthlessness and hopelessness, marred all his efforts. He came to analysis at the age of thirty-five because of a conversion symptom: he suffered from a constant pain in the small of his back and the lower abdomen, which was aggravated by frequent spasms. He described it as "a constant state of childbirth." It appeared in his analysis that the pain started soon after he learned that the wife of his twin brother was pregnant, and he actually came to me for treatment a week before her confinement. He felt that if I could only liberate him from the spasm he would do marvellous things. In his case identification with the pregnant woman, representing the mother, was very obvious, but it was not a happy identification. He felt his mother and the babies inside her had been so completely destroyed by his sadism, and his hope of re-creating them was so slight, that the identification with the pregnant mother meant to him a state of anguish, ruin and abortive pregnancy. Instead of producing the baby, he, like the mother, was destroyed. Feeling destroyed inside and unable to restore the mother, he felt persecuted by her; the internal attacked mother attacked him in turn and robbed him of his babies. Unlike the other three patients described, this one recognized his depression and his reparative drive was therefore very much stronger. The inhibition both in his sexual and artistic achievements was due mainly to a feeling of the inadequacy of his reparative capacity in comparison with the devastation that he felt he had brought about. This feeling of inadequacy made him regress to a paranoid position whenever his anxiety was aroused.

Patient E, a woman writer, was the most disturbed of the patients described here. She was a severe chronic hypochondriac, she suffered from frequent depersonalization and endless phobias, amongst them food phobias leading at times to almost complete anorexia.

She had been a writer, but had not been able to write for a number of years. I want to describe here how her inability to experience depression led to an inhibition of symbolic expression.

One day she told me the following dream: "She was in a Nursing Home and the Matron of this Home, dressed in black, was going to kill a man and a woman. She herself was going to a fancy dress ball. She kept running out of the Nursing Home in various fancy disguises, but somehow something always went wrong, and she had to come back to the Nursing Home, and to meet the Matron. At some point of the dream she was with her friend Joan."

Her friend, Joan, was for my patient the embodiment of mental health and stability. After telling me the dream she said: "Joan was not in a fancy dress, she was undisguised, and I felt her to be so much more vulnerable than me." Then she immediately corrected herself: "Oh, of course I meant she was so much less vulnerable than me." This slip of the patient gave us the key to the dream. The mentally healthy person is more vulnerable than my patient, she wears no disguises and she is vulnerable to illness and death. My patient herself escapes death, represented by the Matron, by using various disguises. Her associations to this dream led us to a review of some of her leading symptoms in terms of her fear of, and attempted escape from, death. The disguises in the dream represented personifications, projective and introjective identifications, all three used by her as means of not living her own life and—in the light of the dream—not dying her own death. She also connected other symptoms of hers with the fear of death. For instance her spending almost half her lifetime lying in bed, "half-dead," was a shamming of death, a way of cheating death. Her phobia of bread, her fear of sex, appeared to her now as ways of escaping full living, which would mean that one day she would have "spent her life" and would have to face death. So far, she had almost lived on "borrowed" life. For instance, she felt extremely well and alive when she was pregnant, she then felt she lived on the baby's life; but immediately after the baby's birth she felt depersonalized and half-dead.

I mention here only some of her more striking symptoms which all pointed in the same direction; to a constant preoccupation with the fear of death. The analyst, represented by the Matron, tears off her disguises one after another, and forces her to lead her own life and so eventually to die.

After some three sessions completely taken up with the elaboration of this theme, she started the next one with what appeared to be a completely new trend of thought. She started complaining of her inability to write. Her associations led her to remember her early dislike of using words. She felt that her dislike was still present and she did not really want to use words at all. Using words, she said, made her break "an endless unity into bits." It was like "chopping up," like "cutting things." It was obviously felt by her as an aggressive act. Besides, using words was "making things finite and separate." To use words meant acknowledging the separateness of the world from herself, and gave her a feeling of loss. She felt that using words made her lose the illusion of possessing and being at one with an endless, undivided world: "When you name a thing you really lose it." [11] It became clear to her that using a symbol (language) meant an acceptance of the separateness of her object from herself, the acknowledgment of her own aggressiveness, "chopping up," "cutting," and finally losing the object.

In this patient the loss of the object was always felt as an imminent threat to her own survival. So we could eventually connect her difficulties in using language with the material of the earlier sessions. Refusing to face this threat of death to her object and to herself, she had to form the various symptoms devised magically to control and avoid death. She also had to give up her creative writing. In order to write again, she would have to be stripped of her disguises, admit reality, and become vulnerable to loss and death.

I shall now describe shortly a session with the same patient two years later.

She had known for some time that she would have to give up her analysis at the end of the term, through external circumstances. She came to this session very sad, for the first time since it became clear that she would end her analysis. In preceding sessions she felt nausea, felt internally persecuted and "all in bits and pieces." She said at the beginning of the session that she could hardly wait to see me for fear that her sadness would turn into a "sickness and badness." She thought of the end of her analysis, wondered if she would be able to go on liking me and how much would she be able to remember me. She also wondered if she in any way resembled me. There were two things she would wish to resemble me in: the truthfulness and the capacity to care for people which she attributed to me. She hoped she may have learned these from me. She also felt I was an ordinary kind of person, and she liked that thought. I interpreted her material as a wish to take me in and identify herself with me as a real "ordinary" feeding breast, in contrast to an earlier situation when an idealized breast was internalized, which subsequently turned into a persecuting one.

She then told me the following dream: "A baby has died—or grown-up—she didn't know which; and as a result her breasts were full of milk. She was feeding a baby of another woman whose breasts were dry."

The transference meaning of that dream was that I weaned her—my breast was dry—but she had acquired a breast and could be a mother herself. The baby who "died or grew up" is herself. The baby dies and the grown woman takes its place. The losing of the analyst is here an experience involving sadness, guilt (about the rivalry with me in relation to the baby), and anxiety (will she be able to go on remembering me). But it is also an experience leading to the enrichment of her ego—she now has the breasts full of milk and therefore need no longer depend on me.

Toward the end of the hour, she said: "Words seem to have a meaning again, they are rich," and she added that she was quite sure she could now write "provided I can go on being sad for a while, without being sick and hating food"—i.e. provided she could mourn me instead of feeling me as an internal persecutor.

Words acquired a meaning and the wish to write returned again when she could give up my breast as an external object and internalize it. This giving up was experienced by her as the death of the breast, which is dried up in the dream and the death of a part of herself—the baby part—which in growing up also dies. In so far as she could mourn me words became rich in meaning.[12]

This patient's material confirmed an impression derived from many other patients, that successful symbol formation is rooted in the depressive position.

One of Freud's greatest contributions to psychology was the discovery that sublimation is the outcome of a successful renunciation of an instinctual aim; I would like to suggest here that such a successful renunciation can only happen through a process of mourning. The giving up of an instinctual aim, or object, is a repetition and at the same time a re-living of the giving up of the breast. It can be successful, like this first situation, if the object to be given up can be assimilated in the ego, by the process of loss and internal restoration. I suggest that such an assimilated object becomes a symbol within the ego. Every aspect of the object, every situation that has to be given up in the process of growing, gives rise to symbol formation.

In this view symbol formation is the outcome of a loss, it is a creative act involving the pain and the whole work of mourning.

If psychic reality is experienced and differentiated from external reality, the symbol is differentiated from the object; it is felt to be created by the self and can be freely used by the self.

I cannot deal here extensively with the problem of symbols. I have brought it up only in so far as it is relevant to my main theme. And it is relevant in that the creation of symbols, the symbolic elaboration of a theme, are the very essence of art.

I should now like to attempt to formulate an answer to the question whether there is a specific factor in the psychology of the successful artist which would differentiate him from the unsuccessful one. In Freud's words: "What distinguishes the poet, the artist, from the neurotic day-dreamer?" In his paper "Formulations Regarding the Two Principles in Mental Functioning," Freud says: "The artist finds a way of returning from the world of phantasy back to reality, with his special gifts he moulds his phantasies into a new kind of reality." Indeed, one could say that the artist has an acute reality sense. He is often neurotic and in many situations may show a complete lack of objectivity, but in two respects, at least, he shows an extremely high reality sense. One is in relation to his own internal reality, and the other in relation to the material of his art. However neurotic Proust was in his attachment to his mother, his homosexuality, his asthma, etc., he had a real insight into the phantastic world of the people inside him, and he knew it was internal, and he knew it was phantasy. He showed an awareness that does not exist in a neurotic who splits off, represses, denies or acts out his phantasy. The second, the reality sense of the artist in relation to his material, is a highly specialized reality assessment of the nature, needs, possibilities and limitations of his material, be it words, sounds, paints or clay. The neurotic uses his material in a magic way, and so does the bad artist. The real artist, being aware of his internal world which he must express, and of the external materials with which he works, can in all consciousness use the material to express the phantasy. He shares with the neurotic all the difficulties of unresolved depression, the constant threat of the collapse of his internal world; but he differs from the neurotic in that he has a greater capacity for tolerating anxiety and depression. The patients I described could not tolerate depressive phantasies and anxieties; they all made use of manic defences leading to a denial of psychic reality. Patient A denied both the loss of her father and his importance to her; Patient B projected his impulses on to an internal bad object, with the result that his ego was split and that he was internally persecuted; Patient C did the same, though to a lesser extent; Patient E regressed to the schizoid mechanisms of splitting and projective identification which led to depersonalization and inhibition in the use of symbols.

In contrast to that, Proust could fully experience depressive mourning. This gave him the possibility of insight into himself, and with it a sense of internal and external reality. Further, this reality sense enabled him to have and to maintain a relationship with other people through the medium of his art. The neurotic's phantasy interferes with his relationships in which he acts it out. The artist withdraws into a world of phantasy, but he can communicate his phantasies and share them. In that way he makes reparation, not only to his own internal objects, but to the external world as well.

I have tried, so far, to show how Melanie Klien's work, especially her concept of the depressive position and the reparative drives that are set in motion by it, and her description of the world of inner objects, throws new light on the psychology of the artist, on the conditions necessary for him to be successful and on those which can inhibit or vitiate his artistic activities. Can this new light on the psychology of the artist help us to understand the aesthetic pleasure experienced by the artist's public? If, for the artist, the work of art is his most complete and satisfactory way of allaying the guilt

and despair arising out of the depressive position and of restoring his destroyed objects, it is but one of the many human ways of achieving this end.
What is it that makes a work of art such a satisfactory experience for the
artist's public? Freud says that he "bribes us with the formal and aesthetic
pleasures."

To begin with, we should distinguish between the aesthetic pleasure and
other incidental pleasures to be found in works of art. For instance, the
satisfaction derived from identification with particular scenes or characters
can also arise in other ways, and it can be derived from bad as well as from
good art. The same would apply to the sentimental interests originating in
memories and associations. The aesthetic pleasure proper, that is, the pleasure derived from a work of art and unique in that it can only be obtained
through a work of art, is due to an identification of ourselves with the work
of art as a whole and with the whole internal world of the artist as represented
by his work. In my view all aesthetic pleasure includes an unconscious re-
living of the artist's experience of creation. In his paper on "The Moses of
Michelangelo," Freud says: "What the artist aims at is to awaken in us
the same mental constellation as that which in him produced the impetus
to create."

We find in Dilthey's philosophy a concept called by him "nach-erleben." [13] This means to him that we can understand other people from
their behaviour and expression, we intuitively reconstruct their mental and
emotional state, we live after them, we re-live them. This process he calls
"nach-erleben." It is, he says, often deeper than introspection can discover.
His concept, I think, is equivalent to unconscious identification. I assume
that this kind of unconscious re-living of the creator's state of mind is the
foundation of all aesthetic pleasure.

To illustrate what I mean I will take as an example the case of "classical"
tragedy. In a tragedy the hero commits a crime: the crime is fated, it is an
"innocent" crime, he is driven to it. Whatever the nature of the crime the
result is always complete destruction—the parental figures and child figures
alike are engulfed by it. That is, at whatever level the conflict starts—
"Oedipus Rex," for instance, states a genital conflict—in the end we arrive
at a picture of the phantasies belonging to the earliest depressive position
where all the objects are destroyed. What is the psychological mechanism of
the listener's "nach-erleben"? As I see it, he makes two identifications. He
identifies himself with the author, and he identifies the whole tragedy with
the author's internal world. He identifies himself with the author while the

latter is facing and expressing his depression. In a simplified way one can summarize the listener's reaction as follows: "The author has, in his hatred, destroyed all his loved objects just as I have done, and like me he felt death and desolation inside him. Yet he can face it and he can make me face it, and despite the ruin and devastation we and the world around us survive. What is more, his objects, which have become evil and were destroyed, have been made alive again and have become immortal by his art. Out of all the chaos and destruction he has created a world which is whole, complete and unified.''

It would appear then that two factors are essential to the excellence of a tragedy: the unshrinking expression of the full horror of the depressive phantasy and the achieving of an impression of wholeness and harmony. The external form of "classical" tragedy is in complete contrast with its content. The formal modes of speech, the unities of time, place and action, the strictness and rigidity of the rules are all, I believe, an unconscious demonstration of the fact that order can emerge out of chaos. Without this formal harmony the depression of the audience would be aroused but not resolved. There can be no aesthetic pleasure without perfect form.[14]

In creating a tragedy I suggest the success of the artist depends on his being able fully to acknowledge and express his depressive phantasies and anxieties. In expressing them he does work similar to the work of mourning in that he internally re-creates a harmonious world which is projected into his work of art.

The reader identifies with the author through the medium of his work of art. In that way he re-experiences his own early depressive anxieties, and through identifying with the artist he experiences a successful mourning, re-establishes his own internal objects and his own internal world, and feels, therefore, re-integrated and enriched.

But is this experience specific to a work of art that is tragic, or is it an essential part of any aesthetic experience? I think I could generalize my argument. To do so I shall have to introduce the more usual terminology of aesthetics and re-state my problems in new terms. The terms I need are "ugly" and "beautiful." For Rickman, in his paper "The Nature of Ugliness and the Creative Impulse,"[15] the "ugly" is the destroyed, the incomplete object. For Ella Sharpe[16] "ugly" is destroyed, arhythmic, and connected with painful tension. I think both these views would be included if we say that "ugliness" is what expresses the state of the internal world in depression. It includes tension, hatred and its results—the destruction of good and whole objects and their change into persecutory fragments. Rickman, however, when he contrasts ugly and beautiful, seems to equate "beautiful" with what is aesthetically satisfying. With that I cannot agree. Ugly and beautiful are two categories of aesthetic experience and, in certain ways, they can be contrasted: but if beautiful is used as synonymous with aesthetically satisfying, then its contradictory is not "ugly," but unaesthetic, or indifferent, or dull. Rickman says that we recoil from the ugly; my contention is that "ugly" is a most important and necessary component of a satisfying aesthetic experience. The concept of ugliness as one element in aesthetic satisfaction is not uncommon in the tradition of philosophical aesthetics; it has been most strikingly expressed, however, by the artists themselves. Rodin writes: "We call ugly that which is formless, unhealthy, which suggests illness, suffering, destruction, which is contrary to regularity—the sign of health. We also call ugly the immoral, the vicious, the criminal and all abnormality which brings evil—the soul of the parricide, the traitor, the self-seeker. But let a great artist get hold of this ugliness; immediately he transfigures it—with a touch of his magic wand he makes it into beauty."

What is "beautiful"? Taking again the beautiful as but one of the categories of the aesthetically satisfying, most writers agree that the main elements of the beautiful—the whole, the complete, and the rhythmical—are in contrast with the ugly. Amongst analytical writers—Rickman equates the beautiful with the whole object; Ella Sharpe considers beauty essentially as rhythm and equates it with the experience of goodness in rhythmical sucking, satisfactory defecation and sexual intercourse. I should add to this rhythmical breathing and the rhythm of our heart-beats. An undisturbed rhythm in a composed whole seems to correspond to the state in which our inner world is at peace. Of non-analytical writers, Herbert Read comes to a similar conclusion when he says that we find rhythmical, simple arithmetical proportions which correspond to the way we are built and our bodies work. But these elements of "beauty" are in themselves insufficient. If they were enough then we would find it most satisfactory to contemplate a circle or listen to a regular tattoo on a drum. I suggest that both beauty, in the narrow sense of the word, and ugliness must be present for a full aesthetic experience.

I would re-word my attempt at analysing the tragic in terms of ugliness and beauty. Broadly speaking, in tragedy "ugly" is the content—the complete ruin and destruction—and "beautiful" is the form. "Ugly" is also an essential part of the comic. The comic here is ugly in that, as in caricature, the overstressing of one or two characteristics ruins the wholeness—the balance—of the character. Ugly and tragic is also the defeat of the comic hero by the sane world. How near the comic hero is to the tragic can be seen from the fact that outstanding comic heroes of past ages are felt, at a later, date, to be mainly tragic figures; few people to-day take Shylock or Falstaff as figures of fun only; we are aware of the tragedy implied. The difference between tragedy and comedy lies then in the comic writer's attempt to dissociate himself from the tragedy of his hero, to feel superior to it in a kind of successful manic defence. But the manic defence is never complete; the original depression is still expressed and it must therefore have been to a large extent acknowledged and lived by the author. The audience re-lives depression, the fear of it, and the aggression against it which are expressed in a comedy and its final successful outcome.

It is easier to discover this pattern of overcoming depression in literature, with its explicit verbal content, than in other forms of art. The further away from literature the more difficult is the task. In music, for instance, we would have to study the introduction of discords, disharmonies, new disorders which are so invariably considered to be ugly before they are universally accepted. New art is considered "difficult," it is resisted, misunderstood, treated with bitter hatred, contempt; or, on the other hand, it may be idealized to such an extent that the apparent admiration defeats its aim and makes its object a butt of ridicule. These prevalent reactions of the public are, I think, manifestations of a manic defence against the depressive anxieties stirred by art. The artists find ever new ways of revealing a repressed and denied depression. The public use against it all their powers of defence until they find the courage to follow the new artist into the depths of his depression, and eventually to share his triumphs.

The idea that ugliness is an essential component of a complete experience seems to be true of the tragic, the comic, the realistic, in fact of all the commonly accepted categories of the aesthetic except one—and this single exception is of great importance.

There is, undoubtedly, a category of art which shows to the greatest extent all the elements of beauty in the narrow sense of the word, and no apparent sign of ugliness; it is often called "classical" beauty. The beauty of the Parthenon, of the Discobolos, is whole, rhythmical, undisturbed. But soul-less imitations of beauty, "pretty" creations are also whole and rhythmical; yet they fail to stir and rouse nothing but boredom. Thus classical beauty must have some other not immediately obvious element.

Returning to the concept of *nach-erleben,* of experiencing along with another, we may say that in order to move us deeply the artist must have embodied in his work some deep experience of his own. And all our analytical experience as well as the knowledge derived from other forms of art suggests that the deep experience must have been what we call, clinically, a depression, and that the stimulus to create such a perfect whole must have lain in the drive to overcome an unusually strong depression. If we consider what is commonly said about beauty by laymen, we find a confirmation of this conclusion. They say that complete beauty makes one both sad and happy at the same time, and that it is a purge for the soul—that it is awe-inspiring. Great artists themselves have been very much aware of the depression and terror embodied in works of classical beauty which are apparently so peaceful. When Faust goes in search of Helen, the perfect classical beauty, he has to face un-named terrors; to go where there is no road:

> Kein Weg! Ins Unbetretene
> Nicht zu Betretende; ein Weg aus Unerbetene,
> Nicht zu Erbittende.

He must face endless emptiness:

> —Nichts Wirst du sehn in ewig leerer Ferne,
> Den Schritt nicht hören den du tust,
> Nichts Festes finden, wo du rühst.

Rilke writes: "Beauty is nothing but the beginning of terror that we are still just able to bear."

Thus to the sensitive onlooker, every work of beauty still embodies the terrifying experience of depression and death. Hanns Sachs, in his book, *Beauty, Life, and Death,* pays particular attention to the awesome aspect of beauty; he says the difficulty is not to understand beauty but to bear it, and he connects this terror with the very peacefulness of the perfect work of art. He calls it the static element; it is peaceful because it seems unchangeable, eternal. And it is terrifying because this eternal unchangeability is the expression of the death instinct—the static element opposed to life and change.

Following quite a different trend of thought I come to similar conclusions about the role of the death instinct in a work of art. Thus far my contention has been that a satisfactory work of art is achieved by a realization and sublimation of the depressive position, and that the effect on the audience is that they unconsciously re-live the artist's experience and share his triumph of achievement and his final detachment. But to realize and symbolically to express depression the artist must acknowledge the death instinct, both in its aggressive and self-destructive aspects, and accept the reality of death for the object and the self. One of the patients I described could not use symbols because of her failure to work through the depressive position; her failure clearly lay in her inability to accept and use her death instinct and to acknowledge death.

Re-stated in terms of instincts, ugliness—destruction—is the expression of the death instinct; beauty—the desire to unite into rhythms and wholes, is that of the life instinct. The achievement of the artist is in giving the fullest expression to the conflict and the union between those two.

This is a conclusion which Freud has brought out in two of his essays, though he did not generalize it as applicable to all art. One of these essays is that on Michelangelo's Moses, where he clearly shows that the latent meaning of this work is the overcoming of wrath. The other essay is his analysis of the theme of the Three Caskets. He shows there that in the choice between the three caskets, or three women, the final choice is always symbolical of death. He interprets Cordelia in *King Lear* as a symbol of death, and for him the solution of the play is Lear's final overcoming of the fear of death and his reconciliation to it. He says: "Thus man overcomes death, which in thought he has acknowledged. No greater triumph of wish-fulfilment is conceivable."

All artists aim at immortality; their objects must not only be brought back to life, but also the life has to be eternal. And of all human activities art comes nearest to achieving immortality; a great work of art is likely to escape destruction and oblivion.

It is tempting to suggest that this is so because in a great work of art the degree of denial of the death instinct is less than in any other human activity, that the death instinct is acknowledged, as fully as can be borne. It is expressed and curbed to the needs of the life instinct and creation.

NOTES

1. Freud (1908). "The Relation of the Poet to Daydreaming," *Collected Papers*, Vol. IV.
2. Freud (1913). "The Theme of the Three Caskets," *Collected Papers*, Vol. IV.
3. E. Jones (1914). "The Conception of the Madonna through the Ear," *Essays in Applied Psycho-Analysis*, Vol. II.
4. M. Klein (1925). "Infantile Anxiety Situations Reflected in a Work of Art and the Creative Impulse." *Contributions to Psycho-Analysis*, 1921–45.

5. Freud (1908). "The Relation of the Poet to Daydreaming," *Collected Papers,* Vol. IV.
6. Freud (1914). "The Moses of Michelangelo." *Collected Papers,* Vol. IV.
7. Freud (1920). *Leonardo da Vinci* (London: Kegan Paul, 1922.)
8. For the description of the preceding phase of development see Melanie Klein's *Contributions to Psycho-Analysis, 1921–1945,* and H. Rosenfeld's paper in *Int. J. Psycho-Anal.* 33 (1952).
9. Melanie Klein (1940). "Mourning and Its Relation to Manic-Depressive States," *Contributions to Psycho-Analysis,* 1921–45.
10. Paula Heimann: "A Contribution to the Problem of Sublimation and its Relation to Processes of Internalization," *Int. J. Psycho-Anal.,* 23, 1942, Part 1.
11. This theme became later linked with the "Rumpelstiltskin" theme of stealing the baby and the penis, but I cannot follow it up here.
12. I have given here only the transference meaning of the dream in order not to detract from my main theme. This transference situation was linked with past experiences of weaning, birth of the new baby and the patient's failure in the past to be a "good" mother to the new baby.
13. *Wilhelm Dilthey,* an Introduction. Hodges.
14. Roger Fry says: "All the essential aesthetic quality has to do with pure form," and I agree, but he adds later: "The odd thing is that it is, apparently, dangerous for the artist to know about this." Roger Fry feels that it is odd, I think, because of an inherent weakness of the formalist school he represents. The formalists discount the importance of emotional factors in art. According to Fry, art must be completely detached from emotions, all emotion is impurity, and the more the form gets freed from the emotional content the nearer it is to the ideal. What the formalists ignore is that form as much as content is in itself an expression of unconscious emotion. What Fry, following Clive Bell, calls "significant form," a term he confesses himself incapable of defining, is form expressing and embodying an unconscious emotional experience. The artist is not trying to produce pretty or even beautiful form, he is engaged on the most important task of re-creating his ruined internal world and the resulting form will depend on how well he succeeds in his task.
15. Rickman (1940). "The Nature of Ugliness and the Creative Impulse," *Int. J. of Psycho-Anal.,* 21, Part 3.
16. Ella Sharpe: "Certain Aspects of Sublimation and Delusion" (1930). "Similar and Divergent Unconscious Determinants Underlying the Sublimations of Pure Art and Pure Science" (1935).

BIBLIOGRAPHY

Bell, C. "Art," 1914.
Ehrenzveig, A. "Unconscious Form Creation in Art," *Brit. J. Med. Psychol,* 21, Parts 2 and 3.
Fairbairn, W. R. D. "The Ultimate Basis of Aesthetic Experience," *Brit. J. Psychol.,* 29, Part 2.
Freud. "The Relation of the Poet to Day-Dreaming," 1908; "Formulations Regarding the Two Principles of Mental Functioning," 1911; "The Theme of the Three Caskets," 1913; "The Moses of Michelangelo," 1914. *Collected Papers,* 4.
Fry, R. "Vision and Design," 1920.
——— "Transformations," 1926.
Heimann, P. "A Contribution to the Problem of Sublimation and Its Relation to Processes of Internalization," *Int. J. Psycho-Anal.,* 23, Part 1.

Jones, E. "The Conception of the Madonna Through the Ear," 1914.

Klein, M. "Infantile Anxiety Situations Reflected in a Work of Art and the Creative Impulse," 1929; "A Contribution to the Psychogenesis of Manic-Depressive States," 1935; "Mourning and its Relation to Manic-Depressive States," 1940. *Contributions to Psycho-Analysis, 1921–45.*

Lee, H. B. "A Critique of the Theory of Sublimation," *Psychiatry,* 2, May 1939.

—— "A Theory Concerning Free Creation in the Inventive Arts," *Psychiatry,* 3, May, 1940.

Listowell. *A Critical History of Modern Aesthetics.* George Allen and Unwin. 1933.

Read, H. "The Meaning of Art," 1931.

—— "Art and Society," 1934.

Rickman, J. "The Nature of Ugliness and the Creative Impulse," *Int. J. Psycho-Anal.,* 21, Part 3.

Sachs, H. "Beauty, Life and Death."

Sharpe, E. "Certain Aspects of Sublimation and Delusion," 1930; "Similar and Divergent Determinants Underlying the Sublimation of Pure Art and Pure Science," 1935. *Collected Papers.*

Introductory Notes to Chapter 27

Rita V. Frankiel

This research was undertaken to provide data that would bear on the impression that, in addition to enduring intense suffering and potentially serious emotional disturbance, those who have experienced parental loss are heavily represented among the extraordinarily creative, powerful, and original figures in the history of civilization. Pollock (1975a, 1975b, 1982, 1989) has published a number of applied analyses of figures in literature, art, music, and political life who suffered early losses, especially of parents or siblings. In studying a variety of eminent figures, Pollock outlined the complex adaptations and resolutions of loss in the gifted.

It is Pollock's idea that object loss and the mourning that follows it can be stimulated by the necessity for adaptation embedded in all transitions and progressions. If resolved, it can be the impetus for a variety of later creative acts and products, depending on the resources and talents of the individual. In the richly endowed, great masterpieces or major contributions that can lead to profound cultural restructurings can result. Pollock (1989) has observed the creative resolution of mourning to be implicated in Freud's completion of "Interpretation of Dreams" (1900), various works by Gustav Mahler, the art works of Kathe Kollwitz, and a host of other creative geniuses. Liebert's (1983) study of Michelangelo presents similar findings. In this study, Michelangelo emerges as someone who was permanently dominated by a sense of maternal inaccessibility and coldness, following early separation from the wet-nurse who raised him and the subsequent death of his biological mother when he was a latency-age child. The work of Hardin (1985) on the effects of the loss of mother surrogates on later personality developments is relevant here.

Few women meet the author's criteria for genius and eminence. It should be noted that he does not take into account the selective gender biases that may well have led to a strikingly low number of women in his sample.

27. Parental Loss and Genius

J. Marvin Eisenstadt

Renewed interest has recently been shown in the study of genius (Albert 1969, 1971, 1975; Besdine 1968a, 1968b; Sorell 1970). Many have tried to explain the development of those who mold civilization. There are leads and there are worthy thoughts on the subject, but few actual facts. Genius was described initially as an act of creativity on the part of the Supreme Creator and until very recently in history was the subject of religious speculation. Beginning in the 1870s, however, scientists attempted to analyze the operational components of genius. Galton believed that the faculty of genius was transmitted through hereditary principles. Lombroso believed in a theory of genius that he based on his work as a psychiatrist. He had observed at close range the many forms of mental deterioration, extreme behavioral manifestations, and emotional disturbances of patients in large institutions for the mentally ill. He believed all forms of genius were the result of psychoses and moral degeneracy, and he offered great numbers of cases to prove his point. There have been many examples of actual insanity among the famous, yet Ellis (1904/1926) reported that mental illness is not found among the famous in anywhere near the proportions which Lombroso stated it would be. A great step forward in the study of the genesis of genius was made by Wilhelm Lange-Eichbaum (1928/1956, 1932). He explained that psychosis does occur in the lives of many geniuses and that even when psychosis is not found, markedly psychopathic traits can be found in a great majority of the eminent. Aside from (a) Galton and his theory of heredity, (b) Lombroso's degenerative-psychosis hypothesis with its modification by Lange-Eichbaum, and (c) the sociological school that cataloged the characteristics of genius (e.g., Bowerman 1947; Cattell 1903; Cox 1926/1959; Ellis

Reprinted by permission of the author and the American Psychological Association from *American Psychologist* 33 (1978):211–23. Copyright © 1978 by the American Psychological Association.

1904/1926; Goertzel and Goertzel 1962; Illingworth and Illingworth 1966; Kenmare 1960), all three of which are acknowledged to be grossly inadequate theories, there is no theoretical position that can explain the phenomenon of eminence or creative genius, and there are no facts to support any generalized theory. In other words, there is as yet no scientific theory to account for the development of a historically eminent individual. The present study attempts a new viewpoint in discussing genius and its origins by relating creative thinking, historical eminence, administrative prowess, and scientific acumen to the variable of loss of the parents by death. The study was an outgrowth of previous work in the area of creativity (Eisenstadt 1966). Genius is defined here as the development of an individual to a high degree of competency and superiority in an occupational field. This is postulated to be due to several factors, including (a) a certain degree of innate, biologically determined characteristics—principally intelligence, physical abilities, and the like; (b) individual development of those capacities by a unique and specific psychological mechanism of interaction within the family unit; and (c) training and educational advancement leading to (d) accomplishment. The unique and specific psychological mechanism focused upon in this study is the bereavement experience and its resolution or, more generally, the problem of orphanhood.

The essential element in orphanhood that uniquely describes it is that no possibility exists for a return to a former family situation. Once a parent dies, whether father or mother, the family unit is permanently altered. A curious fact of the English language is that the word *orphan* is an inexact term. According to the dictionary definition, an orphan is someone who has lost either one parent or both parents. In this study, orphanhood is defined in three aspects: paternal orphanhood—the loss by death of the father; maternal orphanhood—the loss by death of the mother; and full, total, or double orphanhood—the loss by death of both mother and father. I developed the concept of the parental-loss profile to rigorously define the orphanhood situation of any individual. Thus, Sigmund Freud's profile reads F40, M74, meaning that Freud was 40 years old when his father died and 74 years old when his mother died. Charlotte Brontë's profile is F after, M5, S38, which states that her father was still alive when she died at age 38 and that her mother died when she was 5 years old.

In the present study, parental loss by death was the main consideration. Eliminated for the sake of research strategy were sibling loss, the loss of children and its effects on parents, and other loss events including separations, divorces, hospitalizations, mental illness of parents, etc. It seemed expedient from a research point of view to study the most basic form of parental loss—actual loss by death of the parent, or orphanhood. First, when a parental death is studied, it is easier to determine the actual point in time of the loss. Second, the effects should be more prominent and more easily noticed than those of other forms of loss. Third, the information to be obtained is more readily available.

What is the specific relationship between the loss of parents by death and the desire for fame, eminence, and occupational excellence? Certainly one of the important considerations is the nature of the family unit prior to the disruption caused by the death of the parent. The individual whose parents provided defective care and a disturbed family background would be affected quite differently by the death of a parent than the individual with a healthy family background whose parents showed genuine concern. It has already been remarked in the developing parental-loss literature that various facets comprise the crisis of bereavement. Such factors as the age at which the death takes place, the composition of the household at the time of death, the previous psychological and economic relationships that have existed before the loss, and the capacity of the family members to absorb the crisis have been mentioned as contributory factors to the traumatic nature of orphanhood. Thus, parental loss is conceived in two ways: (a) Parental loss by death has a *direct* result, and depending on the age of the child, this result can be specified, and (b) parental loss by death has an *indirect* result depending on the family dynamics existing before the death occurred.

RESEARCHING GENIUS: THE STUDY GROUP AND PARENTAL-LOSS-PROFILE RESULTS

The study of eminence and the criteria used to define the eminent has a well-developed history and can be dated for our purposes as beginning with Sir Francis Galton (1869/1962). The selection of eminent individuals was personally decided upon by him, although he was guided in his choice of judges, statesmen, scientists, poets, and artists by standard reference works available at the time. Galton later selected Fellows of the Royal Society who had won medals for scientific work, had been president of a learned society, had attained membership on the counsel of the society, or were professors at important universities. Havelock Ellis (1904/1926) used the 66 volumes of the *Dictionary of National Biography*. He selected individuals to whom three or more pages were devoted, but he also included those whom he believed to have shown a high order of intellectual ability despite the fewer than three pages of print. He excluded the notorious and members of the nobility regardless of their eminence. Cattell (1903) selected his group of eminent men from six biographical dictionaries or encyclopedias: two French, one German, and three English, including Lippincott's *Biographical Dictionary,* the *Encyclopaedia Britannica,* and Rose's *Biographical Dictionary.* The chosen group was defined by inclusion in at least three of the sources, with the greatest average space allotted determining the magnitude of eminence.

The subjects in the present study were derived from listing all individuals who appeared in the 1963 edition of the *Encyclopaedia Britannica* with one column of space ($\frac{1}{2}$ page) or more and from listing all individuals who were given one column of space ($\frac{1}{2}$ page) or more in the 1964 edition of the *Encyclopedia Americana.* A person with at least one column in each encyclopedia was included; this resulted in a group of 699 individuals, 20 women and 679 men. The famous spanned the ages from Homer to John Kennedy, from the Greek and Roman periods of 500 B.C. through the current eminent of twentieth-century history. Those studied were found to have an average of $1\frac{1}{2}$ pages in the *Encyclopaedia Britannica* ($M = 3.31$ columns, $SD = 3.19$) and an average of 1 page in the *Encyclopedia Americana* ($M = 2.51$ columns, $SD = 2.39$). Thus, the average famous individual in this study was found to have a combined space allocation of slightly less than 3 pages ($M = 5.85$ columns, $SD = 5.18$).

The death dates of the fathers and mothers and the birth and death dates of the eminent individuals themselves were obtained. Subjects were eliminated from statistical computations whenever biographical information was unavailable on the lifespan of the individual or his or her parents. Of the original 699, it was necessary to eliminate 126 (18%) for whom biographical data on parent death dates were unavailable. This left 573 subjects, which constituted the major statistical group. The greatest number of these, 215 (38%), were from the nineteenth century, while 146 (25%) were from the twentieth century. The eighteenth century contributed 75 (13%); the seventeenth century, 55 (10%); the sixteenth century, 39 (7%); and all the others from ancient antiquity through 1499 comprised 43 (7%).

In Cattell's (1903) listing of 1,000 eminent men, the rank order by nationality was France (1), Britain (2), Germany (3), Italy (4), Rome (5), Greece (6), and America (7). If only the top 500 of Cattell's listing are used, the rank order becomes Britain (1), France (2), Greece (3), Germany (4),

Table 27.1
Number and Percentages of Subjects by
Nationality

Nation	%	n
1. Britain	27.8	194
2. America	17.0	119
3. France	12.6	88
4. Italy	8.2	57
5. Germany	6.9	48
6. Greece	4.1	29
7. Rome	4.0	28
8. Russia	2.1	15
9. Biblical	2.0	14
10. Scotland	1.8	13
11. Spain	1.7	12
12. Ireland	1.4	10
13. Austria	1.3	9
14. Combined others	9.1	63

Note. N = 699.

Italy (5), Rome (6), and America (7). The 699 subjects of the present study produced the rank order shown in table 27.1. There were 163 subjects (23%) in this study who "moved up" in individual rank order from Cattell's listing, while 203 subjects (29%) "moved down" in rank order. Almost half, or 333 (48%), of the famous individuals in contemporary history included in the present study were not listed at all in Cattell's study. In the total Cattell group of 1,000, 634 eminent individuals (or 63% of his listing) were not included in the present study. Surprisingly, of those not included in the present study from Cattell's group, 10 individuals appeared in his top 100, 23 in the second 100, 47 in the third 100, 56 in the fourth 100, and at least 70 or more individuals were excluded in each of the subsequent 100s up to 1,000. Thus, we can see the cultural influences and/or prejudices that appear in preparing lists of the eminent.

Each subject in the present study was eminent because of his or her occupational abilities. Some individuals were notable because of exceptional accomplishments in more than one vocation, while some made their mark in one area only. In the total sample of 699 subjects, the largest occupational group was writers, followed by statesmen. Philosophers, poets, and scientists-scholars were given essentially equal prominence. Royalty, soldiers,

Table 27.2
Number and Percentages of Subjects by
Occupational Activity

Occupational Activity	%	n
1. Writers	35.9	251
Poets	13.7	96
Dramatists	6.0	42
Novelists	3.0	21
2. Statesmen	25.3	177
Presidents of the United States	4.7	33
Jurists	2.4	17
Diplomats	1.6	11
Prime ministers	1.3	9
3. Philosophers	15.4	108
4. Scientists, scholars	13.6	95
5. Royalty	9.9	69
6. Founders	9.3	65
7. Soldiers	9.2	64
8. Artists	8.2	57
9. Reformers	5.4	38
10. Composers	3.3	23
11. Explorers	2.7	19

Note. Some individuals were listed in more than one category if they were noted for more than one occupation. $N = 699$.

and a special occupational group, founders, were similarly represented by numbers of individuals. Founders were those who achieved fame through establishing religious societies or some new organizational structure. Another special occupational group, reformers, was separately listed. Table 27.2 gives the numbers and percentages of the various occupational categories found in this study. If individuals were noted for more than one occupation, they were listed in each category of fame. This designation was usually found in the first sentence of the entry in the encyclopedia article. In very few cases was there any question as to the vocational designation to be given each subject.

The subject's age at the time of the death of each parent was considered in relationship to the famous subject's own lifespan. This led to the development of the parental-loss-profile notation used in this study. F and an age indicates the mean age of the eminent individuals when their fathers died. M and an age refers to the mean age of the eminent individuals when their

Table 27.3

Parental-Loss-Profile Results for the Total Group of Famous
Individuals in This Study

Parental-Loss Profile	M (years)	SD	n
Earliest or first parent to die (E)	21.10	14.31	488
Father death (F)	26.50	15.39	546
Mother death (M)	32.86	17.63	466
Last or second parent to die (L)	38.75	14.40	446
Age at death (S)	65.38	14.41	564

mothers died. E and an age refers to the mean age of the subjects when the earliest or first parent died, and L and an age refers to the mean age of the subjects when the last or second parent died. S and an age indicates the mean lifespan of the subjects.

For the total group, the first parent (whether father or mother) died at E21.10 years. The death of the second parent (whether father or mother) occurred at L38.75 years. The subjects lost their fathers at F26.50 years and their mothers at M32.86 years (see table 27.3).

It was determined that 14 fathers (2%) and 42 mothers (7%) outlived their famous children. In 6 cases (1%) both parents outlived their child, while in 50 cases (9%) one parent outlived the child. By age 10, 25.0% of the subjects had one parent dead, and by age 15, 34.5% had one parent dead. By age 10, 3.1% of the subjects had lost both parents, and by age 15, 5.9% had lost both parents. Father death by age 10 was experienced by 17.6%, while mother death by age 10 was experienced by 12.6% of the subjects. By age 15, 24.8% of the subjects had lost their fathers, while 18.5% of the subjects had lost mothers. By age 25, 52.2% had lost one parent, 46.1% had lost their fathers, 28.6% had lost their mothers, and 15.9% had lost both parents. See table 27.4 for the complete results.

There were 497 subjects for whom complete parental-loss information was available. There were 270 subjects (54.3%) whose fathers died before their mothers. They lost their fathers at F21.32 years and their mothers at M41.32 years, or 20 years later. Of these cases, 28% had lost their fathers by age 10, while 37% had lost their fathers by age 15. There were 163 subjects (33.0%) whose mothers died first. In these cases, the loss of the mother occurred at M19.22 years, with the father dying at F33.45 years, or 16 years later. Of

Table 27.4
Five-Year Interval Cumulative Percentages by Age at which Father,
Mother, Earliest Parent, and Last Parent Death Occurred in the
Lifespan of the Famous Individuals in This Study

Age (years)	Earliest or First Parent to Die (E)	Father Death (F)	Mother Death (M)	Last or Second Parent to Die (L)
Before or at birth	4.2	3.1	1.2	0
0–5	13.4	10.8	4.5	.9
6–10	25.0	17.6	12.6	3.1
11–15	34.5	24.8	18.5	5.9
16–20	45.0	36.0	23.2	9.6
21–25	52.2	46.1	28.6	15.9
26–30	61.4	57.1	31.4	20.8
31–35	68.9	65.3	41.9	29.3
36–40	75.4	74.7	50.1	38.2
41–45	80.6	83.8	59.5	50.8
46–50	83.2	89.2	66.7	60.4
51–55	85.0	92.7	74.5	69.1
56–60	85.3	94.8	78.7	74.9
61–65		95.3	80.6	77.3
66–70			80.6	77.3
71–75			81.2	77.3
76–80			81.3	77.7
After	1.0	2.4	7.3	8.7
Unknown	13.6	2.3	11.3	13.6

Note. N = 573.

these subjects, 34% had lost their mothers by age 10, and 50% had lost their mothers by age 15. There were 36 subjects (7.2%) whose mothers died after they did. These subjects lived to the age of S47.72 years, with their fathers dying at F24.56 years. There were only 8 subjects (1.6%) whose fathers died after they did. These subjects lived to the age of S42.50 years, with the mothers dying at M21.12 years. There were six cases (1.2%) in which both the father and the mother died after the subject. These subjects died at the early age of S35.17 years.

The question to be asked is whether these results are unique for the special individuals in the encyclopedia, living in previous centuries when death rates were different, or whether these numbers are average ages at which any group of children and adults lose their parents. The problems in answering such a question are manifold. There are no comparisons to be made between the subjects of 2,500 years of recorded history and any control group. Moreover, insurance-company statistics start in rudimentary fashion only in the nineteenth century. How then to proceed to gain some measure of understanding of the nature of the obtained finding? There are several alternatives. An obvious first step is to compare equal halves of the total group to determine the reliability of the obtained results. Another step is to compare a historical group of individuals not listed in the encyclopedia with the eminent group of this study. Finally, despite numerous methodological problems, base rates of parental loss by death may be ascertained from the literature and used for comparison.

THE ALPHABET TEST

A simple but powerful approach to determining the reliability of the numbers obtained for the total sample is to divide the group into two equal halves. Individuals 1 through 286 (corresponding to last names beginning with the letters A through Kh) were compared with Individuals 287 through 573 (corresponding to last names beginning with the letters Ki through Z) in an alphabetized listing of subjects. No statistically significant differences were determined for any of the ages of death in subject lifespans. These differences ranged from 1.27 years to 2.20 years. The death of the first parent, whether father or mother, occurred at E20.50 years $(SD = 14.29, N = 243)$ in the A to Kh group and at E21.77 years $(SD = 14.24, N = 246)$ in the Ki to Z group. The death of the second parent occurred at L37.96 years $(SD = 15.13, N = 220)$ in the A to Kh group and at L39.56 years in the Ki to Z group. The death of the fathers in the A to Kh and the Ki to Z groups occurred at F25.72 years $(SD = 15.75, N = 271)$ and F27.27 years $(SD = 15.01, N = 275)$, respectively. The death of the mothers occurred at M31.76 years $(SD = 17.65, N = 233)$ in the A to Kh group and at M33.96 years $(SD = 17.58, N = 233)$ in the Ki to Z group. Thus, the results of the alphabet test enable us to have confidence in the numbers found for the group as a whole. They are stable and reliable facts about the eminent individuals of history selected by inclusion in the encyclopedia.

COMPARISONS WITH FATHERS GIVEN OR NOT
GIVEN SPACE IN THE ENCYCLOPAEDIA BRITANNICA

A special group of 51 fathers was found who were famous themselves as well as having eminent children. These fathers had space devoted to them in separate articles in the *Encyclopaedia Britannica* (1968 edition), but not necessarily the amount of space to warrant inclusion in the main eminent group. A major characteristic of these fathers was their short lifespan of S53.92 years. They lost their own fathers at F19.79 years and their own mothers at M30.32 years. They lost their first parent at E13.91 years and their second parent at L34.91 years. This parental loss profile is due primarily to the fact that their first parent to die lived only for an average of 43.95 years. Their fathers lived for an average of 56.18 years and their mothers for an average of 59.71 years. The second parent to die had an average lifespan of 65.86 years.

A separate group of 184 fathers of subjects in this study, who were *not* given space in the *Encyclopedia Britannica* (1968 edition), was available as a control group. They were found to have lived to S65.21 years. Their parental-loss profile was essentially the same as that found before for the study group. They lost their fathers at F26.93 years, their mothers at M34.28 years, their first parent at E19.60 years, and their second parent at L42.07 years. All these findings were not significantly different statistically from those for the total group.

It became possible to compare the group of eminent individuals so designated by inclusion in an encyclopedia with another group from the same periods of history who were not considered eminent. The first step was to see if they were indeed contemporaries. The eminent came from the following centuries: 53% (27 fathers) from the 1600s, 16% (8 fathers) from the 1700s, 27% (14 fathers) from the 1800s, and 4% (2 fathers) from the 1900s. This contrasted with the noneminent fathers as follows: 10% (18 fathers) from the 1600s, 24% (45 fathers) from the 1700s, 56% (106 fathers) from the 1800s, and 10% (18 fathers) from the 1900s. Thus, more of the eminent fathers came from the 1600s, while more of the noneminent fathers came from the 1800s. Any differences between the two groups have to be understood in light of this fact. The very limited numbers of cases are another drawback to these results, but nevertheless some real findings do emerge for interpretation.

Table 27.5

Parental-Loss Data in a Special Group of Eminent Fathers of
the Subjects in This Study Who Were Themselves Given Space
in the *Encyclopaedia Britannica* Compared to a Group of
Fathers Not Given Space

Parental-Loss Profile	M (years)	SD	n
Fathers given space			
(Eminent group)			
Father death (F)	19.79	12.02	48
Mother death (M)	30.32	17.08	34
Earliest or first parent to die (E)	13.91	10.70	33
Last or second parent to die (L)	34.91	13.17	32
Age at own death (S)	53.92	15.36	51
Fathers not given space			
Father death (F)	26.93	16.22	169
Mother death (M)	34.28	19.27	85
Earliest or first parent to die (E)	19.60	14.80	77
Last or second parent to die (L)	42.07	14.66	73
Age at own death (S)	65.21	16.16	184

The parental-loss profile of an average father who was eminent in his
own right was found to be statistically significantly earlier than that of the
noneminent fathers. The earliest parent to die was lost at E13.91 years in the
eminent group, compared to E19.60 years in the noneminent group, a difference of 5.69 years (Z score = 2.27). The father died at F19.79 years in the
eminent group, compared to F26.93 years in the noneminent group, a difference of 7.14 years (Z score = 3.40). In the eminent group, the second parent
to die was lost at L34.91 years, compared to L42.07 years in the noneminent
group, a difference of 7.16 years Z = 2.53). The mother's death occurred
earlier as well, but the difference did not reach statistical significance
(M30.32 years vs. M34.28 years, Z = 1.09). These numbers can be examined
in table 27.5, which also includes the mean lifespans of each father group,
their mothers and fathers, and the parental-loss data. A conclusion may be
made in regard to the parental-loss profile of the eminent-fathers group:
Earlier parental loss is found in an eminent group as compared to a noneminent group. On the basis of these results, genius or eminence appears to be
related to orphanhood factors, as originally proposed. Certainly, some gain

in support for the connection between parental loss and genius was found. The next step is to compare the obtained results with the literature on parental loss.

COMPARISONS WITH THE
PARENTAL-LOSS LITERATURE

Table 27.6 presents a summary of data from the parental-loss literature. The 1921 census data from England and Wales, made useful by Brown (1961), make a good starting point for a comparison between the results of this study and the results reported in the literature. This census stated that in the 0–4 year category, death of one parent was found in 7.86%, death of the father occurred in 6.0%, and death of the mother occurred in 2.16%. In the present study's 0–5 year category, death of one parent occurred in 13.4%, death of the father occurred in 10.8%, and death of the mother in 4.5%. In the 0–9 year category, the census data of 1921 showed the death of one parent to have occurred among 12.4%, the death of the father among 9.4%, and the death of the mother among 3.71%. This contrasts with the 0–10-year category of the present study in which 25.0% had lost one parent, 17.6% had lost the father, and 12.6% had lost the mother. Thus it can be seen that parental loss by age 10 is markedly greater among the eminent subjects of the present study than among the more general population of the census data. In the 0–14-year category, the census data show death of one parent occurring in 16.6%, death of the father in 11.9%, death of the mother in 5.75%, and the death of both parents in 1.2%. This contrasts with the findings of this study in the 0–15-year category in which 34.5% of the eminent had one parent dead, the father's death had occurred in 24.8%, the death of the mother had occurred in 18.5%, and both parents had died in 5.9%. For one parent dead and for father dead, the percentages in the present study are more than twice those from the census data. For both parents dead and for mother dead, the percentages are more than three times greater in this study than in the census data. Naturally, the 2,500 years of recorded history in which the subjects of this study lived had different death rates than found in the England and Wales of 1921. The census population is not meant in any way to be a control group with which the present data can be scientifically compared. Nevertheless, I attempted to make use of the numbers available, and it is readily apparent that orphanhood was essentially more common among the group in the present study.

The Metropolitan Life Insurance Company (1959, 1966) estimates are another source with which a comparison of some significance can be made. In the 0–17-year category for the period 1900–1902, death of the father was estimated to occur for 32.1% of the children born to 50-year-old fathers. If the father was 25 years old at the birth of that child, the chances of losing that father by death were reduced to 12.1%. In the present study, the finding for 0–20 years in the death-of-father category was 36.0%, and in the 0–15-year group, it was 24.8%. These numbers begin to approach, although they do not equal, the estimates made for 1900–1902 by the Metropolitan Life statisticians for children of elderly fathers, but they are greater than the estimates for children of young fathers. Likewise, the death-of-mother estimate at the birth of the child was 21.7% if born to a 45-year-old mother, whereas it was reduced to 9.7% if the child was born to a mother 20 years old during 1900–1902. The corresponding findings in the present study were 23.2% in the 0–20-year category and 18.5% in the 0–15-year category. Once again these numbers are comparable if elderly mothers only are considered.

In the comparisons for the 0–17-year-olds for 1956 and 1964, the estimates for father death were found by Metropolitan Life statisticians to be 32.3% and 33.1%, or essentially the same as that for 1900–1902 for a child born to an elderly 50-year-old father. However, the percentages for loss of mother by death decreased in 1956 and 1964 to 11.5% and 12.4%, respectively, for an elderly mother aged 45 years. Therefore, there was a definite increase in longevity for the mother compared to 1900–1902 estimates.

The study by Petursson (1961) for Icelandic Life Insurance policy holders gives a comparison number of limited value but useful nevertheless. In the period 1921–1930 in the 0–15-year category, 28.5% experienced the death of one parent, which compares to a figure of 34.5% in the 0–15 year group of the present study.

The orphanhood rates for father death, mother death, one parent dead, and both parents dead obtained among the eminent subjects of this study were found to be higher than the general-population results found in the literature. It is clear that the orphanhood rate in the present study is on the high side compared to the rates found in the census data and the Metropolitan Life estimates.

Orphanhood data have also been obtained for specialty groups. Although a specialty group is even less directly comparable to the eminent group in this study, some benefit may be derived by an attempt to compare them. A sub-

Table 27.6

Orphanhood Rates among General Population, Juvenile Delinquents, and Psychiatric Patient Groups

Group	Father Dead (%)	Mother Dead (%)	Both Dead (%)	One or Both Dead (%)
General population				
Brown (1961): 1921 Census				
To age 4	6.00	2.16		7.86
To age 9	9.4	3.71		12.40
To age 14	11.9	5.75	1.2	16.60
Petursson (1961): 1921–1930				
To age 15				28.5
Metropolitan Life Insurance Co. (1959, 1966): 1900–1902				
(estimates; birth depending on age of father or mother)				
To age 17	12.1–32.1	9.7–21.7		
Juvenile delinquents				
Breckinridge and Abbott (1912): 1903–1904	19.9	12.0	4.3	34.0
Rhoades (1907): 1905				
To age 17				35.0
Russell Sage Foundation (1914): 1909				
To age 16	22.7	8.6	5.2	36.5
Shideler (1918)	17.9	12.8	5.7	36.4
Healy and Bronner (1926): 1909–1914				
Chicago	18.0	12.0	3.0	33.0
Boston	15.0	6.5	2.5	24.0
Sullenger (1930): 1922–1927				
To age 17	22.3	16.7	5.5	44.5

Armstrong (1932): 1926–1929	17.7	17.5	3.8	39.0
Brown (1961, 1966, 1968)				
To age 19	31.5	12.25		40.5
Glueck (1950): 1911–1922				35.9
Psychiatric patients				
Barry and Lindemann (1960): 1944–1953				
Males to age 27	17.0	13.66		
Females to age 27	18.01	17.80		
Hill and Price (1967):				
To age 30	36.8			
Beck, Sethi, and Tuthill (1963):				
To age 30				30.3
To age 60				54.8
Brown (1961):				
To age 39	60.8	42.9		

stantial body of orphanhood data has been amassed in the delinquency field. Of the delinquents processed in the Chicago Juvenile Court who were between 8 and 17 years old (average age of 13), 35% had one parent who was dead (Rhoades 1907). In 1925, Healy and Bronner (1926) studied Chicago and Boston juvenile offenders. They found that in the period 1917–1923, 23% of these offenders in Chicago and 29% in Boston had lost one parent. Armstrong (1932) studied the New York City Children's Court during 1926–1929 and found that in a group of 660 runaway boys, 39.0% had lost one parent. Armstrong also described a study of delinquent boys in four penal institutions; 35.6% were found to have lost one parent. The cumulative percentage in the 0–15-year category of the eminent study was 34.5% for the loss of one parent by death. The figure for the loss of both parents obtained in this study was 5.9% in the 0–15-year category, a figure generally reported in the early studies of delinquency as well. For example, in the study by Sullenger (1930) based on the District Court of Omaha, Nebraska, for 1922–1927, it was found that 5.5% of the boys and 5.5% of the girls (combined rate of 5.6%) had lost both parents. Thus, the delinquents of the early twentieth century who found their way into a court or an institution were orphaned at rates comparable to those found in the present study of the eminent.

As to father death, a Russell Sage Foundation (1914/1969) study found a 22.7% rate in a 14–16-year group. Sullenger (1930) reported a figure for father death among 11–17-year-old boys of 22.3%. Similarly, Breckinridge and Abbott (1912) reported that the father-death rate was found to be 19.9% in a special group from 1903 to 1904. Shideler (1918) reported father death of 22.7% in one New York City study. For death of the mother, the Russell Sage Foundation (1914/1969) reported a figure of 8.6% among 14–16-year-olds. Sullenger (1930) reported a corresponding figure of 16.7% for 11–17-year-old boys, while Breckinridge and Abbott (1912) found 9.8% for boys and 20.4% for girls, or a 12% overall rate. Brown (1961, 1966, 1968) and his associates provide some data for comparison with these numbers for ages up to 19: Among women prisoners, death of the father had occurred for 31.5%, while death of the mother had occurred for 12.25%. In another study it was found that 40.5% of the female prisoners 19 years old or younger had lost one parent. In the studies of delinquency by the Gluecks (Glueck 1936, 1959; Glueck and Glueck 1930, 1934a, 1934b, 1950, 1962), the orphanhood rate for the period 1911–1922 among male reformatory prisoners was found to be 35.9%. These results may be compared to the eminent-study findings of 34.5% by age 15 and 45.0% by age 20 for one parent dead. Father death by age 15 occurred among 24.8%; this figure increased to 36.0% by age 20. Mother death by age 15 occurred among 18.5%, and this increased to 23.2% by age 20. Delinquency studies show early-twentieth-century juvenile delinquent populations to have roughly similar orphanhood rates, although they are lower than the rates for the eminent group. Prisoners were also found to have roughly comparable orphanhood experiences. Many studies, however, yielded orphanhood-incidence results much lower than those found among the eminent. Overall, my conclusion is that despite methodological pitfalls inherent in the problems of comparison, it once again appears that the rate of orphanhood among the eminent is even greater than that among delinquents given over to courts and state institutions for care. The reader will have to be the final judge.

While a control group for studying childhood orphanhood rates has been extremely difficult (and perhaps impossible) to construct, constructing one to study adulthood orphanhood rates seems even more impossible. Nevertheless, there are some findings in the literature of orphanhood incidence that were collected in connection with studies of bereavement. In the Barry and Lindemann (1960) study of private patients, 17.0% of the males and 18.01% of the females had lost their fathers by the age of 26. In the same study, 13.66% of the males and 17.8% of the females had lost their mothers by the age of 26. Hill and Price (1967) found that 33.5% of the nondepressed patients and 36.8% of the depressed patients admitted to hospitals in 1958–1963 had lost their fathers by the age of 30. The Beck, Sethi, and Tuthill (1963) study of psychiatric outpatients found cumulative orphanhood rates of 30.3% by age 30 and 54.8% by age 60. Brown (1961) found that of depressed female patients, 60.8% had lost their fathers and 42.9% had lost their mothers by age 39. In the present study of eminence, the findings through age 25 were 46.1% for death of father, 28.6% for death of mother, and 52.2% for death of one parent. Through age 30, the corresponding figures were 57.1% for father death, 31.4% for mother death, and 61.4% for death of one parent, while through age 40 the percentages increased to 74.7% for father death, 50.1% for mother death, and 75.4% for death of one parent. By the age of 60, 85.3% of the eminent subjects had lost one parent by death. There is obviously little scientific connection between any of the foregoing to imply whether the orphanhood rates obtained in this study of eminence are systematically greater (which was found) or are an artifact based on the meager and scattered findings for adulthood in a different century with a group of individuals other than the eminent. However, the rates are provided to arouse the curiosity and interest of the reader.

Review of studies of hospitalized patients indicates that the reliability of these studies is much poorer than the reliability of the studies discussed previously. However, with some exceptions it seems that among a psychotic hospitalized population, as many as 28% may have lost one parent by age 20, compared with 45.0% among the eminent. With numerous exceptions, slightly less than 20% of hospitalized patients have lost their fathers and somewhat less than 15% have lost their mothers. These impressions compare to the figures of 36% and 23% for death of father and death of mother, respectively, obtained among the eminent. The faulty methodology of the literature of hospitalized psychotics has been fairly and extensively scrutinized in the literature, and further comment is not necessary at this point. (See Barry 1949; Beck, Sethi, and Tuthill 1963; Brown 1961; Dennehy 1966; Forrest, Fraser, and Priest 1965; Gay and Tonge 1967; Gregory 1959; Hilgard and Newman 1961, 1963a, 1963b; Hill and Price 1967; Oltman and Friedman 1965; Paffenbarger and Asnes 1966.)

When I examined studies with more specific samples such as depressed or suicidal patients, the percentages reported ranged up to 35% for death of one parent by age 15, which matches the 35% found in the present study. Similarly, father death, with great variations, was found to range from 13% to 28% for adolescents, which again roughly corresponds to the 25% for death of the father by age 15 found in the study of the eminent. With great variations, anywhere from less than 10% to 20% of a severely depressed teenage population had lost their mothers, which can be roughly compared to the 18% of the eminent subjects in this study who had lost their mothers by age 15. Thus, once more we see that in a special group of subjects, in this case the severely depressed, just as was true for seriously delinquent populations, there is a reported incidence of orphanhood which approaches the incidence of orphanhood found among the eminent of the present study. Among the more generalized populations studied, the incidence of orphanhood seemed to be much less than among the eminent. Naturally, the lack of true control groups must be repeatedly emphasized. The present speculations and impressions may or may not be helpful in ascertaining the nature of an orphanhood rate in an average population and how it might compare to the results obtained in this study of eminence. I hope that the difficulties in scientifically studying orphanhood throughout the entire lifespan may be overcome and progress in this field will be made in future work. For further information on the topic of orphanhood, see Barry (1969), Bendiksen and Fulton (1975), Brown (1966), Brown, Epps, and McGlashan (1961), Greer (1966), Gregory (1958, 1965a, 1965b, 1965c, 1966a, 1966b), Hilgard and Newman (1963a, 1963b), Marris (1974), Miller (1972), Moriarty (1967), Neubauer (1960), Oltman and Friedman (1953), and Oltman, McGarry, and Friedman (1952).

IS PARENTAL LOSS A PRIMARY PATHWAY TO CREATIVITY AND EMINENCE?

Parkes (1972) introduced his study of bereavement by reference to Freud's case of Anna O. Her mental illness, including hysterical symptoms of headaches, paralysis, and anaesthesia in her limbs, occurred during the course of her father's terminal illness and became worse upon his death. She was treated during this time (in 1881) by Breuer. Breuer believed Anna O. was helped by talking about these disturbing events of her life—thus the discovery of the link of trauma and symptom. Freud published with Breuer in 1893 (Freud and Breuer, 1893/1947) a description of the case and of the treatment. Anna O. became the first social worker in Germany, founded a periodical, and started several institutes. In the report, trauma and symptom were linked, but trauma and creative productivity and occupational achievement were not linked. One purpose of the present study is to attempt the theory building that would support these overlooked relationships.

The death of a parent in childhood is recognized as a major traumatic event affecting subsequent personality. Not only does the trauma include the separation and loss of the deceased parent but it also alters the relationships with the surviving parent and with other family members. In 1969, Wolfenstein offered a developmental model that helped to explain the relationship between achievement and loss. It is important to know the type of parent surrogate that is identified with following mourning. At times, a child will become his own parent surrogate. If this occurs, an ego ideal may be developed that leads to outstanding accomplishment. Why the child might become his own parent depends on various factors occurring before, during, and after the death. The phase of development at the time of loss, the gruesomeness of the death process if witnessed by the child, and who is available to assume a constructive parent-surrogate role all have to be taken into account. The reaction of rage at being abandoned may assume the proportions of a comprehensive grievance elaborated into an indictment of social justice. This system of thought can then be transformed into either outstanding accomplishment or outstanding antisocial behavior. If there is a need to "wrest from fate a different outcome" and if a repair of faulty reality testing can take place, then positive achievment may be the result. Even if the need to coerce fate has a pathological aspect to it, it still may be reformulated into an ultimately positive statement. Wolfenstein provides a rationale for the beginning of an understanding of how revolutionaries, founders of new societies, and startlingly innovative social critics, who both attack society and hold out a hope for reconciliation through progressive reformation, appear on the scene. The bereavement reaction can be an impetus for creative effort, a force for good, or it can have the effect of stunting personality growth and producing the concomitant antisocial acts, destruction of social relationships, and even the taking of one's own life.

In the creative mourning process there is a sequence of events whereby the loss triggers off a crisis requiring mastery on the part of the bereaved individual. If this crisis is worked through, that is, if the destructive elements and the depressive features of the experience of bereavement are neutralized, then a creative product or a creatively integrated personality can result. It can ultimately mean an elevation in job, a higher social position, or heightened individual social awareness. (See also Kanzer 1953; Rochlin 1961, 1965.)

A theory of bereavement leading to creative output can now begin to be developed. Positive results of the bereavement trauma include the fact that many children are able to assume increased responsibility in the family and adopt a new role based on the new circumstances. Some children are able to begin a differentiation toward a unique personality formation. Attempts at restitution for the parent death require the finding of a suitable replacement. Since fears of worthiness might prevent the establishment of a new relationship, steps are taken to become a more worthwhile person. The idealization of the dead parent leaves many openings for such positive growth. The problem of mastering a changed and changeable environment can be translated into strivings for achievement, accomplishment, and power. This desire to control one's own destiny is frequently seen in children who experience multiple separations either due to long-term illness in the parent or to the inadequacy of surrogate parents. Bereavement may temporarily interfere with intellectual development, but as in other areas, once mastery has occurred, there may be a great motivational desire to excel in intellectual pursuits. If feelings of insecurity, inadequacy, emptiness, and, especially, guilt can inhibit functioning by overwhelming the personality, then the mastery of these feelings may be a springboard of immense compensatory energy. In the mastery of these personal problems and in the previously felt need to master the environment, creative expression may find its deepest roots. The creative effort is thus seen as a restorative act. An attempt is made to produce creative products that will, on the one hand, alleviate those feelings of guilt and apartness and, on the other hand, prove to all the world the individual's essential goodness. The long-term nature of the coping process in bereavement reactions develops a sense of time and persistence that is a fundamental trait necessary in creative effort. The ability to fantasize and the ability to regressively join with a dead parent may lead to a corresponding ruthlessness in dealing with other people. The compensating need for ambition and power of the personally weak but magnetic world leader is obvious. The question of morality and conscience, a hallmark of creativity, enters with the sense of injustice that the child felt and continues to feel in adulthood. The individual, orphaned child was selected by fate or destiny for the bereavement experience while his peers were not. The capacity to endure a self-punishing regimen might enable a creatively gifted individual to pursue creative studies that others might long before have given up. In all of this we are dealing with preexisting patterns upon which the death of a parent is superimposed and from which subsequent relationships will shape a final conclusion.

There are obvious differences between an outstandingly successful, creative individual, that is, a genius, and a disturbed, psychotic individual. However, there are similarities between them that might lead to a restructuring of theory on the nature of psychosis and genius. Among the similarities often found are, first of all, a certain vulnerability and poor ego defenses. Both the creative genius and the psychotic individual can be easily stimulated as a result of their vulnerability, and each can be considered sensitive despite the fact that at times both appear to turn a deaf ear to those trying to gain their attention. Second, both groups have a great energy investment in themselves and in what the self produces (i.e., narcissism). The accomplished genius is rewarded with societal applause. The psychotic, however, is often condemned on the basis of his or her production. Third, both often have disturbed personal relationships with their parents, siblings, and other relatives. Disturbance is also found in their relationships with their spouses or other love partners. A fourth similarity is their apparent ease of regression to more childlike behavior. The creative person seems to have the ability to control this regression, whereas the psychotic individual seems to have no control over it. Both groups have a capacity for suffering and exhibit dissatisfaction and unhappiness with their current circumstances. Corresponding to this dissatisfaction is a desire within both groups to master the environment and to strive for an independent stance. Obviously, one group appears more successful at mastery than the other. However, all those who have seen the inner workings of a large institution for psychotic patients can recognize in these patients a form of mastery over that particular environment. The psychotic individual within narrowly defined environmental limits cannot be coerced or medicated or shocked into doing other than that which he or she chooses to do. This characteristic is also found in outstandingly successful individuals who cannot be coerced by society or their associates into being other than what they choose to be. Both groups are capable of original productions that are statistically infrequent and unique in either thought, behavior, or tangible end results. Sometimes the idiosyncratic product can be useful to society, whereas at other times it can be intolerable to society. There is also the possibility that both positive and negative reactions to the thought or work will be elicted from society at the same time or alternating within a narrow time frame. Both the creative genius and the psychotic individual apparently live in exceedingly complex worlds, with their various personality traits reflective of the complexity of those worlds. In my opinion, the findings of the present study lead to the conclusion that parental loss by death neatly explains these similarities between the genius and the psychotic. However, the parental-loss profile as a research strategy can certainly provide ample opportunity for disproof. Facts can once and for all advance the science of genius and the psychology of the eminent. Its rescue from mysticism and prejudice will not come without struggle. However, I firmly believe that a significant and important beginning has now been made.

REFERENCES

Albert, R. S. Genius: Present-day status of the concept and its implications for the study of creativity and giftedness. *American Psychologist*, 1969, *24*, 743–753.

Albert, R. S. Cognitive development and parental loss among the gifted, the exceptionally gifted and the creative. *Psychological Reports*, 1971, *29*, 19–26.

Albert, R. S. Toward a behavioral definition of genius. *American Psychologist*, 1975, *30*, 140–151.

Armstrong, C. P. *660 runaway boys: Why boys desert their homes*. Boston: Gorham, 1932.

Barry, H., Jr. Significance of maternal bereavement before age of eight in psychiatric patients. *Archives of Neurology and Psychiatry*, 1949, *62*, 630–637.

Barry, H., Jr. Parental deaths: An investigative challenge. *Contemporary Psychology*, 1969, *14*, 102–104.

Barry, H., Jr. & Lindemann, E. Critical ages for maternal bereavement in psychoneurosis. *Psychosomatic Medicine*, 1960, *22*, 166–181.

Beck, A., Sethi, B. & Tuthill, R. Childhood bereavement and adult depression. *Archives of General Psychiatry*, 1963, *9*, 295–302.

Bendiksen, R. & Fulton, R. Childhood bereavement and later behavior disorders: A replication. *Omega*, 1975, *6*, 45–59.

Besdine, M. The Jocasta complex, mothering and genius, part I. *Psychoanalytic Review*, 1968, *55*, 259–277. (a)

Besdine, M. The Jocasta complex, mothering and genius, part II. *Psychoanalytic Review*, 1968, *55*, 574–600. (b)

Bowerman, W. G. *Studies in genius*. New York: Philosophical Library, 1947.

Breckinridge, S. P. & Abbott, E. *The delinquent child and the home*. New York: Russell Sage Foundation, 1912.

Brown, F. Depression and childhood bereavement. *Journal of Mental Science*, 1961, *107*, 754–777.

Brown, F. Childhood bereavement and subsequent psychiatric disorder. *British Journal of Psychiatry*, 1966, *112*, 1035–1041.

Brown, F. Bereavement and lack of a parent in childhood. In E. Miller (Ed.), *Foundations of child psychiatry*. Oxford: Pergamon Press, 1968.

Brown, F. & Epps, P. Childhood bereavement and subsequent crime. *British Journal of Psychiatry*, 1966, *112*, 1043–1048.

Brown, F., Epps, P. & McGlashan, A. The remote and immediate effects of orphanhood. *Proceedings of the Third World Congress of Psychiatry* (Vol. 2). Montreal: McGill University Press, 1961.

Cattell, J. McK. A statistical study of eminent men. *Popular Science Monthly*, 1903, *62*, 359–377.

Census of England and Wales 1921. London: General Register Office, His Majesty's Stationery Office, 1925.

Cox, C. *Genetic studies of genius: II. The early mental traits of 300 geniuses*. Stanford, Calif.: Stanford University Press, 1959. (Originally published, 1926).

Dennehy, C. M. Childhood bereavement and psychiatric illness. *British Journal of Psychiatry*, 1966, *112*, 1049–1069.

Eisenstadt, J. M. Problem-solving ability of creative and non-creative college students. *Journal of Consulting Psychology*, 1966, *30*, 81–83.

Ellis, H. *A study of British genius* (Rev., enlarged ed.). New York: Houghton Mifflin, 1926. (Originally published, 1904.)

Forrest, A. D., Fraser, R. H. & Priest, R. G. Environmental factors in depressive illness. *British Journal of Psychiatry*, 1965, *111*, 243–253.

Freud, S. & Breuer, J. *Studies in hysteria*. New York: Nervous and Mental Disease Publishing, 1947. (Originally published, 1893.)

Galton, F. *Hereditary genius: An inquiry into its laws and consequences*. New York: World, 1962. (Originally published, 1869.)

Gay, M. J. & Tonge, W. L. The late effects of loss of parents in childhood. *British Journal of Psychiatry*, 1967, *113*, 753–759.

Glueck, S. *Crime and justice*. Boston: Little, 1936.

Glueck, S. (Ed.). *The problem of delinquency.* Boston: Houghton Mifflin, 1959.

Glueck, S. & Glueck, E. T. *500 criminal careers.* New York: Knopf, 1930.

Glueck, S. & Glueck, E. T. *500 delinquent women.* New York: Knopf, 1934, (a)

Glueck, S. & Glueck, E. T. *1000 juvenile delinquents* (2nd ed.). Cambridge, Mass.: Harvard University Press, 1934. (b)

Glueck, S. & Glueck, E. T. *Unraveling juvenile delinquency.* Cambridge, Mass.: Harvard University Press, 1950.

Glueck, S. & Glueck, E. T. *Family environment and delinquency.* Boston: Houghton Mifflin, 1962.

Goertzel, V. & Goertzel, M. G. *Cradles of eminence.* Boston: Little, Brown, 1962.

Greer, S. Letter on parental loss and attempted suicide. *British Journal of Psychiatry,* 1966, *112,* 743.

Gregory, I. Studies of parental deprivation in psychiatric patients. *American Journal of Psychiatry,* 1958, *115,* 432–442.

Gregory, I. An analysis of family data on 1000 patients admitted to a Canadian mental hospital. *Acte Genetica et Statistica Medica,* 1959, *9,* 54–96.

Gregory, I. Anterospective data following childhood loss of a parent: I. Delinquency and high school dropout. *Archives of General Psychiatry,* 1965, *13,* 99–109. (a)

Gregory, I. Anterospective data following childhood loss of a parent. II. Pathology, performance, and potential among college students. *Archives of General Psychiatry,* 1965, *13,* 110–120. (b)

Gregory, I. Retrospective estimates of orphanhood from generation life tables. *Milbank Memorial Fund Quarterly,* 1965, *43,* 323–348. (c)

Gregory, I. Retrospective data concerning childhood loss of a parent: I. Actuarial estimates vs. recorded frequencies of orphanhood. *Archives of General Psychiatry,* 1966, *15,* 354–361. (a)

Gregory, I. Retrospective data concerning childhood loss of a parent: II. Category of parental loss by decade of birth, diagnosis, and MMPI. *Archives of General Psychiatry,* 1966, *15,* 362–368. (b)

Healy, W. & Bronner, A. F. *Delinquents and criminals: Their making and unmaking: Studies in two American cities.* New York: Macmillan, 1926.

Hilgard, J. R. & Newman, M. F. Evidence for functional genesis in mental illness: Schizophrenia, depressive psychosis and psychoneurosis. *Journal of Nervous and Mental Diseases,* 1961, *132,* 3–16.

Hilgard, J. R. & Newman, M. F. Early parental deprivation as a functional facctor in the etiology of schizophrenia and alcoholism. *American Journal of Orthopsychiatry,* 1963, *33,* 409–420. (a)

Hilgard, J. R. & Newman, M. F. Parental loss by death in childhood as an etiological factor among schizophrenic and alcoholic patients compared with a non-patient community sample. *Journal of Nervous and Mental Disease,* 1963, *137,* 14–28. (b)

Hill, O. W. & Price, J. S. Childhood bereavement and adult depression. *British Journal of Psychiatry,* 1967, *113,* 743–751.

Illingworth, R. S. & Illingworth, C. M. *Lessons from childhood: Some aspects of the early life of unusual men and women.* Baltimore: Williams & Wilkins, 1966.

Kanzer, M. Writers and the early loss of parents. *Journal of the Hillside Hospital,* 1953, *2,* 148–151.

Kenmare, D. *The nature of genius.* London: Peter Owne, 1960.

Lange-Eichbaum, W. [Genius, insanity and fame] (W. Kurth, Ed.). Munich, Germany: Ernst Reinhardt, 1956. (Originally published, 1928.)

Lange-Eichbaum, W. *The problem of genius.* New York: Macmillan, 1932.

Lombroso, C. *The man of genius.* London: Walter Scott, 1891.

Marris, P. *Loss and change.* New York: Pantheon Books, 1974.

Metropolitan Life Insurance Company. *Family responsibilities increasing* (Statistical Bulletin). New York: Author, April 1959.

Metropolitan Life Insurance Company. *Orphanhood—A continuing problem* (Statistical Bulletin). New York: Author, December 1966.

Miller, J. B. M. Children's reactions to the death of a parent: A review of the psychoanalytic literature. In S. Chess & A. Thomas (Eds.), *Annual progress in child psychiatry and child development.* New York: Brunner/Mazel, 1972.

Moriarty, D. N. (Ed.). *The loss of loved ones: The effects of death in the family on personality development.* Springfield, Ill.: Charles C Thomas, 1967.

Neubauer, P. B. The one-parent child and his oedipal development. *Psychoanalytic Study of the Child,* 1960, *15,* 286–309.

Oltman, J. E. & Friedman, S. A consideration of parental deprivation and other factors in alcohol addicts. *Quarterly Journal of Studies on Alcohol,* 1953, *14,* 49–57.

Oltman, J. E. & Friedman, S. Report of parental deprivation in psychiatric disorders. *Archives of General Psychiatry,* 1965, *12,* 46–56.

Oltman, J., McGarry, J. & Friedman, S. Parental deprivation and the "broken home" in dementia praecox and other mental disorders. *American Journal of Psychiatry,* 1952, *108,* 685–694.

Paffenbarger, R.S., Jr. & Asnes, D. P. Chronic disease in former college students: III. Precursors of suicide in early and middle life. *American Journal of Public Health,* 1966, *56,* 1026–1036.

Parkes, C. M. *Bereavement: Studies of grief in adult life.* New York: International Universities Press, 1972.

Petursson, E. A study of parental deprivation and illness in 291 psychiatric patients. *International Journal of Social Psychiatry,* 1961, *7,* 97–105.

Rhoades, M. C. A case study of delinquent boys in the Juvenile Court of Chicago. *American Journal of Sociology,* 1907, *13,* 56–78.

Rochlin, G. The dread of abandonment: A contribution to the etiology of the loss complex and to depression. *Psychoanalytic Study of the Child,* 1961, *16,* 451–470.

Rochlin, G. *Griefs and discontents: The forces of change.* Boston: Little, Brown, 1965.

Russell Sage Foundation. *Boyhood and lawlessness.* College Park, Md.: McGrath, 1969. (Originally published, 1914.)

Shideler, E. Family disintegration and the delinquent boy in the United States. *Journal of the American Institute of Criminal Law and Criminology,* 1918, *8,* 709–732.

Sorell, W. *The duality of vision: Genius and versatility in the arts.* New York: Bobbs-Merrill, 1970.

Sullenger, T. E. *Social determinants in juvenile delinquency.* Unpublished doctoral dissertation, University of Missouri, 1930.

Wolfenstein, M. Loss, rage, and repetition. *Psychoanalytic Study of the Child,* 1969, *24,* 432–460.

Editor's References

Abraham, K. (1911). Notes on the psycho-analytical investigation and treatment of manic-depressive insanity and allied conditions. In K. Abraham, *Selected Papers of Karl Abraham*. London: Hogarth, 1942. 137–56.

——— (1916). The first pregenital stage of the libido. In K. Abraham, *op. cit.*, 248–79.

——— (1924). A short study of the development of the libido viewed in the light of the mental disorders. In K. Abraham, *op. cit.*, 418–501.

Anthony, E. J. (1973). A working model for family studies. In Anthony, E. J., and Kouperik, C. (eds.), *The Child in His Family: The Impact of Disease and Death*. New York: John Wiley.

Altschul, S. (1988). (Ed.) Childhood bereavement and its aftermath. *Emotions and Behavior Monographs, No. 8*. Madison, Conn.: International Universities Press.

Barnes, M. J. (1964). Reactions to the death of a mother. *Psychoanal. Study Child* 19:334–57.

Becker, D. & Margolin, F. (1967). How surviving parents handled their young children's adaptation to the crisis of loss. *Amer. J. Orthopsychiat.* 37:753–57.

Binswanger, L. (1957). *Sigmund Freud: Reminiscences of a Friendship*. New York: Grune & Stratton.

Bloom-Feshback, J. & S., et al. (1987). *The Psychology of Separation and Loss: Perspectives on Development, Life Transition, and Clinical Practice*. San Francisco: Jossey-Bass.

Bowlby, J. (1944). Forty-four juvenile thieves: Their characters and home life. *Int. J. Psycho-Anal.* 25:19–25 and 107–27.

——— (1951). *Maternal Care and Mental Health*. Geneva: World Health Organization Monograph 2.

——— (1960). Grief and mourning in infancy and early childhood. *Psychoanal. Study Child* 15:9–52.

——— (1961). Processes of mourning. *Int. J. Psycho-Anal.* 44:317–40.

——— (1963). Pathological mourning and childhood mourning. *J. Amer. Psychoanal. Assn.* 11:500–541.

——— (1969, 1973, 1980). *Attachment and Loss*. Vol. I, *Attachment;* Vol. 2, *Separation: Anxiety and Anger;* Vol. 3, *Loss: Sadness and Depression*. New York: Basic Books.

Bowlby, J., Robertson, J. & Rosenbluth, D. (1952). A two-year-old goes to the hospital. *Psychoanal. Study Child* 7:82–94.

Breuer, J. & Freud, S. (1893–95). Studies on hysteria. *S.E.* 2.

Burlingham, D. & Freud, A. (1942). *Young Children in War-Time: A Year's Work in a Residential War Nursery*. London: Allen & Unwin.

Cohler, J. & L. (1991). The charismatic lover: An aspect of unfinished mourning in women with early adolescent maternal loss. Unpublished presidential address, clinical paper and review of the literature. William Alanson White Society, New York City.

Deutsch, H. (1937). Absence of grief. *Psychoanal. Q.* 6:12–22.

Dietrich, D. R. & Shabad, P. C. (1989). *The Problem of Loss and Mourning: Psychoanalytic Perspectives*. Madison, Conn.: International Universities Press.

Eisenstadt, M. (1978). Parental loss and genius. *Amer. Psychol.* 33:211–23.

Engel, G. (1961). Is grief a disease? *Psychosomat. Med.* 23:18–22.

Fleming, J. (1972). Early object deprivation and transference phenomena: The working alliance. *Psychoanal Q.* 41:23–49.

——— (1974). The problem of diagnosis in parent-loss cases. *Contemp. Psychoanal.* 10:439–51.

——— (1975). Some observations on object constancy in the psychoanalysis of adults. *J. Amer. Psychoanal. Assn.* 23:743–59.

——— (1978). Early object deprivation and transference phenomena: Pre-oedipal object need. Unpublished manuscript.

Fleming, J. & Altschul, S. (1963). Activation of mourning and growth by psychoanalysis. *Int. J. Psycho-Anal.* 44:419–31.

Frankiel, R. V. (1984). "Michelangelo, early childhood, and maternal imagery: The sculptor's relation to stone." Unpublished discussion of a paper by Dr. Robert Liebert, presented March 23, 1984, at the William Alanson White Institute, New York.

——— (1993). Hide and seek in the playroom: On object loss and transference in child treatment. *Psychoanal. Rev.*, 80: 340–59.

Frankiel, R. V., Libbey, M., Epstein, L. & Schafer, R. (1989). Preparation for analysis in the face of massive resistance: A clinical symposium. *Psychoanal. Rev.* 76:467–509.

Freud, A. (1958). Adolescence. *Psychoanal. Study Child* 13:255–78.

——— (1960). Discussion of Dr. John Bowlby's paper. *Psychoanal. Study Child* 15:53–62.

——— (1973). Infants without families: Reports on the Hampstead nurseries, 1939–1945. *The Writings of Anna Freud*. Vol. 3. New York: International Universities Press.

Freud, S. (1887–1902). *The Origins of Psycho-Analysis: Letters to Wilhelm Fliess, Drafts and Notes: 1887–1902*. New York: Basic Books, 1954.

——— (1900). The interpretation of dreams. *S.E.* 4 and 5.

——— (1908). Creative writers and daydreaming. *S.E.* 9:143–53.

——— (1909). Notes upon a case of obsessional neurosis. *S.E.* 10:155–249.

——— (1914). On narcissism: An introduction. *S.E.* 14:73–102.

——— (1917). Mourning and melancholia. *S.E.* 14:243–58.

——— (1923). The ego and the id. Part III. *S.E.* 19:28–39.

Freud, S. (1926). Inhibitions, symptoms, and anxiety. *S.E.* 20:77–175.

——— 1927). Fetishism. *S.E.* 21:149–57.

——— (1929). Letter to Binswanger. Letter 239 in E. L. Freud (ed.), *The Letters of Sigmund Freud.* New York: Basic, 1960.

——— (1938a). An outline of psychoanalysis. *S.E.* 23:141–207.

——— (1938b). The splitting of the ego in the process of defense. *S.E.* 23:273–78.

Furman, E. (1974). *A Child's Parent Dies: Studies in Childhood Bereavement.* New Haven: Yale University Press.

——— (1981). Treatment-via-the-parent: A case of bereavement. *J. Child Psychother.* 7:89–102.

——— (1983). Studies in childhood bereavement. *Canad. J. Psychiat.* 28:241–47.

——— (1986). On trauma: When is the death of a parent traumatic? *Psychoanal. Study Child* 41:191–208.

Furman, E. & Furman, R. (1989). Some effects of the one-parent family on personality development. In Dietrich, D. R., and Shabad, P. C. (eds.), *The Problem of Loss and Mourning.* Madison, Conn., International Universities Press. 129–57.

Furman, R. (1964a). Death and the young child: Some preliminary considerations. *Psychoanal. Study Child* 19:321–33.

——— (1964b). Death of a six-year-old's mother during his analysis. *Psychoanal. Study Child* 19:377–97.

——— (1968). Additional remarks on mourning and the young child. *Bull. Phila. Assn. for Psychoanal.* 18:51–64.

——— (1973). A child's capacity for mourning. In Anthony, E. J., and Koupernik, C. (eds.), *The Child in His Family: Impact of Disease and Death. Yearbook of the International Association for Child Psychiatry.* Vol. 2. New York: Wiley. 225–31.

Gay, P. (1988). *Freud: A Life for Our Time.* New York: Norton.

Glenn, J. (1980). Freud's advice to Hans's father: The first supervisory sessions. In M. Kanzer and J. Glenn (eds.), *Freud and His Patients.* New York: Aronson.

Hardin, H. T. (1985). On the vicissitudes of early primary surrogate mothering. *J. Amer. Psychoanal. Assn.* 33:609–29.

Hofer, M. (1984). Relationships as regulators: A psychobiological perspective on bereavement. *Psychosomat. Med.* 46:183–95.

Jacobson, E. (1946). The effect of disappointment on ego and super-ego formation in normal and depressive development. *Psychoanal. Rev.* 33:129–47.

——— (1957). Normal and pathological moods: Their nature and function. *Psychoanal. Study Child* 12:73–113.

——— (1961). Adolescent moods and the remodeling of psychic structures in adolescence. *Psychoanal. Study Child* 16:164–83.

——— (1964). *The Self and the Object World.* New York: International Universities Press.

——— (1965). The return of the lost parent. In M. Schur (ed.), *Drives, Affects, Behavior.* Vol. 2. New York: International Universities Press. 193–211.

Jaques, E. (1965). Death and the mid-life crisis. *Int. J. Psycho-Anal.* 46:502–14.

Katan, A. (1937). The role of 'displacement' in agoraphobia. *Int. J. Psycho-Anal.* 32:41–50, 1951.

Klein, M. (1935). A contribution to the psychogenesis of manic-depressive states. *Int. J. Psycho-Anal.* 16:145–74.

——— (1940). Mourning and its relation to manic-depressive states. *Contributions to Psychoanalysis, 1921–1945.* New York: McGraw-Hill, 1967. 311–33.

Kliman, G. (1965). *Psychological Emergencies of Childhood.* New York: Grune & Stratton.

Lerner, P. (1990). The treatment of early object loss: The need to search. *Psychoanal. Psychol.* 7:79–90.

Liebert, R. S. (1983). *Michelangelo: A Psychoanalytic Study of His Life and Images.* New Haven: Yale University Press.

Lindemann, E. (1944). Symptomatology and management of acute grief. *Amer. J. Psychiatry* 101:141–48.

Loewald, H. W. (1962). Internalization, separation, mourning, and the superego. *Psychoanal. Q.* 31:483–504. Also in H. W. Loewald (ed.), *Papers on Psychoanalysis.* New Haven: Yale University Press, 1980. 257–76.

Lopez, T. & Kliman, G. (1979). Memory, reconstruction and mourning in the analysis of a four-year old child. *Psychoanal. Study Child* 34:235–71.

McCann, M. E. (1974). Mourning accomplished by way of the transference. In M. Harley (ed.), *The Analyst and the Adolescent at Work.* New York: Quadrangle. 110–33. Also in E. Furman, *A Child's Parent Dies, op. cit.,* 69–87.

Meiss, M. (1952). The oedipal problem of a fatherless child. *Psychoanal. Study Child* 7:216–29.

Miller, J. B. M. (1971). Children's reaction to the death of a parent: A review of the psychoanalytic literature. *J. Amer. Psychoanal. Assn.* 19:697–719.

Nagera, H. (1970). Children's reactions to the death of important objects: A developmental approach. *Psychoanal. Study Child* 25:360–400.

Neubauer, P. (1960). The one-parent child and his oedipal development. *Psychoanal. Study Child* 15:286–309.

Osterweis, M., Soloman, F. & Green, M. (1984) (eds.) *Bereavement: Reactions, Consequences, Care.* Washington, D. C.: National Academy Press.

Parkes, C. M. (1987). *Bereavement: Studies of Grief in Adult Life.* 2nd ed. New York: International Universities Press.

Parkes, C. M. & Weiss, R. (1983). *Recovery from Bereavement.* New York: Basic Books.

Parkin, A. (1981). Repetition, mourning, and working through. *Int. J. Psycho-Anal.* 62:271–81.

Pollock, G. H. (1961). Mourning and adaptation. *Int. J. Psycho-Anal.* 42:341–61.

——— (1962). Childhood parent and sibling loss in adult patients: A comparative study. *Arch. Gen. Psychiat.* 7:295–305.

——— (1970). Anniversary reactions: Trauma and mourning. *Psycho-Anal. Q.* 39:347–71.

——— (1971). Temporal anniversary manifestations: Hour, day, holiday. *Psychoanal. Q.* 40:123–31.

Pollock, G. H. (1975a). On mourning, immortality, and utopia. *J. Amer. Psychoanal. Assoc.* 23:334–62.

——— (1975b). Mourning and memorialization through music. *Ann. Psychoanal.* 3:423–36.

——— (1976). Manifestations of abnormal mourning: Homicide and suicide following the death of another. *Annual of Psychoanal.* 4:225–49.

——— (1978a). On siblings, childhood sibling loss, and creativity. *Annual of Psychoanal.* 6:443–81.

——— (1978b). Process and affect: Mourning and grief. *Int. J. Psycho-Anal.* 59:255–76.

——— (1982). The mourning-liberation process and creativity: The case of Kathe Kollwitz. *Annual of Psychoanal.* 10:333–53.

——— (1989). *The Mourning-Liberation Process.* 2 vols. New York: International Universities Press.

Robertson, J. & J. (1971). Young children in brief separation: A fresh look. *Psychoanal. Study Child.* 26:264–315.

Root, N. N. (1957). A neurosis in adolescence. *Psychoanal. Study Child* 12:320–34.

Schafer, R. (1968). The fates of the immortal object. In Schafer, R., *Aspects of Internalization.* New York: International Universities Press. 220–36.

Scharl, A. (1961). Regression and restitution in object loss. *Psychoanal. Study Child* 16:471–80.

Schur, M. (1960). Discussion of John Bowlby's paper. *Psychoanal. Study Child* 15:63–84.

Segal, H. (1952). A psycho-analytical approach to aesthetics. *Int. J. Psycho-Anal.* 33:196–207.

——— (1981). *The Work of Hanna Segal: A Kleinian Approach to Clinical Practice.* London: Free Association Books.

Sekaer, C. (1987). Toward a definition of 'childhood mourning.' *Amer. J. Psychother.* 41:201–19.

Sekaer, C. & Katz, S. (1986). On the concept of mourning in childhood: Reactions of a two-and-one-half-year-old girl to the death of her father. *Psychoanal. Study Child* 41:287–314.

Shambaugh, B. (1961). A study of loss reactions in a seven-year-old. *Psychoanal. Study Child* 16:510–22.

Siggins, L. (1966). Mourning: A critical review of the literature. *Int. J. Psycho-Anal.* 47:14–25.

Spitz, R. (1960). Discussion of John Bowlby's paper. *Psychoanal. Study Child* 15:85–94.

Stein, M., Miller, A. H. & Trestman, R. L. (1991). Depression, the immune system, and health and illness: Findings in search of meaning. *Arch. Gen. Psychiat.* 48:171–77.

Stokes, A. (1965). *The Invitation in Art.* London: Tavistock.

Stolorow, R. D. & Lachmann, F. M. (1975). Early object loss and denial: Developmental considerations. *Psychoanal. Q.* 44:596–611.

Tyson, R. (1983). Some narcissistic consequences of object loss: A developmental view. *Psychoanal. Q.* 52:205–24.

Volkan, V. D. (1972). The linking objects of pathological mourners. *Arch. Gen. Psychiatr.* 27:215–21.

———— (1981). *Linking Objects and Linking Phenomena: A Study of the Forms, Symptoms, Metapsychology, and Therapy of Complicated Mourning.* Madison, Conn.: International Universities Press.

———— (1984–85). Complicated mourning. *Annual of Psychoanal.* 12–13:323–48.

Volkan, V. D., Cillufo, A. F. & Sarvay, T. L. (1975). Re-grief therapy and the function of the linking object as a key to stimulate emotionality. In P. T. Olsen (ed.), *Emotional Flooding.* New York: Human Sciences. 179–224.

Volkan, V. D. & Josephthal, D. (1980). The treatment of established pathological mourners. In B. T. Karasu and L. Bellak (eds.) *Specialized Techniques in Individual Psychotherapy.* New York: 118–42.

Winnicott, D. W. (1965). A child psychiatry case illustrating delayed reaction to loss. In M. Schur (ed.), *Drives, Affects, Behavior.* Vol. 2. New York: International Universities Press.

Wolfenstein, M. (1966). How is mourning possible? *Psychoanal. Study Child* 21:93–123.

———— (1969). Loss, rage, and repetition. *Psychoanal. Study Child* 24:432–46.

Wortman, C. B. & Silver, C. B. (1987). Coping with irrevocable loss. In *Cataclysms, Crises, and Catastrophes: Psychology in Action.* The Master Lecture Series, 6. Washington, D.C.: American Psychological Assn.

Highly Recommended Readings

Grief Observed

Darwin, C. (1872). *The Expression of the Emotions in Man and Animals.* London: John Murray, 80–81, 178–97.

Hofer, M. A. (1984). Relationships as regulators: A psychobiologic perspective on bereavement. *Psychosomatic Medicine* 46:183–95.

Osterweis, M., Solomon, F. & Green, M. (1984) [eds.] *Bereavement: Reactions, Consequences, and Care.* Committee for the Study of the Health Consequences of Bereavement, Washington, D.C.: National Academy Press.

Theoretical Foundations

Bowlby, J. (1961). Processes of mourning. *Int. J. Psycho-Anal.* 42:317–40.

Freud, S. (1914). On narcissism: An introduction. *S.E.* 14:73–102.

———— (1940). Splitting of the ego in the process of defense. *S.E.* 23:271–78.

Jacobson, E. (1957a). Denial and repression. *J. Amer. Psychoanal. Assn.* 5:61–92.

———— (1957b). On normal and pathological moods: Their nature and function. *Psychoanal. Study Child* 12:73–113.

———— (1964). *The Self and the Object World.* New York: International Universities Press.

Klein, M. (1935). A contribution to the psychogenesis of Manic-Depressive states. *Int. J. Psycho-Anal.* 16:145–74.

Mahler, M. S. (1961). On sadness and grief in infancy and childhood: Loss and restoration of the symbiotic love object. *Psychoanal. Study Child* 16:119–20.

———— (1966). Notes on the development of basic moods: the depressive affect. In *The Selected Papers of Margaret S. Mahler, Vol. 2, Separation-Individuation.* New York: Aronson, 1979. 59–75.

Schafer, R. (1968). The fates of the immortal object. In Schafer, R., *Aspects of Internalization.* New York: International Universities Press.

Characteristics of Pathological Mourning

Altschul, S. (1968). Denial and ego arrest. *J. Amer. Psychoanal. Assoc.* 16:301–18.

Fleming, J. (1972). Early object deprivation and transference phenomena: the working alliance. *Psychoanal. Q.* 41:23–49.

———— (1975). Some observations on object constancy in the psychoanalysis of adults. *J. Amer. Psychoanal. Assn.* 23:743–59.

Steiner, J. (1990). Pathological organizations as obstacles to mourning: The role of unbearable guilt. *Int. J. Psycho-Anal.* 71:87–94.
Volkan, V. (1972). The linking objects of pathological mourners. *Arch. Gen. Psychiat.* 27:215–21.

Developmental Perspectives

Bowby, J. (1980). *Loss: Sadness and Depression.* New York: Basic Books.
Freud, A. (1960). Discussion of Dr. John Bowlby's paper. *Psychoanal. Study Child,* 15:53–62.
———— (1973). *Infants Without Families. Reports on the Hampstead Nurseries 1939–1945.* New York: International Universities Press.
Furman, E. (1974). *A Child's Parent Dies: Studies in Childhood Bereavement.* New Haven: Yale University Press.
———— (1986). On trauma: When is the death of a parent traumatic? *Psychoanal. Study Child.* 41:191–208.
———— & Furman, R. (1989). Some effects of the one–parent family on personality development. In Dietrich, D. R., and Shabad, P. C. (eds.) *The Problem of Loss and Mourning.* Madison, Conn.: International Universities Press. 129–57.
Furman, R. (1964). Death and the young child: Some preliminary considerations. *Psychoanal. Study Child* 19:321–33.
Jacobson, E. (1946). The effect of disappointment on ego and superego formation in normal and depressive development. *Psychoanal. Rev.* 33:129–47.
Nagera, H. (1970). Children's reactions to the death of important objects. *Psychoanal. Study Child* 25:360–400.
Sekaer, C. (1987). Toward a definition of "childhood mourning." *Amer. J. Psychother.* 41:201–19.

Case Reports

Furman, R. (1964). Death of a six-year-old's mother during his analysis. *Psychoanal. Study Child* 19:377–97.
Lopez. T. & Kliman, G. (1979). Memory, reconstruction and mourning in the analysis of a 4-year-old child: Maternal bereavement in the second year of life. *Psychoanal. Study Child* 34:235–371.
Meiss, M. (1952). The oedipal problem of a fatherless child. *Psychoanal. Study Child* 7:216–29.
Newbauer, P. B. (1960). The one-parent child and oedipal development. *Psychoanal. Study Child* 15:286–309.
Rochlin, G. (1953). Loss and restitution. *Psychoanal. Study Child* 8:288–309.
Root, N. N. (1957). A neurosis in adolescence. *Psychoanal. Study Child* 12:320–334.
Shambaugh, B. (1961). A study of loss reactions in a seven-year-old. *Psychoanal. Study Child* 16:510–22.

Winnicott, D. W. (1965). A child psychiatry case illustrating delayed reaction to loss. In *Drives, Affects, Behavior*, Vol. 2. M. Shur (ed.) New York: International Universities Press.

Object Loss and the Life Cycle

Leon, I. G. (1990). *When a Baby Dies: Psychotherapy for Pregnancy and Newborn Loss*. New Haven: Yale University Press.

Osterweis, M., Solomon, F. & Green, M. (1984) [eds.] *Bereavement: Reactions, Consequences, and Care*. Committee for the Study of the Health Consequences of Bereavement, Washington, D.C.: National Academy Press.

Parkes, C. M. (1987). *Bereavement: Studies of Grief in Adult Life*. 2nd American edition. Madison, Conn.: International Universities Press.

Parkes, C. M. & Weiss, R. (1983). *Recovery from Bereavement*. New York: Basic Books.

Object Loss and Creativity

Pollock, G. H. (1989). *The Mourning–Liberation Process*. 2 vols. Madison, Conn.: International Universities Press.

Name Index

About the Editor

For over twenty years, Rita V. Frankiel, Ph.D., a member of the International Psychoanalytic Association, has lectured and written about the effects of object loss on children, adolescents, and adults. Across the U.S. and internationally, she has presented papers, led workshops and study groups, and supervised individual treatment focused on the special clinical problems posed by patients who have suffered early loss. Currently, she is Associate Clinical Professor at the New York University Postdoctoral Program in Psychoanalysis and Psychotherapy, where in addition to offering supervision, she gives a course on object loss in clinical practice. She also holds an appointment as Training and Supervising Analyst at the New York Freudian Society; there she has for several years run a study group for Institute graduates on manifestations of early loss in transference and countertransference.

Printed and bound by CPI Group (UK) Ltd, Croydon, CR0 4YY

27/10/2024

14580397-0002